HealthTech Horizons

Charting the Future of Smart Healthcare Innovations, Deepfake and Metaverse

RIVER PUBLISHERS SERIES IN BIOMEDICAL ENGINEERING

Series Editor

DINESH KANT KUMAR
RMIT University, Australia

The "River Publishers Series in Biomedical Engineering" is a series of comprehensive academic and professional books which focus on the engineering and mathematics in medicine and biology. The series presents innovative experimental science and technological development in the biomedical field as well as clinical application of new developments.

Books published in the series include research monographs, edited volumes, handbooks and textbooks. The books provide professionals, researchers, educators, and advanced students in the field with an invaluable insight into the latest research and developments.

Topics covered in the series include, but are by no means restricted to the following:

- Biomedical engineering
- Biomedical physics and applied biophysics
- Bio-informatics
- Bio-metrics
- Bio-signals
- Medical Imaging

For a list of other books in this series, visit www.riverpublishers.com

HealthTech Horizons

Charting the Future of Smart Healthcare Innovations, Deepfake and Metaverse

Editors

Saurav Mallik
Department of Pharmacology & Toxicology,
University of Arizona, Tucson, AZ, USA

Soumita Seth
Department of Computer Science & Engineering,
Future Institute of Engineering and Management,
Narendrapur, Kolkata, West Bengal, India

Ben Othman Soufiene
Computer Science at the Applied College,
King Faisal University, Saudi Arabia

River Publishers

Routledge
Taylor & Francis Group
NEW YORK AND LONDON

Published 2026 by River Publishers
River Publishers
Broagervej 10, 9260 Gistrup, Denmark
www.riverpublishers.com

Distributed exclusively by Routledge
605 Third Avenue, New York, NY 10017, USA
4 Park Square, Milton Park, Abingdon, Oxon OX14 4RN

HealthTech Horizons: Charting the Future of Smart Healthcare Innovations, Deepfake and Metaverse / Saurav Mallik, Soumita Seth and Ben Othman Soufiene.

Routledge is an imprint of the Taylor & Francis Group, an informa business

ISBN 978-87-438-0991-3 (Hardback)
ISBN 978-87-438-0996-8 (Paperback)
ISBN 978-87-438-0993-7 (Ebook)
ISBN 978-87-438-0992-0 (Ebook master)
ISBN 978-87-438-0995-1 (E-pub)

DOI 10.1201/9788743809920

Contents

Preface

This book guides the reader through the emerging frontiers of smart healthcare, deepfake technologies, and the Metaverse. Chapter 1 lays the foundation for exploring the dynamic intersection of healthcare and cutting-edge technologies. It introduces the core themes of the book – smart healthcare innovations, deepfake technology, and the Metaverse – positioning them as pivotal forces reshaping modern medicine. The chapter begins by tracing the evolution of HealthTech, highlighting the paradigm shift from conventional care models to intelligent, data-driven, and immersive healthcare systems. It emphasizes the transformative impact of artificial intelligence, digital twins, and extended reality in diagnosis, treatment, training, and patient engagement. Special attention is given to the emerging roles of deepfake technology in medical education and simulation, and how the Metaverse fosters collaborative care, remote access, and personalized therapeutic experiences. Ethical considerations, data security challenges, and regulatory frameworks are also briefly introduced to underscore the complexity of responsible innovation in this domain. By setting the stage for deeper exploration in subsequent chapters, this introductory chapter provides readers with a comprehensive overview of the technological horizons shaping the future of global healthcare.

Chapter 2 introduces Digital Twins (DTs), a key component of the Metaverse, which are virtual replicas of physical entities. In healthcare, DTs are applied in disease prediction, treatment optimization, and personalized medicine, using technologies such as Cloud computing, AI, and IoT. These digital models enable healthcare providers to create detailed patient profiles, facilitating personalized care and improving patient health outcomes. This chapter explores the diverse applications of DTs, including remote patient monitoring, clinical decision support, drug discovery, and treatment optimization. Additionally, it addresses challenges such as data privacy, security concerns, and computational limitations. Looking forward, the chapter highlights the transformative potential of DTs in revolutionizing healthcare, offering data-driven, personalized solutions that promise to enhance patient care.

Building on this foundation, Chapter 3 examines the rise of deepfake technology, which has garnered significant attention across various industries, including healthcare. This chapter explores the innovative and sometimes challenging applications of deepfakes in medical training, patient education, and telemedicine. By creating realistic simulations and interactive learning experiences, deepfakes have the potential to improve the skills of healthcare professionals and provide patients with a deeper understanding of their health conditions. However, the use of deepfakes also raises important ethical and security concerns, such as the risk of misinformation, consent issues, and the potential for misuse. Through an in-depth review of current literature and case studies, this chapter analyses the benefits and risks of deepfake technology in healthcare, offering insights into necessary regulatory frameworks and best practices. The goal is to provide stakeholders with a comprehensive understanding of the innovative opportunities and the precautions required for the responsible use of deepfakes in health-care.

Chapter 4 shifts the focus to the rapid increase in healthcare innovation, fuelled by technologies such as artificial intelligence algorithms for early disease prediction and personalized treatment planning. Augmented reality is enhancing surgical precision by providing real-time visuals during operations, while virtual reality is transforming physical rehabilitation. Simultaneously, Deepfake technology and the Metaverse have emerged as disruptive forces in healthcare. Deepfakes offer innovative applications in treatment simulations and medical education, while the Metaverse enables telemetry services and collaborative healthcare platforms. However, these advancements also introduce significant challenges, particularly regarding data privacy breaches, misinformation dissemination, and identity theft. To mitigate these risks, robust regulatory measures and ethical guidelines are essential. This chapter explores the roles of the Metaverse and Deepfake technology in smart healthcare, providing an overview of the regulatory landscapes, including Health Insurance Portability and Accountability (HIPAA), General Data Protection Regulation (GDPR), the Food and Drug Administration (FDA), and the European Conformity (CE) Marking. It emphasizes the need for clear policies on data protection, stringent security measures, and the development of ethical standards. By navigating these regulatory frameworks and implementing appropriate measures, healthcare professionals can harness the transformative potential of Deepfakes and the Metaverse while safeguarding patient privacy and security.

Following this, Chapter 5 explores the Metaverse as a transformative technology in emergency response training, offering immersive, real-time, and scalable simulations for healthcare professionals and first responders.

By integrating virtual reality (VR), augmented reality (AR), artificial intelligence (AI), blockchain, and cloud computing, Metaverse environments provide realistic training scenarios for managing pandemics, natural disasters, and mass casualty events. These advanced simulations enable trainees to practice crisis management, triage procedures, and resource allocation in a dynamic and controlled setting, enhancing their decision-making and situational awareness. Furthermore, AI-driven analytics and machine learning algorithms assess trainee performance, providing real-time feedback and personalized training modules. Blockchain technology enhances data security and ensures transparent documentation of certifications and training records. Additionally, 5G and cloud computing facilitate seamless collaboration between trainees and instructors, enabling large-scale, remote emergency training sessions. Despite its vast potential, Metaverse-based training faces challenges such as high implementation costs, technological barriers, the psychological effects of hyper-realistic scenarios, and data security concerns. Addressing these challenges through research, policy development, and technological advancements are key to maximizing the effectiveness of Metaverse-based emergency response training. This chapter examines the core technologies driving Metaverse-based emergency training, highlights real-world applications, identifies existing challenges, and discusses future research directions to optimize the use of Metaverse technologies in emergency preparedness.

Chapter 6 embarks on a rhythmic exploration of the evolution of healthcare, probing the harmonious relationship between artificial intelligence (AI) and medical practitioners in creating a transformative symphony of healing. This chapter unravels the intricate role of AI, focusing on cutting-edge deep learning methodologies that are reshaping the healthcare landscape. It introduces AI as an indispensable partner, seamlessly merging its computational prowess with the nuanced expertise of healthcare professionals. A crescendo unfolds in the field of medical imaging, where advanced neural networks uncover hidden patterns within radiological imagery. This leap beyond human perceptual limitations adds transformative depth to diagnostics, revealing medical images in ways previously unimaginable. The chapter transitions to explore genomics, where AI and deep learning algorithms, much like a virtuoso ensemble, decode the intricate language of our DNA. These algorithms help identify genetic predispositions to diseases and craft personalized treatment strategies tailored to an individual's genetic profile. The narrative further explores the medical consultation process, illustrating the dynamic interplay between healthcare practitioners and intelligent algorithms. Recurrent neural networks, akin to a melodic motif, adapt and learn from patient histories, refining diagnoses and treatment plans in a cyclical, iterative rhythm. At the heart of this evolving symphony is the delicate balance between the technical expertise of AI and the human touch in healthcare, envisioning a harmonious convergence that transforms the medical field. AI, as part of this medical orchestra, contributes to a composition that resonates deeply with the collective heartbeat of humanity.

Building on the evolving role of AI in healthcare, Chapter 7 delves into the challenge of analyzing gene expression datasets, which offer rich insights into biological processes but are often clouded by redundancy and irrelevant features. This chapter emphasizes the importance of effective feature selection (FS) techniques in enhancing the accuracy and precision of gene identification, which is crucial in complex biological datasets. In this context, the chapter introduces a novel hybrid gene selection method, Elephant Herding Optimization with support vector machine (EHOSVM), designed to identify relevant gene subsets for cancer classification. This method is evaluated across four benchmark datasets: breast cancer, central nervous system (CNS), leukemia, and ovarian cancer. By combining the optimization power of the Elephant Herding Optimization algorithm for feature selection with the classification efficiency of support vector machines (SVM), EHOSVM improves classification accuracy. The method is evaluated using performance metrics such as accuracy, precision, recall, F1-score, and AUC-ROC score. The results show that the EHOSVM approach performs exceptionally well, particularly with the leukemia and ovarian cancer datasets, achieving 100% classification accuracy. For the breast cancer dataset, the method achieves 99% accuracy, 98.61% precision, 100% recall, and 99.31% F1-score with 23 selected genes. The method performed less effectively on the CNS dataset, with a lower accuracy of 66%, highlighting the dataset's inherent complexity. Detailed results with varying numbers of selected genes demonstrate the robustness of EHOSVM, consistently delivering high classification metrics across most datasets. In conclusion, EHOSVM proves to be an effective method for identifying relevant gene subsets, showing promise in improving classification accuracy in gene expression datasets. Its ability to achieve perfect accuracy in some cases underscores its potential in high-dimensional biological data. While challenges remain in complex datasets like CNS, this method offers a promising framework for advancing biological data analysis and precision medicine. Future research could focus on refining the method to improve performance in datasets with greater variability and complexity.

Chapter 8 highlights that cancer continues to be a major global health issue, causing a significant number of deaths worldwide. Among the various types of cancer, breast cancer stands out as a pressing health challenge, particularly for women, where it poses a severe threat to their lives. In this context, the timely identification and accurate diagnosis of breast cancer are critical in enabling effective therapeutic interventions and developing personalized treatment strategies. This not only enhances patients' quality of life but also improves survival rates. However, detecting breast cancer through gene expression data is a complex task due to challenges such as high dimensionality and intricate data structures. To address these difficulties, this chapter introduces an innovative deep learning model specifically designed for breast cancer detection, utilizing RNA-Seq gene expression data. What distinguishes this model is its incorporation of a hybrid gene selection approach that combines the strengths of the Harris Hawk and Whale Optimization (HHWO) algorithms with a deep learning architecture. The performance of this novel approach is assessed through a comparative analysis against five conventional algorithms, each integrated with deep learning techniques: Genetic Algorithm (GA), Artificial Bee Colony (ABC), Cuckoo Search (CS), and Particle Swarm Optimization (PSO). The results of our study demonstrate that the proposed model consistently delivers high classification performance, achieving an impressive mean accuracy of 99.0%. These findings highlight the potential of this method as a reliable and accurate tool for early breast cancer detection, which is essential for personalized treatment strategies.

Chapter 9 explores how the integration of advanced technologies in healthcare is ushering in a new era of patient care through the establishment of a sophisticated medical metaverse. This virtual environment allows patients to access remote clinics and hospitals, receive diagnoses, and consult with healthcare providers using virtual avatars, chatbots, and video interactions. AI algorithms further enhance healthcare delivery by analyzing medical data to assist in diagnostic and treatment decisions. The metaverse also provides immersive training for healthcare professionals, enabling them to refine their skills through realistic virtual simulations. With blockchain technology ensuring secure management of health data, patients can maintain control over their medical records while ensuring transparent access. Furthermore, virtual wellness and rehabilitation programs offer personalized therapy sessions, enhancing patient engagement and adherence. Social platforms within the metaverse connect patients with similar health conditions, fostering emotional support and shared experiences. Collaborative research in virtual labs accelerates the development of new treatments, therapies, and medical equipment. The application of big data and machine learning personalizes healthcare experiences, aligning with individual needs and genetic profiles. Ethical and regulatory frameworks protect patient privacy and ensure

Aims and Objectives

Aims of the Book

1. To explore the transformative impact of emerging technologies – such as HealthTech, artificial intelligence, deepfake, and the metaverse [u1.1]– on modern healthcare systems.
2. To provide a comprehensive understanding of innovative digital solutions like virtual healthcare, Digital Twins, and immersive technologies.
3. To examine the ethical, regulatory, and privacy challenges associated with the integration of AI, Deepfake, and Metaverse in healthcare.
4. To bridge the gap between healthcare innovation and practical applications, highlighting both clinical and business perspectives.

Objectives of the Book

1. Introduce readers to the core concepts of smart healthcare, HealthTech, Deepfake technology, and the Metaverse.
2. Explain how AI, machine learning, and immersive technologies are revolutionizing diagnostics, treatment, and patient engagement.
3. Analyze regulatory frameworks, ethical guidelines, and data privacy concerns in emerging healthcare technologies.
4. Present case studies and practical examples of precision medicine, digital twins, virtual reality, and blockchain applications in healthcare.
5. Equip researchers, practitioners, and students with knowledge to critically evaluate and adopt innovative healthcare solutions.
6. Highlight future trends and research directions at the intersection of technology and healthcare innovation.

List of Contributors

Ahmed, Saboor Uddin, *VIT Bhopal University, India*

Atanga, Roger, *University of Arizona, Tucson, AZ, USA*

Aziz, Rabia Musheer, *State Planning Institute, India*

Bandyopadhyay, Anjan, *Kalinga Institute of Industrial Technology, India*

Bhat, Mohd Abas, *University of Kashmir, India*

Budhathoki, Ram Kaji, *Kathmandu University, Nepal*

C., Chandru Vignesh, *Vellore Institute of Technology, India*

Chetana, V Lakshmi, *Amrita Vishwa Vidyapeetham, India*

Das, Aryan, *VIT Bhopal University, India*

Dinda, Sushil Kr., *Kalinga Institute of Industrial Technology, India*

Ghosh, Joyita, *Meghnad Saha Institute of Technlogy, India*

Gulzar, Yonis, *King Faisal University, Saudi Arabia*

Hu, Ruifeng, *Harvard Medical School, USA*

J., Alfred Daniel, *Karpagam Academy of Higher Education, India*

Jaganathan, Dharani, *KPR Institute of Engineering and Technology, India*

Juneja, Sapna, *KIET Group of Institutions, India*

Katti, Amogh, *GITAM University, India*

Kundu, Sayantan, *Kalinga Institute of Industrial Technology, India*

Lakshmi, R. Vijaya, *Amrita Vishwa Vidyapeetham, India*

Li., Aimin, *Xi'an University of Technology, China*

M., Arun Anoop, *AJ Institute of Engineering and Technology, India*

M., Saradha, *REVA University, India*

Mahmoud, Amena, *Kafrelsheikh University, Egypt; Sophia University, Japan*

Mahto, Rajul, *VIT Bhopal University, India*

Mallik, Saurav, *Harvard T H Chan School of Public Health, USA; The University of Arizona, Tucson, AZ, USA*

Mathivanan, Sandeep Kumar, *Galgotias University, India*

Mishra, Pradeep Kumar, *VIT Bhopal University, India*

Muthukumaran, V., *SRM Institute of Science and Technology, India*

N., Krishnaraj, *Vellore Institute of Technology, India*

Narmadha, R.P., *KIT – Kalaignar Karunanidhi Institute of Technology, India*

Naved, Mohd Inshal, *VIT Bhopal University, India*

Onyema, Edeh Michael, *Saveetha Institute of Medical and Technical Sciences, India*

P., Karthikeyan, *Velammal College of Engineering & Technology, India*

Pradhan, Tejaswini, *Kalinga University, India*

Rao, G.V.V. Jagannadha, *Kalinga University, India*

S., Ben Othman Soufiene, *King Faisal University, Saudi Arabia*

Seth, Soumita, *Future Institute of Engineering and Management, India; Aliah University, India*

Sett, Songita, *Maulana Abul Kalam Azad University of Technology, India*

Sree, Sure Divya, *REVA University, India*

Suman, Preetam, *VIT Bhopal University, India*

Verma, Navneet Kumar, *VIT Bhopal University's School of Advanced Science and Language, India*

Yaqoob, Abrar, *VIT Bhopal University's School of Advanced Science and Language, India*

List of Figures

List of Tables

List of Abbreviations

ABC	Artificial bee colony
AI	Artificial intelligence
AR	Augmented reality
ARTG	Australian register of therapeutic goods
ASM	Angular second moment
AUC	Area under the curve
BAM	Binary alignment map
BAT	Bat-inspired algorithm
CA	Classification accuracy
CAD	Computer-aided detection
CCU	Critical care units
cDNA	Complementary DNA
CDS	Clinical decision support
cffDNA	Cell-free fetal DNA
CNN	Convolutional neural network
CNS	Central nervous system
CS	Cuckoo search
DCE	Dynamic contrast-enhanced
DPIAs	Data protection impact assessments
DT	Decision tree
DTs	Digital twins
EHO	Elephant herding optimization
EHOSVM	Optimization with support vector machine
EHRs	Electronic health records
ELM	Extreme learning machine
EMA	European medicines agency
FDA	U.S. Food and drug administration
FN	False negatives
FP	False positives
FPR	False positive rate
GA	Genetic algorithm
GANs	General adversarial networks

GDPR	General data protection regulation
GLCM	Gray-level co-occurrence matrix
GLDZM	Gray level distance zone matrix
GLGM	Gray level and gradient magnitude
GLLV	Gray level-local variance
GLSC	Gray level spatial correlation
GLSZM	Gray level size zone matrix
GMP	Good manufacturing practice
GTF	Gene transfer format
GWAS	Genome-wide association studies
GWF	Gray weber features
GWO	Grey wolf optimizer
HazMat	Hazardous materials
HHO	Harris hawk optimization
HHWO	Harris hawk whale optimization
HIPAA	Health insurance portability and accountability act
HPV	Human papillomavirus
ICU	Intensive care units
ID	Intellectual disability
IDM	Inverse difference moments
IoMT	Internet of medical things
IoT	Internet of things
IVDR	In vitro diagnostic regulation
KNN	K-nearest neighbors
LBP	Local binary pattern
LCOS	Low cardiac output syndrome
LOOCV	Leave-one-out cross-validation
LSTM	Long short-term memory
MCIs	Mass casualty events
MDR	Medical devices regulation
MGLSZ	Multiple gray level size-zone
MHRA	Medicines and healthcare products regulatory agency
MIL	Multiple instance learning
ML	Machine learning
MR	Mixed reality
MRMR	Minimum redundancy maximum relevance
NB	Naive bayes
NDRF	National disaster response force
NGLDM	Neighborhood gray level dependence matrix
NGS	Next-generation sequencing

NGTDM	Neighborhood gray tone difference matrix
NLP	Natural language processing
NMPA	China's national medical products administration
OSA	Obstructive sleep apnea
PCR	Pathological complete response
PCR	Polymerase chain reaction
PFS	Progression-free survival
PMA	Premarket approval
PPV	Positive predictivity value
PR	Precision–recall
PSO	Particle swarm optimization
PTSD	Post-traumatic stress disorder
QNN	Quantum neural networks
RBM	Restricted boltzmann machine
RCB	Residual cancer burden
ResNets	Residual networks
RL	Reinforcement learning
RNA-seq	RNA sequencing
RNNs	Recurrent neural networks
ROC	Receiver operating characteristic
SAM	Sequence alignment map
SL	Supervised learning
SMO	Spider monkey optimization
SRA	Sequence read archive
SSA	Salp swarm algorithm
SSL	Semi-supervised learning
SVM	Support vector machines
TGA	Therapeutic goods administration
TN	True negatives
TP	True positives
TPR	True positive rate
UKCA	UK conformity assessed
VAEs	Variational autoencoders
VR	Virtual reality
VUS	Variants of unknown significance
WGLv	Weber gray local variants
WHO	World health organization
WOA	Whale optimization algorithm
WSI	Whole-slide images
WSL	Windows subsystem for linux

1

Introduction: Fundamentals of HealthTech Horizons with Smart Healthcare Innovations, Deepfake, and the Metaverse

Songita Sett[1], Soumita Seth[2,3], Saurav Mallik[4,5] and Roger Atanga[5]

[1]Maulana Abul Kalam Azad University of Technology, India.
[2]Future Institute of Engineering and Management, India.
[3]Aliah University, India.
[4]Harvard T H Chan School of Public Health, USA.
[5]University of Arizona, Tucson, AZ, USA.

Email: songita.sett@gmail.com; soumita.seth@teamfuture.in; soumita.seth@gmail.com; sauravmtech2@gmail.com; smallik@arizona.edu; ratanga@arizona.edu

Abstract

This chapter lays the foundation for exploring the dynamic intersection of healthcare and cutting-edge technologies. It introduces the core themes of the book – smart healthcare innovations, deepfake technology, and the Metaverse – positioning them as pivotal forces reshaping modern medicine. The chapter begins by tracing the evolution of HealthTech, highlighting the paradigm shift from conventional care models to intelligent, data-driven, and immersive healthcare systems. It emphasizes the transformative impact of artificial intelligence, digital twins, and extended reality in diagnosis, treatment, training, and patient engagement. Special attention is given to the emerging roles of deepfake technology in medical education and simulation, and how the Metaverse fosters collaborative care, remote access, and

DOI: 10.1201/9788743809920-1

personalized therapeutic experiences. Ethical considerations, data security challenges, and regulatory frameworks are also briefly introduced to underscore the complexity of responsible innovation in this domain. By setting the stage for deeper exploration in subsequent chapters, this introductory chapter provides readers with a comprehensive overview of the technological horizons shaping the future of global healthcare.

1.1 The Transformation of Healthcare

Healthcare has always been a domain shaped by innovation, but never before has the pace of change been so swift, nor its potential so profound. Today, we are witnessing a monumental shift – one where technology is no longer an accessory to healthcare but a driving force at its core. Artificial intelligence, the internet of medical things (IoMT), virtual reality, and data-driven diagnostics are transforming the way we understand, deliver, and experience care [1].

This evolution is not happening in isolation. Broader societal changes – such as the rise of remote work, increasing digital literacy, and the explosion of wearable technologies – are making smart healthcare more accessible, more personalized, and more integral to everyday life. What was once futuristic is now becoming foundational [2].

1.2 The Rise of Deepfake and Synthetic Media in Healthcare

Parallel to the explosion of smart healthcare technologies is the controversial yet powerful growth of deepfake and synthetic media technologies. While often discussed in the context of misinformation, deepfake tools also present transformative possibilities for healthcare when applied ethically [3].

From creating realistic patient simulations for medical training to developing advanced therapeutic interventions, synthetic media could help bridge gaps in education, accessibility, and communication. As these technologies mature, they offer a new kind of storytelling – one that can deepen empathy, improve patient engagement, and support complex medical decisions in dynamic ways [4].

However, with such power comes responsibility. The healthcare sector must ensure that synthetic media technologies are developed and deployed with the utmost regard for authenticity, consent, and the preservation of trust – values that are foundational to medicine [5].

1.3 Healthcare in the Metaverse: New Dimensions of Care

The Metaverse, a collective virtual space combining digital realities, is beginning to open new frontiers for healthcare innovation. In these immersive environments, patients and providers can interact beyond physical limitations. Virtual hospitals, rehabilitation programs, mental health communities, and training simulations are already taking form within this new digital realm [6].

The Metaverse offers potential for truly patient-centered care – where personalized, continuous, and engaging healthcare journeys become the norm. From enabling remote surgical collaborations to hosting decentralized clinical trials, the possibilities for more efficient, accessible, and immersive healthcare experiences are expanding rapidly.

Yet, navigating healthcare in the Metaverse requires a rethinking of regulation, security, ethical norms, and even the traditional definitions of clinical spaces. As healthcare expands into these virtual dimensions, striking the right balance between technological freedom and human-centered care will be crucial.

1.4 Challenges and Responsibilities Ahead

The convergence of smart technologies, deepfake media, and the Metaverse in healthcare brings extraordinary promise – but it also carries significant challenges. Privacy concerns, digital inequality, cybersecurity threats, and ethical dilemmas are already emerging as central issues.

Healthcare systems must address not just the technological questions of "what" is possible, but also the societal questions of "why" and "for whom." Innovation must serve humanity, not widen gaps in access, trust, or quality. Equity, transparency, empathy, and safety must guide every step forward.

Policy makers, technologists, clinicians, educators, and patients themselves all have roles to play in shaping a future where technology elevates health outcomes rather than creating new vulnerabilities [7].

1.5 A New Horizon of Hope and Innovation

At its heart, the future of healthcare is about more than technology; it is about human lives, dignity, and well-being. As we stand at this crossroads, we are presented with an extraordinary opportunity: to imagine, design, and build healthcare systems that are smarter, more inclusive, more compassionate, and profoundly more effective.

The path ahead demands bold vision, careful stewardship, and a collective commitment to align innovation with humanity's deepest values. By harnessing the best of smart healthcare innovations, synthetic media, and immersive virtual realities, we can move toward a future where health and technology are partners – not competitors – in the service of life.

The horizon is bright, and the journey has just begun.

1.6 Translating Innovation into Clinical Reality

While technological possibilities abound, the translation of HealthTech innovation into real-world clinical practice is a nuanced process. Healthcare systems are complex and deeply human-centric. Integrating technologies like AI, digital twins, and the Metaverse requires **behavioral change, policy readiness**, and **trust-building** among users. For example, introducing AI-based diagnostics into radiology departments demands [7]:

- Clinician training to interpret model outputs
- Regulatory clearance to ensure compliance with health safety laws
- IT support for integration with hospital information systems
- Ethical review to prevent biases in decision-making

A 2023 survey conducted across 150 global hospitals (see Table 1.1) revealed that over 60% of technology pilots fail not because of the algorithm's performance but due to poor workflow integration, lack of clinician buy-in, and data quality issues.

Table 1.1 Top barriers to implementing HealthTech in hospitals.

Barrier	Percentage affected
Lack of workflow integration	63%
Low clinician trust	59%
Data privacy concerns	48%
High implementation costs	45%
Unclear regulatory guidelines	42%
Poor digital infrastructure	38%

Conventional era →	**Digital augmentation →**	**Immersive simulation**
Lectures, books	Online courses, AI MCQs	VR, digital twins, deepfake patients
Cadaver dissection	3D models	Haptic feedback simulations
Observation-based	Case libraries	Adaptive AI tutors

Figure 1.1 Evolution of medical education in the HealthTech age.

1.7 Rethinking Medical Education in the Digital Era

Health Tech doesn't just change how we treat diseases – it transforms how we teach medicine. The traditional model of lectures, dissection labs, and apprenticeship is rapidly evolving. In its place emerges a digitally enriched, simulation- driven, and AI-supported educational ecosystem [8]. Medical students today are being trained with:

- VR/AR-based anatomical learning
- AI-powered personalized quizzes
- Metaverse-based collaborative simulations
- Deepfake-based dynamic patient interactions

These innovations enable exposure to rare diseases, difficult conversations, and emergency scenarios that would be hard to replicate in the real world (Figure 1.1).

1.8 Ethical Imperatives in the HealthTech Age

Ethics in HealthTech is not a side note – it is central. Technologies like deepfakes and AI not only challenge clinical norms but also redefine **truth, consent, and autonomy** in healthcare [9]. Key ethical questions in emerging HealthTech:

- Can synthetic medical data be used without disclosing its origin to trainees?
- Who is legally accountable for an AI's misdiagnosis?
- Should patients be allowed to "opt out" of digital twin modelling?
- How do we ensure emotional safety in hyper-realistic Metaverse environments?

Table 1.2 Four-layer ethical framework for HealthTech.

Ethical layer	Description
Data ethics	Consent, transparency, anonymization
Algorithmic ethics	Fairness, explainability, reproducibility
Interface ethics	Avatar behavior, user psychology
Social ethics	Access, equity, digital divide

A 4-layer ethical framework is emerging in global discourse, outlining key principles that guide responsible innovation in HealthTech, as summarized in Table 1.2.

1.9 Toward a Humane and Inclusive Future

HealthTech's promise lies in **personalization, precision, and participation** – but its true success will be measured by how **inclusively and humanely** it is applied. We must ensure:

- Cultural sensitivity in digital design
- Inclusion for the elderly and disabled
- Low-bandwidth compatibility for rural populations
- Ethical data use across demographic boundaries

In this way, the future becomes not just smarter, but fairer – bringing the benefits of HealthTech to both the world's elite institutions and its most underserved clinics.

1.10 Conclusion

The HealthTech revolution is more than a convergence of technology and medicine – it is the emergence of a new philosophy of care. One that is immersive, data-driven, ethically aware, and centered on human dignity. As we move deeper into this landscape, we must proceed with equal measures of curiosity and caution, speed and sensitivity, invention and introspection. This chapter lays the foundation not only for exploring tools like AI, deepfakes, and the Metaverse – but for reimagining care itself. The horizon is bright, but it is the wisdom of our steps that will determine whether we build a system that heals both the body and the soul.

Building upon this conceptual foundation, the subsequent chapters expand into focused domains where these transformative technologies are actively shaping the future of healthcare. From the use of digital twins in disease prediction and personalized treatment optimization, to the application of deepfake technologies in medical training, simulation, and patient education, each chapter explores how once-speculative tools are now embedded in practical and experimental workflows. Several chapters investigate how advanced deep learning techniques are revolutionizing medical imaging, genomic diagnostics, and precision oncology – unlocking patterns in high-dimensional gene expression data that were previously too complex to decipher. Attention is also given to the clinical integration of hybrid optimization methods, such as nature-inspired algorithms and ensemble classifiers, which have shown remarkable success in feature selection and disease classification. The book further delves into the ethical and security implications of medical image manipulation, proposing AI-driven frameworks to detect forgery and ensure image authenticity in diagnostic contexts. Emergency response is reimagined through immersive Metaverse platforms, offering virtual simulations that prepare first responders and clinicians for high-risk scenarios using real-time feedback, blockchain-secured records, and AI-guided decision-making. As the narrative unfolds, the reader is guided through a multidimensional landscape – spanning chronic disease prediction, virtual therapy, telemedicine interfaces, and computational models for colorectal and breast cancer – each case revealing how digital health technologies are evolving from experimental to essential. Together, the chapters demonstrate not only the promise but also the complexity of building a responsible, intelligent, and inclusive digital health future – anchored in ethical design, clinical utility, and patient-centered care.

"Technology will change the tools of healing, but never its purpose."

References

[1] Topol, E. J. (2019). High-performance medicine: the convergence of human and artificial intelligence. *Nature Medicine*, **25**(1), 44–56.

[2] Esteva, A., Robicquet, A., Ramsundar, B., et al. (2021). A guide to deep learning in healthcare. *Nature Medicine*, **25**(1), 24–29.

[3] Sharif, W., Khan, M. U., Haider, S. (2020). A Deepfake bot for teaching medical communication: a proof-of-concept study. *Artificial Intelligence in Medicine*, **108**, 101962.

[4] Yu, L., et al. (2019). Medical image synthesis for data augmentation and anonymization using generative adversarial networks. *Medical Image Analysis*, **55**, 93–101.
[5] Van der Meer, T., Younesi, E. (2020). Digital twins: applications in health care and the challenges ahead. *npj Digital Medicine*, **3**, 1–5.
[6] Saini, P., Chouhan, V., & Mehta, D. (2023). Application and challenges of a metaverse in medicine. *Frontiers in Robotics and AI*, **10**, 1291199. https: //doi.org/10.3389/frobt.2023.1291199.
[7] Mesko, B. (2020). The future of medicine is digital health and smart tech- nology. *Journal of Clinical Medicine*, **9**(2), 279.
[8] Bandyopadhyay, A., Sarkar, A., Swain, S., Banik, D., Hassanien, A. E., Mallik, S., Li, A., Qin, H., "A Game Theoretic Approach For Rendering Immersive Experiences In The Metaverse", Special issue of "Mathematical Modelling in Biology", Mathematics, 2023, 11(6), 1286; https://doi.org/ 10.3390/math11061286.
[9] Morley, J., Machado, C.C.V., Burr, C., Cowls, J., Joshi, I., Taddeo, M., & Floridi, L. (2020). The ethics of AI in health care: A mapping re- view. Social Science & Medicine, 260, 113172. https://doi.org/10.1016/ j.socscimed.2020.113172.

2

Health Digital Twins: A New Era in Healthcare

V Lakshmi Chetana[1], Amogh Katti[2], Saurav Mallik[3] and Ruifeng Hu[4]

[1]School of Computing, Amrita Vishwa Vidyapeetham, Amaravati Campus, Kuragallu Village, Andhra Pradesh, India.
[2]GITAM University, Hyderabad, Telangana, India.
[3]University of Arizona, Tucson, AZ 85721, USA.
[4]Harvard Medical School, Boston, MA 02115, USA.

Email: s_lakshmichetana@av.amrita.edu; akatti@gitam.edu; sauravmtech2@gmail.com; huruifeng.cn@hotmail.com

Abstract

Digital twins (DTs), an umbrella of metaverse, are the virtual representations of physical entities, which are applied in disease prediction, treatment optimization, and personalized medicine domains. They use technologies like Cloud, AI, IoT, etc., to create detailed patient models, enable healthcare providers to facilitate tailored patient care, and further improve patient health conditions. This chapter presents the applications of DTs in healthcare domain, like personalized medicine, remote patient monitoring, treatment optimization, clinical decision support, and drug discovery. It also highlights the challenges of digital twins, like data privacy, security, and computational limitations. It also highlights the promising future of DTs in revolutionizing healthcare by providing personalized, data-driven solutions and improving patient outcomes.

2.1 Introduction

One of the newest ideas shaping the future of the internet is Web 3.0. Often called the Semantic Web, Web 3.0 is a big change in how we use the internet.

DOI: 10.1201/9788743809920-2

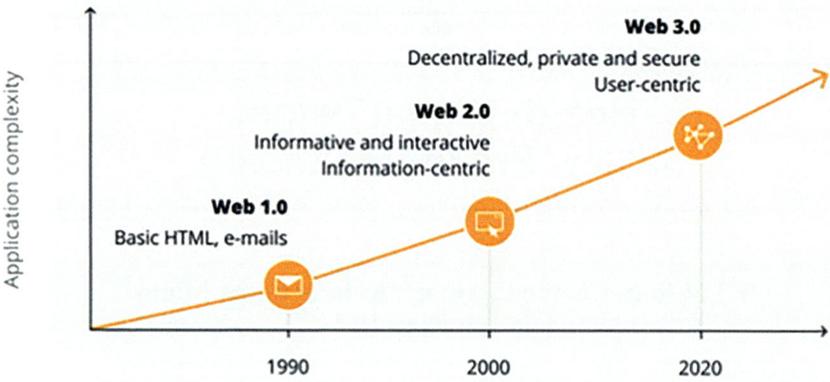

Figure 2.1 Evolution of Web 3.0 [6] (Source: 101 Blockchain).

Figure 2.1 shows the evolution of Web 3.0. In the past, we used Web 1.0 (static web), where we could only read things online, like simple web pages. Then came Web 2.0, which made the internet more fun. We could create and share content using social media, blogs, and videos. Here, technologies allow for decentralization, meaning that users have more authority over their activities and data on the internet [1–3]. Instead of relying on big organizations, Web 3.0 utilizes blockchain as a means to decentralize control. In this context, metaverse is a perfect example of what the next generation of internet is going to look like. The metaverse is decentralized, as it is based on the principles of Web 3.0. Thus, it empowers users and turns all that we do on the internet into virtual reality worlds. Therefore, the metaverse is a part of the "new" internet in that it goes beyond everyday technologies and makes for a vast environment for users to give a try to something innovative and unfamiliar [2]. Metaverse is a combination of several innovative technologies, including blockchain, artificial intelligence (AI), virtual reality (VR), and augmented reality (AR) [3–5].

The metaverse has the potential to revolutionize various industries. In entertainment and gaming, immersive virtual environments can enhance social experiences and create new economic opportunities [7]. Educational institutions leverage metaverse for collaborative learning, virtual classrooms, and simulations [1]. E-commerce platforms offer a unique shopping experience to their customers to search and buy items in a virtual environment. Businesses can benefit from virtual meetings, conferences, and collaborative workspaces, facilitating global connections. Healthcare providers use metaverse for virtual training, remote consultations, and therapeutic interventions. Real estate can also benefit from virtual property tours, events, and business meetings. The metaverse's versatility extends across multiple domains, reforming how we interact, learn, work, and play.

The metaverse is a boon for healthcare domain, particularly during the challenges posed by the COVID-19 pandemic. As healthcare systems worldwide grapple with the strain of the crisis, innovative approaches are essential to ensure continuous care, engage patients, and minimize physical contact. The metaverse offers a compelling platform for virtual healthcare delivery, facilitating remote consultations, telemedicine services, and immersive medical training experiences. VR and AR technologies empower individuals to conveniently access healthcare facilities from their homes [1], minimizing the risk of virus transmission and easing the burden on strained healthcare facilities. Furthermore, the metaverse fosters virtual support communities and educational resources, promoting collaboration and knowledge sharing among healthcare practitioners and researchers globally. Ultimately, integrating the metaverse into healthcare infrastructure provides a transformative opportunity to enhance accessibility, effectiveness, and adaptability in addressing public health emergencies like the COVID-19 pandemic [8].

Digital twins (DTs) revolutionize modelling and simulation by creating virtual replicas of real-world entities within a virtual environment. These digital counterparts enable in-depth analysis, monitoring, and experimentation in an immersive and interactive manner [9]. In the healthcare sector, DTs serve as invaluable tools for generating personalized patient models. These models allow healthcare professionals to track health conditions, predict potential complications, and tailor treatments with greater accuracy. This innovative approach marks a significant shift toward patient-centered, inclusive, and data-driven healthcare. The metaverse, with its immersive capabilities, plays a vital role in enabling this transformation, enhancing healthcare delivery and accessibility [10]. As a result, patients can actively manage their health more effectively, while healthcare providers can deliver personalized and efficient care. This chapter delves into the concepts of health digital twins, exploring their potential to enhance patient outcomes and healthcare service delivery [11]. It delves into the necessary technologies for digital twin implementation, explores their various applications and advantages, and scrutinizes their adaptability across different healthcare scenarios. Additionally, it highlights the challenges in integrating digital twin technology into healthcare and suggests potential remedies [12].

2.2 Digital Twin Technology

The term "digital twin (DT)" was coined by Michael Grieves at the Michigan University in 2003 in the manufacturing and engineering sectors [7]. It was initially conceived as a method to digitally replicate physical objects or systems for analysis and optimization. Digital twins, initially employed for simulation and analysis in manufacturing, have expanded their applications across diverse fields like healthcare, transportation, energy, and urban planning. Advances in IoT, cloud, data analytics, and AI have accelerated their adoption. Organizations are now utilizing digital twins to predict maintenance needs, optimize operations, and make data-driven decisions. Digital twins in healthcare are virtual representations of patients or physiological systems, revolutionizing healthcare delivery and management. By integrating data from diverse sources, like genetic information, medical imaging, electronic health records, and wearable technology, these digital twins create intricate models for each patient [11]. Figure 2.2 illustrates a patient's digital twin. Through advanced analytics and simulation, healthcare providers gain a profound understanding of patient conditions, predict disease progression, and optimize treatment strategies [13]. This technology enables personalized medicine, tailoring interventions to individual patient characteristics and enhancing clinical outcomes. Digital twins allow patients to enthusiastically participate in their healthcare journey, delivering valuable insights into their health status and treatment options [13]. As the healthcare sector continues to evolve, digital twins are indispensable for driving innovation, optimizing processes, and delivering patient-centered care.

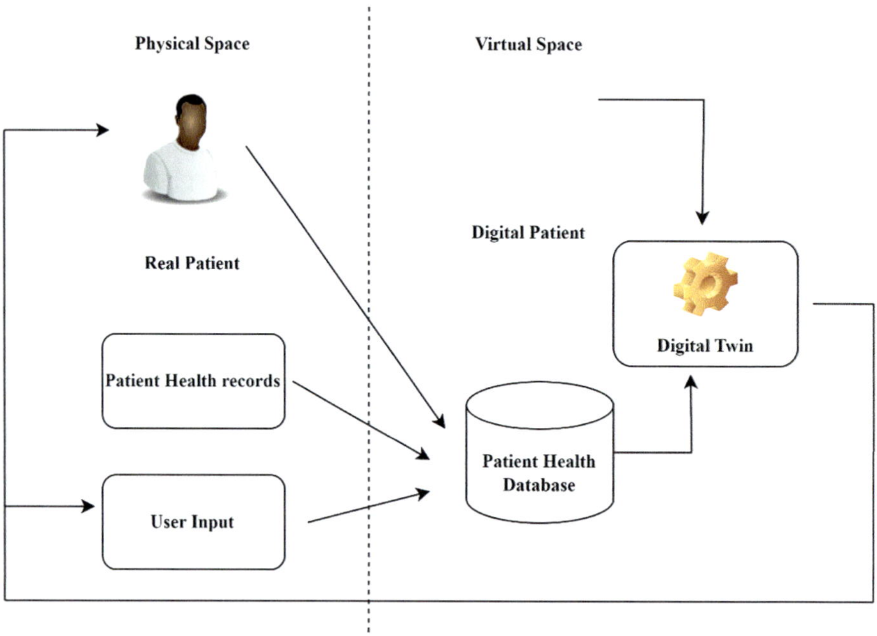

Figure 2.2 An illustration of a patient's digital twin.

2.2.1 Foundations of digital twin technology

Digital twins utilize a mixture of technologies to create virtual representations of physical objects. Figure 2.3 depicts some of the key technologies employed in digital twins, such as:

1. ***Internet of Things:*** Utilizing sensors and actuators, the IoT collects data from physical objects and environments. Digital twins use this for analysis and monitoring [14, 9].

2. ***Cloud Computing:*** Cloud platforms offer necessary computational and storage capabilities to handle the large datasets produced by digital twins [8, 15].

3. ***Big Data Analytics:*** Employing AI and ML techniques, big data analytics examines data from sensors and various sources, extracting valuable insights and identifying patterns.

4. ***VR and AR:*** VR and AR provide immersive visualization capabilities, permitting users to interact with and explore digital twins in three-dimensional environments.

5. ***Blockchain:*** This technology ensures the security, integrity, and transparency of data stored in digital twins, especially in healthcare and

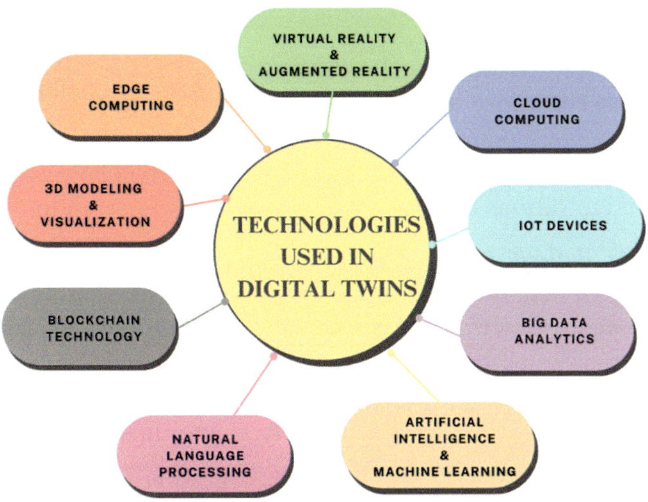

Figure 2.3 Technologies used in health digital twins.

supply chain management domains where data privacy and provenance are crucial.

6. ***Edge Computing:*** This approach enables processing of data nearer to its origin, which reduces latency in distributed digital twin environments.
7. ***3D Modelling and Visualization:*** In some cases, 3D printing technology is used to create physical replicas of digital twin models for further analysis or validation.
8. ***AI and ML:*** Usage of these techniques analyze data, optimize models, and enable autonomous decision-making, improving prediction and adaptability in digital twin environments.
9. ***Natural Language Processing:*** NLP allows digital twins to understand, communicate, and extract insights from textual data, enhancing their effectiveness.

By integrating these technologies, digital twins can accurately replicate and simulate the behavior of complex physical entities, providing valuable insights and supporting informed decision-making in areas like manufacturing, healthcare, transportation, and smart cities.

2.2.2 Health digital twin applications

Digital twins are being used in myriad ways in different sectors of healthcare, as shown in Figure 2.4. These encompass:

1. ***Personalized Medicine:*** Health digital twins enable healthcare providers to customize treatment plans based on patient's distinct genetic makeup, past medical records, lifestyle, and environmental factors. By analyzing this comprehensive data, DTs can predict how a patient might respond to various therapies, medications, and interventions [13].
2. ***Remote Patient Monitoring:*** Because of continuous collection and analysis of health records from wearable devices, sensors, and mobile applications [16], digital twins allow healthcare specialists to distantly observe patients' behavior toward a medicine, and their overall well-being. By promptly alerting healthcare teams to potential health concerns, these digital representations facilitate timely interventions and reduce frequent in-person visits.
3. ***Treatment Optimization:*** By leveraging personalized patient data, digital twins simulate various scenarios and predict their potential outcomes, aiding healthcare providers in optimizing treatments. By assessing the

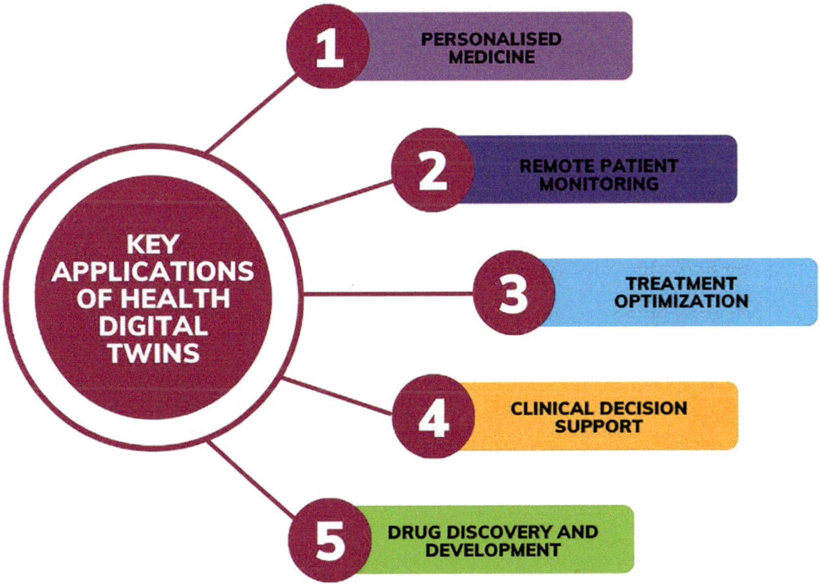

Figure 2.4 Applications of health digital twins.

efficacy of different treatment options, adjusting medication dosages, and tailoring therapy plans, clinicians can maximize patient outcomes while minimizing adverse effects and risks.

4. ***Clinical Decision Support (CDS):*** By integrating patient-specific data with clinical protocols and scholarly resources, these digital representations enable clinicians to make informed decisions regarding diagnosis, treatment strategies, and overall patient care.

5. ***Drug Discovery and Development:*** Digital twins play a pivotal role in drug development and discovery by simulating the effects of potential drug candidates on virtual patient models. These digital replicas enable pharmaceutical firms to predict drug reactions, identify patient groups likely to benefit from specific therapies, and optimize clinical trial designs to improve drug efficacy and safety.

2.3 Recent works on Digital Twins in Healthcare

This section provides a literature survey on digital twins in healthcare involving a review of research articles, conference papers, and other scholarly sources to assess the current advancements, as outlined in Table 2.1.

Table 2.1 Current developments in digital twin technology for health care.

Paper	Year	Contributions
[13]	2023	• The authors proposed that DT technology could significantly transform healthcare. • They envision DTs as virtual representations of patients, organs, or even entire hospitals. • By combining data from multiple sources like wearable devices, electronic health records (EHRs), etc., these digital replicas could provide real-time insights for tailored treatment plans, enhanced clinical care, and predictive analytics. • However, the paper highlights the challenges of integrating diverse data sources and ensuring data privacy and security.
[17]	2023	• This work provides a thorough outline of current research going on in the field of health digital twins. • It highlights its applications like individualized treatment plans, predictive modelling, medical education, remote patient monitoring, drug discovery, and optimizing healthcare systems.
[18]	2023	• This research explores the potential of health DTs. The authors examine how DTs can enhance patient care, personalize treatments, and improve healthcare education in this virtual environment. • While the study highlights the benefits of DTs, it could delve deeper into the technical challenges and limitations of their implementation.
[19]	2023	• This work provides the revolutionary potential of DTs in healthcare. • It showcases a few of its applications, like personalized medicine, predictive analytics, remote monitoring, and healthcare system optimization. • It also highlights the advantages of DTs in optimizing healthcare administration, patient results, and expediting advancements in medical research and innovation.
[20]	2022	• This paper outlines how digital twins revolutionize healthcare. This work discusses applications like remote monitoring, personalized medicine, predictive analytics, drug development, and healthcare system optimization.

[21]	2022	• This work outlines the potential impact of metaverse on personal healthcare. • It explores how the metaverse could facilitate innovative healthcare solutions, such as personalized health tracking, virtual medical consultations, interactive health education, and game-based wellness experiences. • The paper highlights concerns related to data privacy and security in virtual spaces, unequal access to metaverse technologies, potential ethical issues with virtual health interventions, and the necessity for regulatory frameworks to ensure the safety and efficacy of metaverse-based healthcare solutions.
[22]	2023	• The authors concentrated on constructing virtual patient replicas to assist in diagnosis, treatment planning, and resource management. Machine learning and modelling approaches are investigated to forecast disease progression and create decision-support tools. • While the paper likely emphasizes the advantages of DTs, it may not extensively explore the ethical considerations of utilizing personal patient information or the difficulties associated with data privacy. • Furthermore, the technical challenges of integrating various healthcare data sources into a unified DT system may not be fully addressed.
[23]	2022	• This research examines the technological foundations of digital twins, including IoT, cloud computing, AI, and data analytics. It underscores the advantages of digital twins in predictive maintenance, optimization, and decision-making. • Additionally, the study addresses challenges such as data security and privacy, standardization, and integration with existing systems. Finally, it explores emerging trends and future applications of digital twins across various industries.
[24]	2023	• This work investigates the potential of DTs in personalized medicine. It explores applications in patient monitoring, disease diagnosis, and the development of tailored treatment plans. • The paper underscores the importance of integrating diverse data sources, including omics data and AI, to create comprehensive digital twins. • However, it also acknowledges challenges such as data integration complexities, computational limitations for handling complex models, and patient privacy concerns. The study suggests that overcoming these obstacles could lead to a future of revolutionary healthcare with personalized solutions.

(*Continued*)

Table 2.1 *Continued.*

Paper	Year	Contributions
[25]	2023	• This study examines the increasing use of digital twin technology in personalized healthcare. It discusses its potential benefits in diagnosing diseases, planning treatments, and managing hospitals. • However, the authors recognize the need for accurate data to create effective simulations and the difficulties of using this technology in real-world medical settings
[26]	2023	• This study explores the growing impact of digital twins in various industries. They offer many benefits, including faster product development, better maintenance planning, and smoother operations. • The research shows case studies in areas like manufacturing, shipping, and city planning. • However, the authors also point out challenges such as data security, the complexity of creating and maintaining digital twins, and the need for standard ways of working.
[27]	2020	• This paper delves into digital twins, which are virtual counterparts of real-world entities, investigating the fundamental technologies underpinning DTs such as AI, IoT, and cloud computing. • It emphasizes the advantages of DTs across different sectors for predictive maintenance and performance optimization. • Nevertheless, it recognizes hurdles like establishing a sturdy IT infrastructure for data management and the necessity for more exploration in aspects like DT standardization and security.
[28]	2024	• The paper explores the potential of DTs in revolutionizing the healthcare domain. • DTs offers a promising approach to personalized medicine by leveraging data collected from wearable devices. They also help in predicting disease progression, optimizing treatment plans, and enabling remote patient monitoring. • However, they suffer from issues like data privacy, model accuracy, and ethical considerations.
[29]	2024	• This work explores the DT's potential in medicine by improving patient health, reducing costs, and enhancing self-management. • It proposes a four-level ontological model for creating patient-centric digital twins, aiming to optimize disease therapy and healthcare decision-making. • It highlights the challenges like data privacy, ethical considerations, and the complexity of accurately modelling human physiology, highlighting the need for further research to address these limitations [30].

2.4 Role of Digital Twins among Different Healthcare Contexts

Digital twin technology can be used in a wide range of healthcare contexts. Some of the contexts include:

2.4.1 For COVID patients

The COVID-19 outbreak presented unprecedented challenges to healthcare systems worldwide, necessitating innovative solutions for its effective management and control. In this context, DT technology has emerged as a valuable tool, that offers healthcare professionals real-time insights, predictive analytics, and simulation capabilities. This technology plays a critical role in remotely monitoring patients, facilitating the real-time tracking and analysis of health data. With the help of DTs, healthcare providers made informed decisions and adjustments to treatment plans without the need for in-person visits. Overall, their implementation during the COVID pandemic, highlighted the significance and potential of digital health technologies in revolutionizing the way healthcare is delivered.

2.4.2 For intellectual disability (ID) people

People with intellectual disabilities need special help to overcome their challenges and live better lives. Regular ways of caring for them might not work for everyone. Digital twins, which are like digital copies of people, can help caregivers understand their needs, likes, and what they can do. This can lead to better care plans, easier communication, and a better quality of life. As digital twins get better, they can help people with intellectual disabilities a lot and make society more inclusive.

2.4.3 For cancer patients

Cancer remains a major cause of illness and death worldwide, posing significant challenges for healthcare systems and individuals. Traditional cancer treatments often use a one-size-fits-all method, which may not take each patient's profile into consideration. Digital twin, a new technology, can create personalized virtual models of a patient's cancer [31]. This allows doctors to test different treatments on a digital copy of the tumor before using them in real life. This helps doctors predict how a cancer will respond to different therapies, leading to more personalized and effective treatment plans.

Digital twins can also track the progress of the cancer in real time, providing valuable information for adjusting treatment as needed. As cancer treatment moves toward more personalized approaches, digital twins offer a promising tool for improving patient outcomes.2.4.4 For critical care units (CCU) and intensive care units (ICU) patients: CCUs and ICUs are essential for treating very sick patients. These patients need constant watching, quick help, and special care. DT technology makes ICUs better by creating virtual copies of patients. This lets doctors see what's happening in real time, predict problems, and plan the best care. It also lets them try different treatments and see what works best. Using DT, doctors can track important signs, see problems coming, and change treatments to help patients get better faster and leave the ICU sooner.

2.4.5 For patients with chronic disease conditions

Chronic diseases, like diabetes, heart problems, and lung conditions, are putting a strain on healthcare systems around the world. To manage these diseases effectively, doctors need to create personalized treatment plans, monitor patients regularly, and step in quickly to prevent complications. Digital twin technology can help by creating virtual copies of each patient. This allows doctors to tailor treatment plans and improve patient care, especially for people with chronic illnesses.

2.5 Challenges of Health Digital Twins

Table 2.2 lists the key issues faced by health digital twins and their possible solutions to overcome.

Table 2.2 Key challenges and its possible solutions for health digital twins.

Challenge	Description	Possible solution
Data privacy and security	Protecting sensitive health data from breaches and unauthorized access.	• Implement strong cybersecurity measures, data encryption, and access control. • Educate healthcare providers and patients on data privacy practices. • Develop clear legal frameworks for data ownership and usage.

Challenge	Description	Possible solution
Data integration and interoperability	Ensuring data quality, consistency, and seamless integration from various sources (wearables, medical records, etc.).	• Standardize data formats, perform regular data audits and cleansing, utilize data harmonization tools, and invest in secure data platforms.
Data quality and accuracy	Inaccurate data leads to unreliable predictions.	• Implement data validation, cleansing, and governance procedures. • Use AI-powered tools for anomaly detection and data cleaning. • Encourage patients to actively participate in data verification.
Computational power and cost	Requiring significant processing power and storage for complex models and real-time updates.	• Explore cloud computing solutions, optimize algorithms, and leverage distributed computing systems. • Develop cost-effective approaches and prioritize essential functionalities.
Model development and maintenance	Creating high-fidelity models that accurately represent individual patient physiology and respond to interventions.	• Utilize advanced AI and machine learning techniques, integrate multi-scale and multi-physics models, and validate models with real-world data. • Establish standardized development and maintenance processes.
Model complexity and explainability	Complex models can be difficult to interpret and trust.	• Develop explainable AI (XAI) techniques that elucidate model decisions. • Encourage collaboration between clinicians and data scientists to build clinically relevant models.
User acceptance and adoption	Healthcare providers and patients need to be comfortable using digital twins.	• Provide detailed information on the benefits and risks of using digital twins. • Conduct training and awareness campaigns. • Demonstrate the value proposition of digital twins through pilot projects and real-world examples.

(Continued)

Table 2.2 *Continued.*

Challenge	Description	Possible solution
Ethical considerations	Addressing concerns about potential biases, discrimination, and misuse of patient data.	• Develop clear ethical guidelines and transparency protocols. • Ensure user control over data access and use. • Promote responsible AI development and deployment.
Legal and regulatory landscape	Navigating evolving regulations and data privacy laws.	• Advocate for clear and adaptable regulatory frameworks for digital twins in healthcare. • Collaborate with policymakers and legal experts to address emerging challenges.

2.6 Conclusion

Metaverse, a digital space, is a key concept in Web 3.0, integrates the concepts of cloud, blockchain, virtual and augmented reality, and artificial intelligence. This blurs the line between physical and digital realities, offering immersive virtual worlds and interactive experiences across industries. Digital twins, enable real-time interaction, personalization, and persistence in immersive digital environments. Digital twins are now present across multiple sectors, like energy, healthcare, urban planning, and transportation. They enable healthcare providers to gain deeper insights into patient conditions, predict disease progression, and optimize treatment strategies. However, challenges like data privacy, security concerns, disparities in access to metaverse technologies, and potential ethical issues must be addressed. Solutions for implementing digital twins in healthcare include strong cybersecurity measures, data encryption, access control, data quality and accuracy, cloud computing solutions, explainable AI techniques, user acceptance and adoption, addressing potential biases, discrimination, and misuse of patient data, and navigating evolving regulations and data privacy laws.

References

[1] G. Chhabra and K. Kaushik, *Understanding the Metaverse : applications, challenges, and the future*. Springer, 2025.

[2] "Metaverse Development Company - Shaping Virtual Realities for Limitless Adventures and Creating Infinite Realities for Tomorrow |

The Chain." [Online]. Available: https://vocal.media/theChain/metaverse-development-company-shaping-virtual-realities-for-limitless-adventures-and-creating-infinite-realities-for-tomorrow. [Accessed: 23-Jul-2024].

[3] Maria Megia Cardenoso, "Digital Twins in Civil Engineering : Conceptual Framework and Real-World Implementations," 2024.

[4] Y.-S. Seo, Hyo-Min Kim, and Austin Kang, "ANALYSIS OF MEDIA DISCOURSE ON INTELLECTUAL PROPERTY RIGHTS RELATED TO METAVERSE IN KOREA," *Int. J. Secur. Priv. Trust Manag.*, vol. 13, no. 2, 2024.

[5] C. Song, S. Shin, and Kwang-Seong Shin, "Exploring the Key Characteristics and Theoretical Framework for Research on the Metaverse," *Appl. Sci.*, vol. 13, 2023.

[6] D. Kukreja, S. Gupta, D. Patel, and J. N. Rai, "Scientometric review of Web 3.0," *https://doi.org/10.1177/01655515231182073*, Jun. 2023.

[7] E. TUR, "Harnessing the Power of Digital Twins for Enhanced Material Behavior Prediction and Manufacturing Process Optimization in Materials Engineering," *Bayburt Üniversitesi Fen Bilim. Derg.*, vol. 6, no. 2, pp. 172–190, 2023.

[8] K. Mondal, O. Martinez, and P. Jain, "Advanced manufacturing and digital twin technology for nuclear energy," *Front. Energy Res.*, vol. 12, no. February, pp. 1–20, 2024.

[9] S. Rani, P. Bhambri, S. Kumar, P. K. Pareek, and A. A. Elngar, *AI-Driven Digital Twin and Industry 4.0: A Conceptual Framework with Applications*. CRC Press, 2024.

[10] A. Shachar, *Introduction to Algogens*. 2024.

[11] Y. M. Patil, P. V. Chintalapati, B. Kandasamy, and S. Balasubramanian, *Exploring digital twin technologies to examine transformation in healthcare systems*. IGI Global, 2024.

[12] D. Menon, B. Anand, and C. L. Chowdhary, "Digital Twin: Exploring the Intersection of Virtual and Physical Worlds," *IEEE Access*, vol. 11, pp. 75152–75172, 2023.

[13] A. Vallée, "Digital twin for healthcare systems," *Front. Digit. Heal.*, vol. 5, no. September, pp. 1–6, 2023.

[14] H. Gong, D. Su, S. Zeng, and X. Chen, "Advancements in digital twin modeling for underground spaces and lightweight geometric modeling technologies," *Autom. Constr.*, vol. 165, no. 3688, p. 105578, 2024.

[15] S. Attaran, M. Attaran, and B. G. Celik, "Digital Twins and Industrial Internet of Things: Uncovering operational intelligence in industry 4.0," *Decis. Anal. J.*, vol. 10, no. October 2023, 2024.

3.1 Introduction

Artificial intelligence-based deepfake technology, named after deep learning and fake, was first developed to manipulate the facial images and voices of celebrities. Before deepfake technology, a simple and time-consuming process was used to produce fake videos by editing sound and images mixer. Based on the outstanding growth of artificial intelligence and deep learning, generation equipment with a higher quality and an easier deepfake algorithm has been created [1]. Deepfake algorithm begins automatically by processing the AI program with a set of facial photos, creating a facial recognition model to map these photos and generate a source model as a reference for the replacement video. To generate a more realistic visual effect, it is efficient to use a GAN model that distinguishes real with fake video, refining it until it is almost undone [2].

The expansion of the deepfake technology has drastically curved the reflection of fake contents from a variety of fields, threatening the multimedia and politics industries. In particular, killing videos and speeches with imitations of national authority figures have been distributed intensely, and deepfake accident news has increased the anxiety of disinformation. The K-pop group AOA has recently been subjected to false accusations by malicious editing of a video, which accused the member, Chanmi, a school bully victim. In court, despite the publication of the unedited original video, it was virtually impossible to prove the distorted evidence. An increasing amount of fake content in the industry leads to consumers of video news questioning all videos, and the viewers' divided belief regarding an authentic video has amplified the difficulty of identifying it. In the same light, it is necessary to contemplate algorithmic developments regarding the detection of deep-forged manufacturing technology. Still, its technological improvement can mitigate the societal hazards caused by deepfakes. What is critical may be the capacity to enhance the method of detecting the fabrications by continuously monitoring the deep-fake creation environment and platforms [3, 4].

3.2 Historical Context and Development

Despite the recent public and policy interest in image and video tampering, manipulated media has a long history. As soon as people invented photography, they exploited this new technology to fabricate images. The invention of the camera in the early 19th century not only revolutionized portraiture but also heralded a new age of faked photographs. Photo editing even predated the invention of photography. The earliest known, credible doctored picture

The Chain." [Online]. Available: https://vocal.media/theChain/metaverse-development-company-shaping-virtual-realities-for-limitless-adventures-and-creating-infinite-realities-for-tomorrow. [Accessed: 23-Jul-2024].

[3] Maria Megia Cardenoso, "Digital Twins in Civil Engineering : Conceptual Framework and Real-World Implementations," 2024.

[4] Y.-S. Seo, Hyo-Min Kim, and Austin Kang, "ANALYSIS OF MEDIA DISCOURSE ON INTELLECTUAL PROPERTY RIGHTS RELATED TO METAVERSE IN KOREA," *Int. J. Secur. Priv. Trust Manag.*, vol. 13, no. 2, 2024.

[5] C. Song, S. Shin, and Kwang-Seong Shin, "Exploring the Key Characteristics and Theoretical Framework for Research on the Metaverse," *Appl. Sci.*, vol. 13, 2023.

[6] D. Kukreja, S. Gupta, D. Patel, and J. N. Rai, "Scientometric review of Web 3.0," *https://doi.org/10.1177/01655515231182073*, Jun. 2023.

[7] E. TUR, "Harnessing the Power of Digital Twins for Enhanced Material Behavior Prediction and Manufacturing Process Optimization in Materials Engineering," *Bayburt Üniversitesi Fen Bilim. Derg.*, vol. 6, no. 2, pp. 172–190, 2023.

[8] K. Mondal, O. Martinez, and P. Jain, "Advanced manufacturing and digital twin technology for nuclear energy," *Front. Energy Res.*, vol. 12, no. February, pp. 1–20, 2024.

[9] S. Rani, P. Bhambri, S. Kumar, P. K. Pareek, and A. A. Elngar, *AI-Driven Digital Twin and Industry 4.0: A Conceptual Framework with Applications*. CRC Press, 2024.

[10] A. Shachar, *Introduction to Algogens*. 2024.

[11] Y. M. Patil, P. V. Chintalapati, B. Kandasamy, and S. Balasubramanian, *Exploring digital twin technologies to examine transformation in healthcare systems*. IGI Global, 2024.

[12] D. Menon, B. Anand, and C. L. Chowdhary, "Digital Twin: Exploring the Intersection of Virtual and Physical Worlds," *IEEE Access*, vol. 11, pp. 75152–75172, 2023.

[13] A. Vallée, "Digital twin for healthcare systems," *Front. Digit. Heal.*, vol. 5, no. September, pp. 1–6, 2023.

[14] H. Gong, D. Su, S. Zeng, and X. Chen, "Advancements in digital twin modeling for underground spaces and lightweight geometric modeling technologies," *Autom. Constr.*, vol. 165, no. 3688, p. 105578, 2024.

[15] S. Attaran, M. Attaran, and B. G. Celik, "Digital Twins and Industrial Internet of Things: Uncovering operational intelligence in industry 4.0," *Decis. Anal. J.*, vol. 10, no. October 2023, 2024.

3.1 Introduction

Artificial intelligence-based deepfake technology, named after deep learning and fake, was first developed to manipulate the facial images and voices of celebrities. Before deepfake technology, a simple and time-consuming process was used to produce fake videos by editing sound and images mixer. Based on the outstanding growth of artificial intelligence and deep learning, generation equipment with a higher quality and an easier deepfake algorithm has been created [1]. Deepfake algorithm begins automatically by processing the AI program with a set of facial photos, creating a facial recognition model to map these photos and generate a source model as a reference for the replacement video. To generate a more realistic visual effect, it is efficient to use a GAN model that distinguishes real with fake video, refining it until it is almost undone [2].

The expansion of the deepfake technology has drastically curved the reflection of fake contents from a variety of fields, threatening the multimedia and politics industries. In particular, killing videos and speeches with imitations of national authority figures have been distributed intensely, and deepfake accident news has increased the anxiety of disinformation. The K-pop group AOA has recently been subjected to false accusations by malicious editing of a video, which accused the member, Chanmi, a school bully victim. In court, despite the publication of the unedited original video, it was virtually impossible to prove the distorted evidence. An increasing amount of fake content in the industry leads to consumers of video news questioning all videos, and the viewers' divided belief regarding an authentic video has amplified the difficulty of identifying it. In the same light, it is necessary to contemplate algorithmic developments regarding the detection of deep-forged manufacturing technology. Still, its technological improvement can mitigate the societal hazards caused by deepfakes. What is critical may be the capacity to enhance the method of detecting the fabrications by continuously monitoring the deep-fake creation environment and platforms [3, 4].

3.2 Historical Context and Development

Despite the recent public and policy interest in image and video tampering, manipulated media has a long history. As soon as people invented photography, they exploited this new technology to fabricate images. The invention of the camera in the early 19th century not only revolutionized portraiture but also heralded a new age of faked photographs. Photo editing even predated the invention of photography. The earliest known, credible doctored picture

The Chain." [Online]. Available: https://vocal.media/theChain/metaverse-development-company-shaping-virtual-realities-for-limitless-adventures-and-creating-infinite-realities-for-tomorrow. [Accessed: 23-Jul-2024].

[3] Maria Megia Cardenoso, "Digital Twins in Civil Engineering : Conceptual Framework and Real-World Implementations," 2024.

[4] Y.-S. Seo, Hyo-Min Kim, and Austin Kang, "ANALYSIS OF MEDIA DISCOURSE ON INTELLECTUAL PROPERTY RIGHTS RELATED TO METAVERSE IN KOREA," *Int. J. Secur. Priv. Trust Manag.*, vol. 13, no. 2, 2024.

[5] C. Song, S. Shin, and Kwang-Seong Shin, "Exploring the Key Characteristics and Theoretical Framework for Research on the Metaverse," *Appl. Sci.*, vol. 13, 2023.

[6] D. Kukreja, S. Gupta, D. Patel, and J. N. Rai, "Scientometric review of Web 3.0," *https://doi.org/10.1177/01655515231182073*, Jun. 2023.

[7] E. TUR, "Harnessing the Power of Digital Twins for Enhanced Material Behavior Prediction and Manufacturing Process Optimization in Materials Engineering," *Bayburt Üniversitesi Fen Bilim. Derg.*, vol. 6, no. 2, pp. 172–190, 2023.

[8] K. Mondal, O. Martinez, and P. Jain, "Advanced manufacturing and digital twin technology for nuclear energy," *Front. Energy Res.*, vol. 12, no. February, pp. 1–20, 2024.

[9] S. Rani, P. Bhambri, S. Kumar, P. K. Pareek, and A. A. Elngar, *AI-Driven Digital Twin and Industry 4.0: A Conceptual Framework with Applications*. CRC Press, 2024.

[10] A. Shachar, *Introduction to Algogens*. 2024.

[11] Y. M. Patil, P. V. Chintalapati, B. Kandasamy, and S. Balasubramanian, *Exploring digital twin technologies to examine transformation in healthcare systems*. IGI Global, 2024.

[12] D. Menon, B. Anand, and C. L. Chowdhary, "Digital Twin: Exploring the Intersection of Virtual and Physical Worlds," *IEEE Access*, vol. 11, pp. 75152–75172, 2023.

[13] A. Vallée, "Digital twin for healthcare systems," *Front. Digit. Heal.*, vol. 5, no. September, pp. 1–6, 2023.

[14] H. Gong, D. Su, S. Zeng, and X. Chen, "Advancements in digital twin modeling for underground spaces and lightweight geometric modeling technologies," *Autom. Constr.*, vol. 165, no. 3688, p. 105578, 2024.

[15] S. Attaran, M. Attaran, and B. G. Celik, "Digital Twins and Industrial Internet of Things: Uncovering operational intelligence in industry 4.0," *Decis. Anal. J.*, vol. 10, no. October 2023, 2024.

[16] N. Peladarinos, D. Piromalis, V. Cheimaras, E. Tserepas, R. A. Munteanu, and P. Papageorgas, "Enhancing Smart Agriculture by Implementing Digital Twins : A Comprehensive Review," *Sensors*, vol. 23, pp. 1–38, 2023.

[17] T. M. Machado and F. T. Berssaneti, "Literature review of digital twin in healthcare," *Heliyon*, vol. 9, no. 9, 2023.

[18] M. Turab and S. Jamil, "A Comprehensive Survey of Digital Twins in Healthcare in the Era of Metaverse," *BioMedInformatics*, vol. 3, pp. 563–584, 2023.

[19] A. Haleem, M. Javaid, R. Pratap, and R. Suman, "Biomedical Technology Exploring the revolution in healthcare systems through the applications of digital twin technology," *Biomed. Technol.*, vol. 4, no. January, pp. 28–38, 2023.

[20] T. Sun, X. He, X. Song, L. Shu, and Z. Li, "The Digital Twin in Medicine : A Key to the Future of Healthcare ?," *Front. Med.*, vol. 9, no. July, pp. 1–8, 2022.

[21] Yeong-Tae Song and Jiachen Qin, "Metaverse and Personal Healthcare," in *The 12th International Conference on Current and Future Trends of Information and Communication Technologies in Healthcare (ICTH 2022) Communica ion Technologies in Healthcare (ICTH 2022)*, 2022, vol. 210, pp. 189–197.

[22] S. Ghatti, L. A. Yurish, H. Shen, K. Rheuban, and K. B. En, "Digital Twins in Healthcare : A Survey of Current Methods," *Arch. Clin. Biomed. Res.*, vol. 7, no. 3, pp. 365–381, 2023.

[23] S. Mihai *et al.*, "Digital Twins : A Survey on Enabling Technologies, Challenges, Trends and Future Prospects," *IEEE Commun. Surv. Tutorials*, vol. 24, no. 4, pp. 2255–2291, 2022.

[24] C. Meijer, H. Uh, and S. Bouhaddani, "Digital Twins in Healthcare : Methodological Challenges and Opportunities," *J. Pers. Med.*, vol. 13, no. 1522, 2023.

[25] T. Sun, X. He, and Z. Li, "Digital twin in healthcare : Recent updates and challenges," *Digit. Heal.*, vol. 9, pp. 1–13, 2023.

[26] M. Attaran and B. Gokhan, "Digital Twin : Benefits, use cases, challenges, and opportunities," *Decis. Anal. J.*, vol. 6, no. January, p. 100165, 2023.

[27] A. Fuller, S. Member, Z. Fan, C. Day, and C. Barlow, "Digital Twin : Enabling Technologies, Challenges and Open Research," *IEEE Access*, vol. 8, pp. 108952–108971, 2020.

[28] Z. Johnson and M. J. Saikia, "Digital Twins for Healthcare Using Wearables," *Bioengineering*, vol. 11, no. 6, p. 606, 2024.

[29] A. Ahmadova, "Applications of digital twins in medicine and the ontological model of medical digital twins," *Probl. Inf. Soc.*, vol. 15, no. 1, pp. 98–105, 2024.

[30] I. U. Khan, M. Ouaissa, M. Ouaissa, M. Fayaz, and R. Ullah, "Artificial Intelligence for Intelligent Systems: Fundamentals, Challenges, and Applications," *Artif. Intell. Intell. Syst. Fundam. Challenges, Appl.*, pp. 1–344, Jul. 2024.

[31] M. S. Rodrigo, D. Rivera, J. I. Moreno, S. Member, M. Álvarez-campana, and D. R. López, "Digital Twins for 5G Networks : A Modeling and Deployment Methodology," *IEEE Access*, vol. 11, no. March, pp. 38112–38126, 2023.

3

Exploring Deepfake Technology in Healthcare: Innovations, Applications, and Challenges

Amena Mahmoud[1,2], Yonis Gulzar[3] and Sapna Juneja[4]

[1]Kafrelsheikh University, Egypt.
[2]Sophia University, Japan.
[3]King Faisal University, Saudi Arabia.
[4]Krishna Institute of Engineering and Technology (KIET), Ghaziabad, India.

Email: Amena_mahmoud@fci.kfs.edu.eg, ygulzar@kfu.edu.sa; sapnajuneja1983@gmail.com

Abstract

The advent of deepfake technology has sparked significant interest across various sectors, including healthcare, where its potential applications and implications are both innovative and challenging. This paper explores the transformative role of deepfake technology in healthcare, highlighting its applications in medical training, patient education, and telemedicine. By creating realistic simulations and enhancing interactive learning experiences, deepfakes can improve the proficiency of healthcare professionals and empower patients with a better understanding of their conditions. However, the use of deepfake technology also raises critical ethical and security concerns, including misinformation, consent issues, and the potential for misuse. Through a comprehensive review of current literature and case studies, this study examines the benefits and risks associated with deepfake technology in healthcare, providing insights into regulatory frameworks and best practices. Ultimately, this paper aims to inform stakeholders about the innovative possibilities and the necessary precautions to ensure the responsible implementation of deepfake technology in the healthcare sector.

DOI: 10.1201/9788743809920-3

3.1 Introduction

Artificial intelligence-based deepfake technology, named after deep learning and fake, was first developed to manipulate the facial images and voices of celebrities. Before deepfake technology, a simple and time-consuming process was used to produce fake videos by editing sound and images mixer. Based on the outstanding growth of artificial intelligence and deep learning, generation equipment with a higher quality and an easier deepfake algorithm has been created [1]. Deepfake algorithm begins automatically by processing the AI program with a set of facial photos, creating a facial recognition model to map these photos and generate a source model as a reference for the replacement video. To generate a more realistic visual effect, it is efficient to use a GAN model that distinguishes real with fake video, refining it until it is almost undone [2].

The expansion of the deepfake technology has drastically curved the reflection of fake contents from a variety of fields, threatening the multimedia and politics industries. In particular, killing videos and speeches with imitations of national authority figures have been distributed intensely, and deepfake accident news has increased the anxiety of disinformation. The K-pop group AOA has recently been subjected to false accusations by malicious editing of a video, which accused the member, Chanmi, a school bully victim. In court, despite the publication of the unedited original video, it was virtually impossible to prove the distorted evidence. An increasing amount of fake content in the industry leads to consumers of video news questioning all videos, and the viewers' divided belief regarding an authentic video has amplified the difficulty of identifying it. In the same light, it is necessary to contemplate algorithmic developments regarding the detection of deep-forged manufacturing technology. Still, its technological improvement can mitigate the societal hazards caused by deepfakes. What is critical may be the capacity to enhance the method of detecting the fabrications by continuously monitoring the deep-fake creation environment and platforms [3, 4].

3.2 Historical Context and Development

Despite the recent public and policy interest in image and video tampering, manipulated media has a long history. As soon as people invented photography, they exploited this new technology to fabricate images. The invention of the camera in the early 19th century not only revolutionized portraiture but also heralded a new age of faked photographs. Photo editing even predated the invention of photography. The earliest known, credible doctored picture

was the portrait of U.S. President Abraham Lincoln, whose head was taken from a photograph and transposed onto the image of John Calhoun from a lithograph. And so, photo manipulation was born. The transition from analog to digital imagery made the process of image tampering much easier. The ubiquity and advances in computer software and hardware have enhanced the capabilities of creating fake images and videos even for laypeople [1]. The latest breakthroughs in artificial intelligence (AI) and machine learning have provided a suite of tools that can "generate high-quality deepfake videos and photos with little data and would be increasingly difficult to detect" [5].

Historically, there were natural images and mastered images, which were hard to differentiate. Nevertheless, as the creation of mastered fakes (deepfakes) increases, so does the capability to build deep learning and novel forensic techniques to identify deepfakes. Understanding deepfake's historical context and current level of development in healthcare will illustrate the multifaceted nature of this threat. Viewing the deepfake healthcare applications and challenges as the targeted entity within the entire deepfake creation-detection-using cycle, several socio-technical interfaces must be addressed and tackled between each phase to lower the readiness of professional and laymen deepfakers to fabricate and distribute deepfakes and their detectability afterward. Beyond the bare existence of deepfakes, it is reflected upon how, as such, they can frame several healthcare-related tasks, from the impersonation of pathogens and side effects to the heated steering of the visualized treatment of dermal herpes [6].

3.3 Technical Foundations of Deepfake Technology

Deepfake technology refers to computer-generated or edited audiovisual content that convincingly imitates real-world events. It is produced by means of highly sophisticated algorithms, often involving artificial intelligence and machine learning. The technological foundation of deepfakes can be divided into synthesis and detection. DeEpFakes are an advanced use of general adversarial networks (GANs) techniques applied to deep neural networks, which are unique in their high seeding quality in terms of both image and voice, and have an appearance of very fine synchrony. At the most advanced level, deepfakes involve a combination of text-to-speech models rhythmically synchronized with lip movements in a face-swap video. All these three domains become the technical factors shaping the future of malicious deepfakes. Amid the COVID-19 pandemic, advanced deepfake technology makes it possible to fake the authorship of text, to imitate famous people's written style with just a small amount of textual prolonging. It is expected that future deepfakes converged with medical search-related issues may hinder the efforts of healthcare workers and policymakers [7].

Social media has also significantly emphasized sensational headlines, which can sometimes transmit false or misrepresented information far away. Most of the platforms are equipped with fact-checking mechanisms, which makes the dissemination of text-based misinformation through those channels less efficient. Because of this, misleading narratives are expected to be transmitted through advanced deepfake technology. Currently, the video deepfakes are taking the lead; however, the emergence of ultra-realistic voice and text deepfakes should not be undermined. Besides the common imagination, a "reverse engineering" deepfake platform is also coming in the near horizon, allowing the public app to generate indistinguishable super-resolution fake videos. Therefore, it is crucial to pay attention to safeguards and mechanisms that can substantially put deepfakes to good use and limit their harmful potential [8].

3.3.1 Machine learning algorithms

Deepfake technology has been successfully applied to generating fake audio, image, and video content [1]. The appearance of realistically manipulated content generated by deepfake has raised many challenges. Current imaging advances also facilitate the generation of deepfake health images, and one should be vigilant. Because the result of such an attack may have a significant impact on disease diagnosis and treatment, a comprehensive review of the advances in deepfake technology, applications related to health, and detection methods in health imaging is given. In future research, it is suggested that the privacy and data security risks of health index applications caused by deepfakes should be highly valued, and a robust detection method should be developed. Advances in machine learning algorithms for tampered medical image deepfake detection are addressed [6].

A structured case study regarding the comparative effect of eight machine learning models, including support vector machine, random forest, and decision tree, and five deep learning models, DenseNet121, DenseNet201, ResNet50, ResNet101, VGG19, is put forward. For deep learning models, feature extraction is done via the five models, and fine-tuning is then executed for each pre-trained model. Epoch training is performed for the feature extraction and fine-tuned models employing 125–100 epochs with an 11/3-6/1 separation ratio for a training/testing process. Six feature extraction models result in nearly perfect categorization of tampered and untampered instances with accuracy in the range of 99–100%. The fine-tuned models do not outperform the feature extraction models, suggesting a potentially too aggressive training strategy [9].

3.3.2 Data requirements and processing

Deepfake technology has developed in recent years, thanks to the growth of digital capture of the world in the form of multimedia content, as well as the advancement in AI generation techniques. The current arsenal of deepfake content includes videos, images, audio, and text, and a wide range of different technologies, with deep learning variations like GANs and transformer models leading the current state-of-the-art for implementation [10]. Generation of deepfake video content requires preparation of an initial video dataset, technical knowledge of deep learning and computer vision pipelines, specialized hardware requirements in the form of GPUs, a powerful server or cloud environment, encoding and decoding algorithms, video editing software, and a variety of open-source or self-developed scripts and libraries for asset preparation [11].

Challenges arise regarding video preparation, computing resources, choice of deepfake method, and distribution of the final visual content. A dearth of high-quality video data makes first-time video makers usually rely on their personal footage, often inadequately lit and filmed on consumer equipment. Conversely, professional video data is costly and hard to acquire. Video deepfake software requires complex installation as a part of prerequisites, but results in easy and automated scripts and a graphical interface. Similarly to the challenges of making original content, campaigning across platforms to reach a wider audience is difficult for a newcomer in the field. Moreover, success on this scale may target corporate interests and little financial gain. Measurement of good metrics is vital, and first-time experiences offer little insight. Trial and error are often slow, while detailed clarifications regarding improvement methods are nonexistent. In turn, following tutorials and guidance by seasoned manipulators breaches copyright agreements. This complex environment hampers the ability to make a difference and ultimately fades interest.

3.4 Innovations in Healthcare

In order for deepfake technologies and their applications to be fully explored, the negative stigma on technology must be addressed first [12]. People are naturally hesitant and scared due to the immense implications fake media can have when used to manipulate certain individuals or scenarios. Generally, society views the possibilities and risks of technology long before the tech itself becomes truly viable. Neither the legal system nor the general populace was prepared for the deepfake wave of the last couple of years. As it stands, the legal framework has yet to catch up with the proliferation of deepfakes, but the establishment of a comprehensive legal framework would be one of the most important steps toward enabling the deepfake recognition software to outcompete deepfake media creation, ensuring that fake can always be recognized from reality. Therefore, in order to facilitate the development of deepfake technologies, as well as their applications in a range of different fields of science, the promotion of creative solutions to change the negative outlook on possibilities opened by deepfakes is necessary.

Deepfake technology, for better or for worse, can revolutionize a range of different sectors, from journalism to politics, entertainment, marketing, criminal justice, and healthcare, with the primary benefit being the prevention of manipulated and wrongful accusations or coerced false confessions. If both officials and suspects had access to deepfake tech, any interrogation could proceed on equal footing. People accused of a crime, if innocent, could create fake evidence of their whereabouts, alibis, or proof of being maligned. In healthcare, deepfakes could be used very efficiently by teaching hospitals to recreate medical cases offered to students [9].

Other potential applications include the synthetic generation of various voice elements, like improving speech quality or helping stroke patients with dysphasia regain some of their lost capabilities. However, regardless of the application, the use of deepfake technology requires a recognized and well-established legal and ethical framework. On the one hand, the inherent nature of deepfake technologies is to create fake content, which can then be used to deceive, so the relevant ethical consequences would have to be addressed by professionals from different disciplines in order to allow a broad understanding of the possible consequences of using deepfake. On the other hand, adequate measures need to be undertaken to protect the potential targets of possible abuse of deepfake technology by offering a means to detect fake content [13].

3.4.1 Medical training and simulation

Whether one is embarking on medical training, completing life support training, or trialing new techniques, simulation is essential. Simulation can range from a group-based practice in managing a significant incident to individual immersion in a newly implemented process through the use of a screen-based virtual reality. This review will introduce and argue innovative simulations in the world of healthcare, sharing the simulation techniques that have recently been explored or embarked on [14].

Simulation-based medical teaching and learning is becoming progressively popular around the globe. In the past year, simulation-based training was attempted and explored extensively not only for medical personnel performing procedures but also for the individuals experiencing the steps [15]. The primary goal was to minimize the gap between individuals perceiving a particular step and actively conducting it. Defining this as a process-based definition, it has provided researchers with the flexibility to interpret learning in a variety of ways open to examination. Simulation-based research in healthcare extends beyond recognizing incidental learning to include reflective learning, discovery learning, and whiteboard understanding, to name but a few variations [16]. Simulation-based techniques in medical science include models of medical procedure trainers, multimedia simulations, virtual reality training, eminent persons, standard patient playing, and educational games.

Simulation largely relies upon the alignment of simulation type or method chosen with the learning goals and objectives. This is a fundamental principle of good practice outlined by professional bodies and higher education educators. Simulation exercises can range from screen-based virtual reality games providing interactive discovery learning activities through to live simulations such as responding to an anaphylaxis allergic reaction. Simulation-based training is a process in which a measurement is made of performance for a defined procedure, a controlled learning experience is offered, and then another measure of performance is made of the same procedure under controlled conditions. This basic structure can be and has been expanded upon, including the refinement of performance indicators, timings, and educational interventions. For the sake of this review, simulation-based training is the process of stepping in and out until competency has been successfully assessed [17].

3.4.2 Patient education and engagement

Considering the vast potential that deepfakes may have for the undermining of trust in evidence in legal settings, what is the research being done to account for the limitations in this context specifically? What could be the proactive politic–legal measures to ameliorate or abate the damage that deepfakes can inflict in decontextualized settings, even if there is eventual public understanding and awareness of the errors made by the algorithm? [18].

Artificial intelligence (AI) has its roots in the 1950s, but the disjunction between AI policy tools and the rapidly expanding AI transformations in many sectors of the economy and society has prompted a reassessment of government responsibility for these changes. A priority for national AI strategies should be to ensure that these policies assume a better stance in terms of understanding and assessing other AI-induced changes and impact both the potential opportunities and threats – on a more sophisticated and nuanced view of AI transformation. AI applications are rapidly increasing their footprint across a broader array of sectors, from fisheries and livestock farming to e-commerce and healthcare [12]. And as AI applications become more diverse and pervasive, more sectors are affected by them, gaining increased visibility in the public narrative. Moreover, the pace of AI application is also accelerating markedly, as ever more AI-based devices – drones, sensors, robots, and the like – are developed and deployed. AI's core technology, machine learning, again has been sharply trending toward complexity.

AI is not only transforming productivity, services, and employment, but also dramatically restructuring many sectors and manifesting entirely new implications for regulating and governance [19]. Deepfakes are a big challenge in a context where AI is widely used to create fake content, exacerbating the spread of mis- and disinformation. Deepfake technologies are growing fast as a form of synthetic media creation using deep learning algorithms to combine real and fake images or recordings, often with the intent to deceive an audience. Since the development of deepfake videos became widely known in 2017, there have been numerous public pronouncements bewailing their misuse. However, on account of research on deepfake technology, taking into account these public pronouncements finds that legal-context research vastly outnumbers other forms of research. In order to provide empirical perspectives on technology and its implications, academic research on deepfakes is connected to illustrative examples within the fields of media law, media psychology, and political sciences, while also highlighting the limitations of existing and ongoing research.

3.5 Applications of Deepfake Technology in Healthcare

Impressive advancements in healthcare technology have been made in the past few decades, providing a great benefit to both patients and staff of the healthcare sector. Recently, a rising topic that links to the technology of healthcare is becoming attractive, given that healthcare workers and the public expect further exploration of deepfake technology in the future. Deepfake technology falls into the category of artificial intelligence, which is capable of mapping facial features onto a prerecorded video clip [12]. Within the capacity of this technology, some potential directions are offered for exploration. This viewpoint not only discusses challenges posed by the misuse of deepfake technology but also highlights its possibly fruitful application in healthcare, profiting from its capacity.

Deepfake technology was created using autoencoders, generating an imposter of someone in an authentic video. It was primarily used to swap videos but has expanded into face editing. By 2020, this technology created a flood of revenue from the manufacturing of fake content. Over unique accounts have viewed fake media, and there is an increase in the use of less expensive and easier to obtain synthetic media by the media company. Deepfakes have become more readily accessible to the public in using social media, providing it as political commentary or investigative journalism; the public perceives this media as a reliable source of information. In order for deepfake technologies and their applications to be fully explored, it is important that the negative stigma on the technology is addressed first. Many people are hesitant and scared due to the immense implications fake media can have when used to manipulate, misinterpret, or abuse [20].

3.5.1 Telemedicine enhancements

The COVID-19 pandemic has had a significant impact on healthcare, including non-emergency care, as services transition to telemedicine. Challenges in telemedicine include a reduced ability to conduct physical examinations and visually examine patients. The creation and rapid evolution of deepfake technology has the potential to alleviate these concerns. Given the increasing availability and ease of use, deepfake technology is quickly becoming not only more accessible, but also potentially more reliable. A multi-center cohort study on healthcare utilization during the COVID-19 pandemic found that substantial reductions occurred in new outpatient visits, including primary and specialty care, suggesting the use of telemedicine as an alternative [21].

Efforts to overcome the challenges associated with telemedicine have seen the use of deep learning and AI in tasks such as patient monitoring and image analysis when physical examination is not possible, typically in intensive care and remote areas with limited resources. Additionally, and more commonly, AI models are used in consultation with healthcare professionals by providing analysis and insights to help diagnose or treat patients. In telemedicine, this can be extended to the synchronous analysis and interpretation of patients' and healthcare providers' video streams, potentially simulating a physical examination. This would clearly be a valuable addition to the telemedicine service. Deepfake technology could enhance the AI model by providing high-quality, high-fidelity responses in a visual, rather than just an informational, form. This would provide an experience more akin to a real physical examination and could help mitigate the observed decrease in new patient visits during the pandemic [22].

3.5.2 Mental health interventions

In 2032, depression is anticipated to be the second leading exacerbation of disease, a condition affecting an estimated 848 million individuals (10.4% of the worldwide population) [23]. In 2017, the number one source of mental healthcare treatment gaps was low-income and middle-income countries. Statistically, their findings propose using the digital model to screen individuals demonstrating severe mental illness with an accuracy rate of 81.00%. Nevertheless, they accent a vulnerability where their volunteers are medical students ($n = 56$). Consequently, despite their necessity to improve knowledge about psychopathology and investigate the efficiency of specialist assistance, their volunteer population may be more informed about psychopathology because of their education. Thus, this circumstance potentially limits the generality of their search findings.

Burnout and high workloads dominantly influence medical students and practitioners' emotional and mental condition, potentially leading to fragile mental health. This situation generally leads to increased suicidal attempts, because of particularly vulnerable behavior demonstrated by healthcare specialists. In the case of the United States, suicides were the cause of 400 to 800 fatalities amongst physicians. The search domain is service sector employees that include medical universities. The confirmation and significance of research extend the understanding of mental health difficulties, stay up to date, and react to relevant changes. Regarding the requirement to counter challenges established by Mental Healthcare Personnel, these apprehensions are beneficial to establish facilities fostering mental health recovery [24].

In 2019, it was declared that mental health difficulties would grow to be the major cause of morbidity. This disease is anticipated to rise by 50% by 2030. The probability of getting clinically crucial psychological disturbances (i.e., depression) is large for the community. The near future has to expect the complete understaffing of the current medical system of the country because of them attempting to care for a considerable number of people. For example, in the case of the delineated above, only 0.13% of potentially depressed individuals might consult a professional. Strategically, the imminent spreading of AI is the reason to foresee and make efforts for applicable alterations. Discussions generally talk about development, identification, and current focus, nevertheless, overlooking the recognizing aspect. Because of this gap, the present study is concentrated on how satisfactorily AI can recognize mental health concerns. In connection with the present course of applications and requests, AI could be used for impeccable diagnosis and recognizing cases of severe mental health difficulties.

3.5.3 Surgical planning and visualization

Deepfakes technology is an innovative synthesis of AI, image, video, and voice processing technologies to create or alter recorded content. Deepfakes consist of two main technologies: generative adversarial networks, for realistic video generation and transformer models, for synthetic voice generation. The clinical diagnosis and monitoring of sleep disorders, such as obstructive sleep apnea (OSA), typically involve assessing patients' video-recorded sleep study for their sleep-related symptoms and breathing patterns. Wearable sensors and mobile devices record the patient's sleep study video, which is subsequently analyzed by healthcare professionals – a clinician or a computer algorithm [25].

It can also be used to determine potential complications and challenges that could occur during the surgery, allowing the surgical team to develop contingency plans to address such issues. A surgeon may use scenario modeling to identify the optimal incision points during dissection for minimally invasive cardiac surgery while considering the anatomical structure of the patient's ribs and internal organs. Once surgery has been successfully performed, the digital twin feature in the AI-XR surgical metaverse will allow surgeons to simulate the impact of postoperative care in real-time and optimize treatment decisions. Patients are prescribed inotropes to improve hemodynamic function and avoid hypotension and low cardiac output syndrome (LCOS) after heart surgery. The prescribing surgeons can simulate the impact of various doses of inotropes in the AI-XR surgical metaverse and visualize risks to determine the most optimal dosages [26].

3.6 Ethical Considerations

Deepfake technology has gained popularity in the healthcare sector due to the rising phenomenon of deepfake audio and video. It involves the alteration of original multimedia data by embedding new data. The alterations could be natural and subtle or unnatural and obvious, depending on the application and the motivation behind the making and use of deepfakes. Deepfake voice technology could benefit individuals with motor problems, while deepfake video technology could benefit individuals with language-compartmentalized lesions by aiding in comprehension. Moreover, it could be used for training medical students and caregivers in a safe and ethical environment where they can interact with a digital patient. A patient questionnaire revealed that interviewees consider deepfake technology is trustworthy for medical education, useful for learning about diseases and treatment options, ethical for treating patients under supervision, and beneficial for practicing patient communication. Nevertheless, many interviewees are concerned about safety, data privacy, and specific healthcare scenarios when they meet deepfake technology [27].

The current state of deepfake technology in primary care settings and surgical training influenced the balance of technology applications and patient well-being. One interviewee proposed selectively upgrading deepfake capabilities to maximize its benefits, while another suggested focusing on early disease detection. Patients believe deepfake technology could alter how healthcare professionals treat them and straightforwardly voice skeptical opinions. They contemplate learning more about the feasibility of deepfake technology and discussing its impact with healthcare providers. There is a decisive need for the preservation of ethical breaches because public knowledge of these could prevent egregious abuses. The more advanced public understanding is of the unique characteristics and likely sources of deepfake media replication and fabrication. Here, and over the mid-term, there is a clear need for the public to be testimonial to technical advances that will aid public, corporate, and governmental entities in not being deceived by deepfake video, audio, and personalized text threats. In summary, it cannot be overstated that the focus in research, development, and application should be to prevent and combat deepfake media rather than to generate it, even when benign or with a benevolent intent [28, 29].

3.6.1 Consent and privacy issues

Deepfake technology is an AI-based innovation that uses deep learning algorithms to create videos that manipulate people's facial mannerisms, draft videos of people saying something they never said, or set them in different environments. Rapid advancement in deep learning technology and the exponential growth of data generation in the digital era have bolstered the development and application of deep learning in various domains, including the creation and detection of deepfake videos. Deepfake detection technology uses high-level machine learning algorithms, as possible differences between authentic and deepfake footage are either not discernible or can be meticulously disguised. In preparation for future innovators and healthcare providers, this review summarizes the current research and applications of deepfake technology in healthcare and discusses probable innovations, applications, and challenges of deepfake technology in the healthcare industry.

Half a million people worldwide, including around 140,000 in the USA, live an additional five years past their initial prognosis threshold each year. Deep learning analysis of medical imaging may have the most potential to access a rigorous stance in the subset of medical specialties formalized by medical imaging. Both Radiology and Mental Health, Medicine's IT-native kin, benefit vastly from the high-dimensional detail provided by a digital read. Despite the complexity and objective nature of the human body, the diagnosis of a particular pathophysiologic state is sometimes discernible visually and often forms the basis of medical imaging generally. Moreover, most diseases have distinct stages where medical imaging captures gross cellular disparity visible in training data, and detection of these states can have a dramatic effect on prognosis and treatment. There appear to be eighteen diseases in all medicine that have demonstrated digital read prognostication approximation capable of achieving clinical validation [30].

3.6.2 Misinformation and trust

Attacks of misinformation and Deepfake videos online have led to a lack of trust in news circulating on social media. This fear about deep video technology and the perception of misinformation is threatening the information ecosystem. Online media sources aim to convince consumers, intentionally providing accurate and unjust information as a result of engagement with potential audiences about current social preferences. Since the information ecosystem requires the active contribution of service providers to prevent the publication of inaccurate information and also includes numerous actors with distinct roles, there is a need for taking more proactive measures instead of acting on the basis of incident-specific reactions to new misrepresentative content on social media that reaches news organizations. Misinterpreting the information is making the fake video credible. Credibility only happens if virtual understanding is possible; so, if misinformation is the understanding of the provided information in a manner that differs from the intended purposes, it demonstrates that the individual is truly misled [31].

There is an actress pretending to cut off the baby's head. The speech of the baby's head is a response to the question "What are you going to do?" From the understanding perspective, this appears to be deliberate because a three-year-old cannot engage in such a beheading act. This iconic goal in this instance is the act of metaphorical decapitation. It is clearly shown to be impossible. There seems to be an organizational surplus; when the intent is established as an iconic act of this size, it contains excess production. But the provided information also has more meaning than it appears [32].

3.7 Regulatory and Legal Challenges

Advancing increasingly rapidly, AI-assisted diagnostic software systems can be applied effectively for the creation of a deepfake healthcare occurrence [33]. Furthermore, in the deepfake healthcare model, AI-based incentive-laden chatbots can be expected to take an increasing index within the forge. In terms of recurrent revenue, the focus of interest will move toward how capital requirements may vary according to integration within incentives. It is found that the incentive structure, for the possibility of drawbacks, that an increasing rate of incentives might very quickly begin to work against promotion. Further, as incentives based on AI-powered chatbots become more prevalent, care should turn to how the dominance of a market player that can afford large numbers of AI-promoted prompts would skew the adoption, and barriers to entry for new chatbot integration players. On the groundwork of chatlogs from an AI-promoted AI-powered chatbot, implement the rate of prompts in a conversation, highlighting the presence of AI-promoted, and uncovering its impact on the rates of negative conversational developments.

AI use in healthcare deepfakes can potentially create a range of practical applications. The applications of deepfake technologies to surgery in surgery room, medical education, and consultation between medical staff could take advantage of AI technologies in the way that can better manage hospital or clinic and provide opportunities to expand the access to healthcare in rural areas. The main reason is that deepfake technology not yet been widely applied to healthcare, despite the growing trend, will be an increased empathetic intelligent approach to improve and nurture. Nevertheless, the finding that a large portion of the insight published recently using the empathy intellectual approach other than established techniques, it is apparent that a general unawareness of empathy intelligence is not to issue holding back its adoption and healthcare use deepfake. Introducing some unique applications in how it could be used interconnectedly, deepfake and empathy intelligence in the healthcare context, presented in ways that have been only rarely shown in literature [6, 13].

3.7.1 Current regulations

Artificial Intelligence (AI) and machine learning have seen massive adoption across different sectors due to high computational power. Classification, clustering, and prediction tasks can now be performed with increased efficiency. Since deep learning's introduction in 2010, the combination of cloud storage and computing power was an essential advantage. Deep learning further refined AI capabilities and eventually powered deepfake creation. Deep learning's essence is pattern recognition through the handling of processed data, including text, images, video, and audio. The representation of knowledge by data enables algorithms to conduct a wide array of complicated functions: original implementation (like filtering or noise removal), translation to a different domain (like translating scripts or face-id matching), or content alteration, like superimposition of media. Deepfakes exploit convolutional neural networks (CNN), an AI type developed for image and video processing. Currently, CNNs store knowledge from frames and recreate the signal of a previously given output. Recordings or uploads are then used to inform models to rebuild media, allowing background modification or object replacement [34].

Several nations have passed fitness and falsification-related restrictions, banning deepfake applications against pornography, bulimia, hatred, hoaxes, and conservation. Nonetheless, ethical and legal inquiries remain in terms of art, politics, and realistic misinformation. Open-research endeavors generated 'fingerprints' through deepfake recognition to detect content alterations by other AI. Nonetheless, adapted synthetic material is continuously upgrading. Being volatile and innovative, lawmakers lag in determining what should be taboo. Yet, democratic countries have considered legislative change to tackle three fronts: truth validation, copyrighted item creation, and the illegal publication of adapted content.

In the medical field, deepfake tech has also grown; hospitals have used it to assist patients in palliative and terminal conditions. However, despite improving communication and understanding, the creation of new deepfake forms has developed an important and controversial moral and legal basis in singular claims. There is no set approach for screening, monitoring, or preventing deepfakes. Nonetheless, AI identifying AI and a conservatorship system have begun to develop. Regarding well-being, creators should research the potential damage and provide resources to mitigate them. But developing technology should provide resources to eliminate bad, not counter good, ventures. In conclusion, while there are numerous uses for deepfakes in the fields, the moral and legal issues surrounding acknowledge deepfakes are crucial. Unfortunately, the task at hand to prevent these problems is equally ethically and legally challenging [35].

3.7.2 Future legal frameworks

Today, synthetic media generation has recently witnessed a boom, with deep learning models powered by large datasets purporting to generate text, images, videos, and audio files of unprecedented quality. Among these models, Generative Adversarial Networks and others have been widely adopted to create natural-looking visual and audio content – a demonstration of all these model's colossal potential in film production; video games and entertainment; the creation of avatars for disease diagnosis; various scientific, medical, and other research; as well as their applications in computer graphics, design, fashion, and art.

The increasing prevalence of deepfake technologies in the generation of fake audio and video content, coupled with the difficulties in detecting and preventing this type of malicious attack, poses new challenges for counterfeit protection, the verification of evidence integrity, and the ability to maintain trust in digital media. Some novel classified image alteration techniques with improved robustness have been proposed, while newly devised phase estimation-based solutions show promising results in detecting face warping artifacts through computational visual forensics analysis. Past work offers various solutions based on multimedia forensics and machine learning analysis to better combat voice synthesis. Digital liveness detection systems using deep learning models offer the potential to distinguish deepfake records from real videos, forgery, and legitimate content. Unfortunately, most forgery detection models available treat generated pharmaceutical data as a form of counterfeiting modification, relying primarily on the underlying data; these methods are not suitable for other types of fake media forms or modifications.

3.8 Technical Challenges and Limitations

In recent years, deepfake technology has advanced to a stage where creating highly realistic fake media is easy, even without professional knowledge. Fake media includes images, videos, and audio. Although it is commonly used in pornographic contents, it can also be used in other fields. Since the emergence of fake media, healthcare has taken an interest in it. It has recognized the effectiveness and innovation of using fake media and the evolution of deepfakes, which are easy to generate and difficult to distinguish.

The innovations in the healthcare field that use deepfakes, as demonstrated in COVID-19, are as follows. First, an outbreak of infectious disease like COVID-19 threatens public health and safety with high transmission and mortality rates. It may also have negative economic effects. Therefore, rapid response is important. However, detecting patients with a certain type of infectious disease takes time, cost, and confidentiality issues for a professional healthcare worker. In this regard, it is desirable to detect a candidate patient using only publicly available resources. Second, if a person finds out that they have been in contact with an infected person, that person goes to a healthcare provider to check for the disease, but it is costly and causes emotional tension. However, it is known that a person's body temperature rises when infected with an infectious disease. So, this work heats up the false video that a person has to be infected for a while and outputs it in a video similar to reality.

3.8.1 Quality and authenticity of deepfakes

This article approaches the topic of digital deepfake technology from the perspectives of quality and authenticity of deepfake images and videos, associated detection and verification methods, pragmatic consequences or manipulations based on deepfakes, and pertinent regulatory efforts. Although deepfakes have elicited widespread concerns about their misuse, it is emphasized that not all fakes are bad and may even be used for socially beneficial purposes when properly labeled and accompanied by necessary disclaimers.

Quality and authenticity of deepfake images and videos are explored, especially focusing on the extent and ways spatio-temporal artifacts persist in synthesized deepfake videos and contribute to vulnerabilities in detection authenticity. Observations of detection errors are shown to concentrate on distorted regions, while spatial artifacts conspicuously affect classification results. A method to align spatial and historical characteristics is explored, which leads to a noticeable decrease in detection and classification performance, especially for models trained on high-quality data.

Having spread deepfake images and videos across the Internet, confidence in digital content has been profoundly undermined, especially in contexts of news reporting or political canvassing. A new generation of deep network models is proposed to synthesize faces via various procedures, including feature transformation, 3D projection, and inference network adaptation, permitting effective induction of the desired facial angle, translation, and identity. This task follows an exploration of the persuasiveness of deepfake videos viewed in countries with minimal technology infrastructure. Given that deepfake videos generally require access to at least some level of technology, a degree of expected video quality and fidelity may limit real-world applicability in regions without advanced technology infrastructure, particularly viewers residing in remote or developing and less developed nations. Since 2019, intense debates have been held about the impacts of deepfake technology on subjects such as cybersecurity, information integrity, and interpersonal trust.

3.8.2 Integration with existing systems

Deepfake technologies are an innovative approach to voice and video synthesis, allowing the generation of photo-realistic synthetic movies of people who are not actually present in the scene. Though deepfake technology has been widely deployed for various aspects since its appearance in 2017, research on its applications and broader implications is still nascent. For example, in the healthcare industry, with the integration of recent progress in deepfake technologies, real-time patient simulations based on their historical medical data and lifestyle can be rendered. This opens up a realm of completely new validation methodologies, the development of which warrants a good understanding of deepfake technologies. Systems and tests need to be developed to differentiate between classic automation tools, such as VFX editing from the output of deepfake algorithms. Owing to the synchronized advancement of new technologies and innovations, misinformation has become harder and harder to detect. The current era of civilization faces an 'infodemic,' paving the way for future endeavors to spread it and take full advantage. The main challenge concerns how deepfake technologies can best be utilized to reach the end goal. Compatible hardware is continuously developing further potential. The ability to scan people is not prohibited legally in most parts of the world, although there are some concerning data protection and privacy issues associated.

The ability to generate deepfakes using commonly available equipment has empowered both the casual creative and those with malign intentions. There is therefore a need for this to be counterbalanced. The first step is to provide deepfake recognition software. The second step would then be to prosecute those who make deepfake porn. Such actions are meant to act as a deterrent. In order to combine two clips, it is necessary for them to be synchronous. An overlapping start or completion to adjacent sentences is a feature of normal dialogue, yet is rarely found in a premeditated spam message recording. Therefore, a validation check could include both speakers diving into words or talking over the top of one another.

3.9 Case Studies

With recent advancements in deep generative networks, the ability to generate almost perfect fakes of any digital media has exponentially increased in quality over the past year. This has garnered a negative spotlight for fake news and celebrity face-swapping on mainstream media, forcing large companies to act on these issues by developing deepfake detection pipelines. However, deepfake technology has far more applications than controversial face-swapping videos, which are not widely addressed in the deepfake research community. There are numerous benign and advantageous applications that experts in the subject have thought of in the areas of filmmaking, teaching, and many others [36].

A brief examination on deepfakes could guide social media companies to change this emerging technology and shape it in a more socially responsible way. Shallow and fake news detection are two of the most active industries in the field of deepfake research. There will undoubtedly be an improvement in developing deepfakes for malicious purposes, thereby escalating the arms race between the fake creators and detectors. Yet, as deepfakes continue to proliferate, there are countless avenues for the growth of application domains. This paper explicates an approach for a deep learning model that can classify fake detection papers into eight different areas.

Deep generative networks in recent years have reinforced the need for caution while consuming various modalities of digital information. A common way deepfake objects are created is by fine-tuning generative adversarial networks (GANs) with a source video and a target face to leverage the lip and facial actions of the source faces on the real-time target [37]. One of the subgenres of fake videos leveraging this technology consists of generating hate speech and provocation from politicians. Indeed, this latter type was detected and recovered by algorithms on multiple occasions. Another, far less studied, one consists of generating deepfakes of medical experts. One obvious extension of this is the deepfake creation of videos informing people that they are clear from viruses when they are not. Furthermore, fake creators may generate fake statements from doctors mentioning the wrongdoing of a hospital. Failure to detect these fake videos can have large ramifications, such as consummation of hospital preparation resources for legitimate accidents or even loss of life.

3.9.1 Successful implementations

Advances in polymerase chain reaction (PCR) test technology and the introduction of deep learning algorithms allowed for the recognition of the challenge. Subsequently, many techniques using deep learning and deepfake have been developed and applied not only in images but also in various fields, for example, speech, video, gesture, etc. In addition, current challenges and ethical issues related to deep fake technology are discussed. Deepfake technology is advancing at a rapid pace, but its practical implementation has been limited to very few applications globally. In order to fully explore this technological advancement, it is first important to address the negative stigma surrounding it, and the legal aspects need to be fully developed and established. This section discusses the successful implementation of deep fake technology as well as its applications, ongoing work in healthcare, and the potential hurdles in implementing health-related applications [12].

3.9.2 Failures and lessons learned

Due to a significant amount of visual processing being observed, it is speculated that smartphone users may upload their videos to a site where a server does the bulk of the processing. It is difficult to distinguish exactly where the majority of creations occurred since a significant number of entries were submitted using public computers, and the data card does not have a computer at their location. This potentially points transparently to the Cloud as a growing market. However, these visuals are technically edited, so the figure is a gross underestimate of the total market share. At its core, deepfakes consist of models compressed into nearly MB sized. These deepfakes, given appropriate conditions, can be ported anywhere, including a smartphone, and edited from there. Deepfakes are also distributed as still image sets and video clips, which can be transferred by simply dragging and dropping the files. This could indicate that people in areas with poorer internet infrastructure are more likely to use a SoC or they prefer heavy video editing establishments similar to Cybercafes. Potentially a result of feeding more cut-and-paste edits, like changing the face of the shadow puppet. Regardless, this practice could stem from a burnout of making deepfake-family videos instead of posting the original setting where they are generated. The proliferation of user-friendly datasets and tools will allow the creation of deepfakes in a matter of minutes.

It is crucial to keep in mind that the first deepfake iteration posted in the open-ended pilot study was not a hit. None of the other rules, including the last three, were initially followed. Because of the competition, the majority of participants decided to try creating a deepfake anyway, in most cases choosing a scene with an abundance of images at nearly the same time. Still, almost one in four randomly selected participants managed to generate a deepfake. The capability to make various predictions about deepfake creation accessibility, depending on the interpretation of related statistics, could make this hobby less feasible. Here are some key takeaways from the open starter kit and paid versions: The largest difference in money spent involved buying the continuous video or downloading high-resolution video. Foreign participants most likely needed to pay for video streaming.

3.10 Future Trends and Research Directions

In recent years, deep learning has emerged to address a range of complex issues, impacting everything from big data analysis to computer vision and natural language processing. But it has also raised challenges to the privacy, democracy, and national security of individuals. Recent work often refers to deepfake technology, one striking instance of this. Deepfakes refer to media generated by deep learning technologies and formed by the fusion of a set of facial features of a person into a different image or video. Deepfakes technology can also manipulate the expression, make-up, and hairstyle of the people in the content. Technologies for detecting and evaluating the authenticity of digital visual media have garnered interest as a natural technology to secure digital visual media content and guard against the propagation of digital content with a synthetic appearance edited by deep learning [1]. Several algorithms have been proposed to create deepfakes, in addition to many proposed approaches improving deepfakes detection algorithms [38]. This paper presents a concise study of employed deep learning algorithms to craft deep fake content and an extensive discussion of algorithms to pinpoint deep fake content. Key challenges, research tendencies, and future guidance for deepfake technologies are reviewed in the survey. This paper is structured as follows. Background on deepfakes and advanced anticipations for detecting them. An overview of the most recent works associated with creating and detecting deepfakes. Advantages of current techniques and points to expected future research adjustments and deepfake technology development. For the longer term, a number of thoughts and forecasts on the progress of deep learning the means of anticipating and defending against technologies are presented.

3.10.1 Advancements in technology

AI-synthesized or digitally manipulated face samples, commonly known as DeepFakes, imperil the dependability of face recognition systems and the reliability of video data on the Internet. The coronavirus-2019 (COVID-19) pandemic has prompted the wider acceptance of telemedicine for remote treatment of patients. Alongside other decision-making methods, the advent of DeepFakes footage in medical practices has recently been presented as a realistic threat. Deepfake technology might manipulate symptoms to have a precursor unfavorable patient outcome. Also, ultrasonic facial authentication methods can be deceived in sophisticated operative scenarios with synthetic facial films, namely, DeepFakes, of the legal operator. The fusion of synced facial videos with Exceptional Patient Encounter Footage may intercept these Anomaly Videos and help detect DeepFakes.

Further, potential pathways are envisaged to safeguard DeepFakes detection. With the advances in generative adversarial networks, video altering is not hardwired or automated within smartphone apps anymore, but gives way to subtle admiration of lips or facial signs. Encouraging technical advances in video clip reassignment makes video evidence more prone to alteration. Techniques such as the new "DeepNudes" app testify not merely to the storyline and audible events, but also that they are vulnerable to counterfeiting. To make a video seem true, a mid-like residue pair of movement edit is superimposed on the original footage as a movable mask. Meanwhile, the established mechanics of enforcement upholding will cast doubts on footage, perceivably demonstrating brutality or inappropriate overall takeout, possibly on a grand scale. Career-threatening and even obscure stories could be sparked on the Internet, where the charity of reality will be nearly insufferable to establish [39].

3.10.2 Potential new applications

Fake news is a serious threat to democracies worldwide in the age of digital media. More advanced algorithms, frequently based on machine learning approaches, and increasing computational performance allow the production of deepfakes that are barely distinguishable from authentic media. So far, the detection algorithms are one step behind the fakes; hence, it is valuable to deepen the public understanding to preserve the effectiveness and minimize false consequences. On the other side, there are only a few positive examples of applications that use the same technology for good purposes, such as the possibility to continue "hearing" a deceased poet's poetic voice to analyze his/her life's work using artificial sound [12].

3.11 Conclusion

Blending digital video copied as a fake onto a general video clip, deepfake technology enables super-realistic counterfeit videos. Notwithstanding numerous ethical and legal concerns related to their misuse, various and diverse applications are continuously being discovered across multiple sectors. In veterinary medical training, the production and distribution of animal biology training videos could be simplified, expanded, and up-to-date thanks to the creation and sharing of deepfakes mimicking animal diseases. Long-term treatment progress of pet animals and livestock animals could be monitored by acoustic deepfake video footage, detecting audible abnormal fluctuations in the respiratory output sound, and comparing the audio with historic deepfake sounds. Cows, pigs, and poultry frequently display abrupt health problems that, if unnoticed, would generate large financial losses to the farm and require expensive intervention. The application of increasingly popular animals as pets and the recent disinvestment in poultry farm incomes will increase investments and interest in livestock farming-related AI technologies, including deepfake monitoring systems and specifically crafted try-on detection livestock breeds.

Acknowledgment

This work was supported by the Deanship of Scientific Research, the Vice Presidency for Graduate Studies and Scientific Research, King Faisal University, Saudi Arabia, under the project KFU251304

References

[1] T. Thi Nguyen, Q. Viet Hung Nguyen, D. Tien Nguyen, D. Thanh Nguyen et al., "Deep Learning for Deepfakes Creation and Detection: A Survey," 2019. [PDF]

[2] M. Masood, M. Nawaz, K. M. Malik, A. Javed, A. Irtaza, "Deepfakes generation and detection: State-of-the-art, open challenges, countermeasures, and way forward," *Applied Sciences*, vol. 2023, Springer. [PDF]

[3] M. A. Farouk and B. M. Fahmi, "Deepfakes and media integrity: Navigating the new reality of synthetic content," Journal of Media and Interdisciplinary, 2024.

[4] Amena Mahmoud and Eiko Takaoka. " An enhanced machine learning approach with stacking ensemble learner for accurate liver cancer diagnosis using feature selection and gene expression data," Healthcare Analytics, Elsevier, vol. 6, 2025.

[5] S. Nasiri and A. Hashemzadeh, "The Evolution of Disinformation from Fake News Propaganda to AI-driven Narratives as Deepfake," Journal of Cyberspace Studies, 2025. ut.ac.ir
[6] Amena Mahmoud, Musaed Alhussein, Khursheed Aurangzeb, and Eiko Takaoka. " Breast Cancer Survival Prediction Modelling Based on Genomic Data: An Improved Prognosis-Driven Deep Learning Approach," IEEE Access, vol. 12, 2024.
[7] A. Uchendu, T. Le, and D. Lee, "Topformer: Topology-aware authorship attribution of deepfake texts with diverse writing styles," ECAI 2024, 2024. iospress.nl
[8] A. Uchendu, S. Venkatraman, T. Le, "Catch me if you gpt: Tutorial on deepfake texts," in *Proceedings of the Conference on Language Technologies*, 2024. aclanthology.org
[9] K. Chandrappa and K. K. Shankar, "Combating deep fakes by the power of artificial intelligence and block chain in healthcare applications," in *Proceedings of Blockchain Technology for Healthcare*, 2023, Elsevier. [HTML]
[10] P. Cantero-Arjona and A. Sánchez-Macián, "Deepfake Detection and the Impact of Limited Computing Capabilities," 2024. [PDF]
[11] R. Shad, J. P. Cunningham, E. A. Ashley, C. P. Langlotz et al., "Medical Imaging and Machine Learning," 2021. [PDF]
[12] S. Neethirajan, "Is Seeing Still Believing? Leveraging Deepfake Technology for Livestock Farming," 2021. ncbi.nlm.nih.gov
[13] J. Qureshi and S. Khan, "Artificial Intelligence (AI) Deepfakes in Healthcare Systems: A Double-Edged Sword? Balancing Opportunities and Navigating Risks," 2024. researchgate.net
[14] C. Elendu, D. C. Amaechi, A. U. Okatta, E. C. Amaechi, "The impact of simulation-based training in medical education: A review," Medicine, 2024. lww.com
[15] E. Yates, R. Chirurgi, F. Adamakos, R. Habal et al., "Development and Utilization of 3D Printed Material for Thoracotomy Simulation," 2018. ncbi.nlm.nih.gov
[16] S. Gupta, K. Wilcocks, C. Matava, J. Wiegelmann et al., "Creating a Successful Virtual Reality–Based Medical Simulation Environment: Tutorial," 2023. ncbi.nlm.nih.gov
[17] C. Toale, M. Morris, and D. O. Kavanagh, "Perspectives on simulation-based assessment of operative skill in surgical training," Medical Teacher, 2023. [HTML]
[18] Surjeet Dalal, Pallavi Goel, Edeh Michael Onyema, Adnan Alharbi, Amena Mahmoud, Majed A. Algarni, Halifa Awal; "Application of Machine Learning for Cardiovascular Disease Risk Prediction", Computational

Intelligence and Neuroscience, (Special issue: Exploration of Human Cognition using Artificial Intelligence in Healthcare), ID: 9418666, 2023.
[19] L. Naamati-Schneider, "Enhancing AI competence in health management: students' experiences with ChatGPT as a learning Tool," 2024. ncbi.nlm.nih.gov
[20] Amena Mahmoud, Nancy Awadallah Awad, Najah Alsubaie, Syed Immamul Ansarullah, Mohammed S. Alqahtani, Mohamed Abbas, Mohammed Usman, Ben Othman Soufiene, and Abeer Saber; "Advanced Deep Learning Approaches for Accurate Brain Tumor Classification in Medical Imaging," Symmetry, Vol 15(3), pp: 571, 2023.
[21] S. Alanazi, S. Asif, A. Caird-Daley, and I. Moulitsas, "Unmasking deepfakes: a multidisciplinary examination of social impacts and regulatory responses," Human-Intelligent Systems, 2025. springer.com
[22] Y. Zhang, Z. Pang, S. Huang, C. Wang et al., "Unmasking AI-Created Visual Content: A Review of Generated Images and Deepfake Detection Technologies," 2025. preprints.org
[23] Sarang Sharma, Sheifali Gupta, Deepali Gupta, Sapna Juneja, Amena Mahmoud, Shaker El-sappagh, and KYUNG-SUP KWAK. "Transfer Learning based Modified Inception Model for Diagnosis of Alzheimer's Disease," Frontiers in Computational Neuroscience: pp. 119, 2022.
[24] C. Zimmermann, S. Strohmaier, T. Niederkrotenthaler, and others, "Suicide mortality among physicians, dentists, veterinarians, and pharmacists as well as other high-skilled occupations in Austria from 1986 through 2020," *Psychiatry*, vol. 2023, Elsevier. sciencedirect.com
[25] A. Qayyum, M. Bilal, M. Hadi, P. Capik et al., "Can We Revitalize Interventional Healthcare with AI-XR Surgical Metaverses?," 2023. [PDF]
[26] J. Cylwik, M. Celińska-Spodar, and M. Dudzic, "Hypotension Prediction Index Software and the Dynamics of Troponin and NTproBNP Concentration Changes in Patients Undergoing Oncological Abdominal Surgery," *Journal of Personalized Medicine*, vol. 2024. mdpi.com
[27] S. Pasricha, "AI Ethics in Smart Healthcare," 2022. [PDF]
[28] O. Navarro Martínez and D. Fernández-García, "Possible Health Benefits and Risks of DeepFake Videos: A Qualitative Study in Nursing Students," Nursing Reports, vol. 2024. mdpi.com
[29] Ali Tariq Nagi, Mazhar Javed Awan, Mazin Abed Mohammed, Amena Mahmoud, Arnab Majumdar, and Orawit Thinnukool; "Performance Analysis for COVID-19 Diagnosis Using Custom and State-of-the-Art Deep Learning Models", Applied Sciences, Vol 12(13), 2022.
[30] J. M. Dennis, K. G. Young, P. Cardoso, L. M. Güdemann, et al., "A five-drug class model using routinely available clinical features to optimise

prescribing in type 2 diabetes: a prediction model development and validation study," The Lancet, 2025. thelancet.com

[31] A. D. Samuel-Okon, O. I. Akinola, and O. O. Olaniyi, "Assessing the effectiveness of network security tools in mitigating the impact of deepfakes AI on public trust in media," 2024. ssrn.com

[32] J. Twomey, D. Ching, M. P. Aylett, M. Quayle, C. Linehan, "Do deepfake videos undermine our epistemic trust? A thematic analysis of tweets that discuss deepfakes in the Russian invasion of Ukraine," PLOS ONE, 2023. plos.org

[33] C. Mennella, U. Maniscalco, G. De Pietro, and M. Esposito, "Ethical and regulatory challenges of AI technologies in healthcare: A narrative review," 2024. ncbi.nlm.nih.gov

[34] A. H. Khalifa, N. A. Zaher, A. S. Abdallah, and M. W. Fakhr, "Convolutional neural network based on diverse Gabor filters for deepfake recognition," IEEE Access, 2022. ieee.org

[35] S. Hoek, S. Metselaar, C. Ploem, and M. Bak, "Promising for patients or deeply disturbing? The ethical and legal aspects of deepfake therapy," Journal of Medical Ethics, 2024. bmj.com

[36] D. Giri and E. Brady, "Exploring outlooks towards generative AI-based assistive technologies for people with Autism," 2023. [PDF]

[37] S. Solaiyappan and Y. Wen, "Machine Learning based Medical Image Deepfake Detection: A Comparative Study," 2021. [PDF]

[38] S. Zobaed, M. Fazle Rabby, M. Istiaq Hossain, E. Hossain et al., "DeepFakes: Detecting Forged and Synthetic Media Content Using Machine Learning," 2021. [PDF]

[39] Z. Akhtar, "Deepfakes Generation and Detection: A Short Survey," 2023. ncbi.nlm.nih.gov

[40] Dhiman, Gaurav, et al. "Federated learning approach to protect healthcare data over big data scenario." *Sustainability* 14.5 (2022): 2500.

[41] Chawla, Paras, et al. "Artificial intelligent systems in smart medical healthcare: Current trends." *Int. J. Adv. Sci. Technol* 29.10 (2020): 1476-1484.

[42] Singh, Shailendra Pratap, et al. "Dual adaption based evolutionary algorithm for optimized the smart healthcare communication service of the Internet of Things in smart city." *Physical Communication* 55 (2022): 101893.

[43] Anand, Rohit, et al. "Building integrated systems for healthcare considering mobile computing and IoT." *Integration of IoT with Cloud Computing for Smart Applications.* Chapman and Hall/CRC, 2023. 203-225.

4

Regulatory Frameworks and Ethics in Smart Healthcare Innovations: Deepfakes and the Metaverse

Ben Othman Soufiene S.[1], R.P. Narmadha[2], Dharani Jaganathan[3], Ram Kaji Budhathoki[4] and Soumita Seth[5,6]

[1]King Faisal University, Saudi Arabia.
[2]KIT – Kalaignar Karunanidhi Institute of Technology, India.
[3]KPR Institute of Engineering and Technology, India.
[4]Kathmandu University, Nepal
[5]Future Institute of Engineering and Management, India.
[6]Aliah University, India.

Email: sbenothman@kfu.edu.sa; nammu14@gmail.com; dharaniijagan92@gmail.com; soumita.seth@teamfuture.in

Abstract

The pace of innovation in healthcare has accelerated rapidly, driven by technologies such as artificial intelligence (AI) for early disease prediction and personalized treatment, augmented reality (AR) for real-time surgical visualization, and virtual reality (VR) for physical rehabilitation. In parallel, deepfake technology and the metaverse have emerged as disruptive forces, offering novel applications across clinical and educational domains. Deepfakes provide opportunities for realistic treatment simulations and interactive medical training, while the metaverse supports telemedicine and collaborative healthcare platforms. However, these advances pose significant challenges: deepfakes risk propagating misinformation, identity theft, and manipulated content, while metaverse environments introduce vulnerabilities related to data privacy, security, and consent. To address these concerns, robust regulatory frameworks and ethical governance are essential.

DOI: 10.1201/9788743809920-4

This chapter explores the roles of deepfake technology and the metaverse in smart healthcare, examining established regulatory standards such as the Health Insurance Portability and Accountability Act (HIPAA), General Data Protection Regulation (GDPR), U.S. Food and Drug Administration (FDA) guidelines, and European CE Marking. It emphasizes the need for clear policies to ensure data protection, enforce strict security measures, and uphold ethical standards. By aligning innovation with regulation, healthcare professionals can harness the transformative potential of deepfakes and the metaverse while safeguarding privacy, security, and trust.

4.1 Introduction

The healthcare industry has undergone a significant transformation due to rapid technological advancements. Smart healthcare integrates various advanced tools and technologies such as artificial intelligence (AI), the internet of things (IoT), big data analytics, and wearable devices. These innovations contribute to enhanced operational efficiency, improved patient care, and more effective health management. The evolution of smart healthcare can be traced through key technological milestones and shifts in clinical practices, as illustrated in Table 4.1 [1].

4.1.1 Importance of regulatory frameworks and ethical considerations

The development of smart healthcare technologies requires robust regulatory frameworks and ethical guidelines to ensure their safety, efficacy, and responsible use. These measures are essential to retain public trust and protect patient rights. Regulatory bodies play a key role in evaluating and approving new healthcare technologies through rigorous assessments. They are also responsible for post-market surveillance, setting standards for device development, manufacturing, and testing, and enforcing compliance through inspections, audits, and penalties [2].

4.2 Understanding Deepfakes in Healthcare

Deepfakes refer to the creation of highly realistic but synthetic media using deep learning techniques, primarily through artificial neural networks. These systems manipulate or superimpose images, videos, or audio onto existing content by learning and replicating facial features, gestures, and vocal tones from large datasets, typically comprised of images or videos. One of the

Table 4.1 Evolution of smart health care.

Innovation	Definition	Key technologies	Applications
Telemedicine and telehealth **1990s–2000s**	Digital tools for providing healthcare services remotely	Video conferencing, mobile apps, and remote monitoring devices	Remote consultations, follow-up visits, teletherapy, and telemonitoring
Wearable health devices **starts from 2010 to as of now**	Devices worn to continuously monitor health metrics	Smartwatches, fitness trackers, and implantable sensors	Tracking physical activity, heart rate, sleep patterns, and glucose levels
Artificial intelligence (AI) and Machine learning (ML) **2010s–present**	Algorithms and data analytics mimicking human intelligence	Natural language processing, predictive analytics, and image recognition	Diagnostic tools, predictive healthcare, personalized treatment plans, and administrative automation
Bin data analytics **2010s–present**	Processing and analyzing large datasets to extract insights	Data mining, predictive analytics, cloud computing	Population health management, disease outbreak prediction, and clinical decision support
Deepfakes **starts at 2020s**	AI-generated synthetic media creates realistic but fake images or videos	Generative adversarial networks (GANs)	Medical training simulations, patient education, and realistic virtual patient interactions
The Metaverse **starts at 2020s**	Virtual shared space merging physical reality with virtual space	Virtual reality (VR), augmented reality (AR), and mixed reality (MR)	Virtual clinics, medical training, patient support groups, and immersive therapy sessions
Robotics **starts in the 2020s**	Machines capable of performing complex actions autonomously	Surgical robots, robotic exoskeletons, and automated pharmacy dispensing systems	Minimally invasive surgery, rehabilitation, and automated medication dispensing

most common techniques used to generate deepfake content is the generative adversarial network (GAN), which synthesizes media by integrating the characteristics of a target person into various contexts.

A GAN consists of two neural networks: the generator (*G*) and the discriminator (*D*), trained simultaneously with opposing objectives. The generator produces synthetic data ($G(z)$) from random noise (z), aiming to make it indistinguishable from real data (x). Conversely, the discriminator evaluates both real and fake data to differentiate between them.

Accurate training of GANs requires careful calculation of loss functions, which guide the learning process of both networks. The discriminator loss (L_D) measures how effectively the discriminator distinguishes real data from the fake data generated by the generator. It is defined as follows [3]:

$$L_D = -E_{x \sim p_{data}}(x)\left[\log\left(1 - D\left(G\left(z\right)\right)\right)\right] \tag{4.1}$$

The above eqn (4.1) helps the ability of *D* to classify real and fake data samples by minimizing the loss. Meanwhile, the generator loss, measures how well generator can fool discriminator and is given by

$$L_G = -E_{z \sim p_z}(z)\left[\log\left(D\left(G\left(z\right)\right)\right)\right] \tag{4.2}$$

Minimizing the generator loss (L_G) encourages the generator (*G*) to produce increasingly realistic synthetic data. This adversarial process – driven by the minimization of both (L_G) and (L_D) using gradient descent algorithms—ensures that the generator becomes more skilled at producing lifelike outputs, while the discriminator (*D*) continues improving its ability to distinguish real data from fake. In the final stages of deepfake creation, developers further refine the output by adjusting facial expressions, lip movement, and other subtle details to enhance realism.

4.2.1 Potential benefits of deepfakes in healthcare

Deepfakes offer transformative possibilities across multiple domains of healthcare, as illustrated in Figure 4.1. In medical training and education, deepfakes enable the creation of virtual patients that closely resemble real individuals, including those presenting with rare conditions. Medical students can interact with these lifelike deepfake patients through simulated video consultations, offering a highly interactive and immersive learning experience. Furthermore, deepfake models can provide real-time feedback

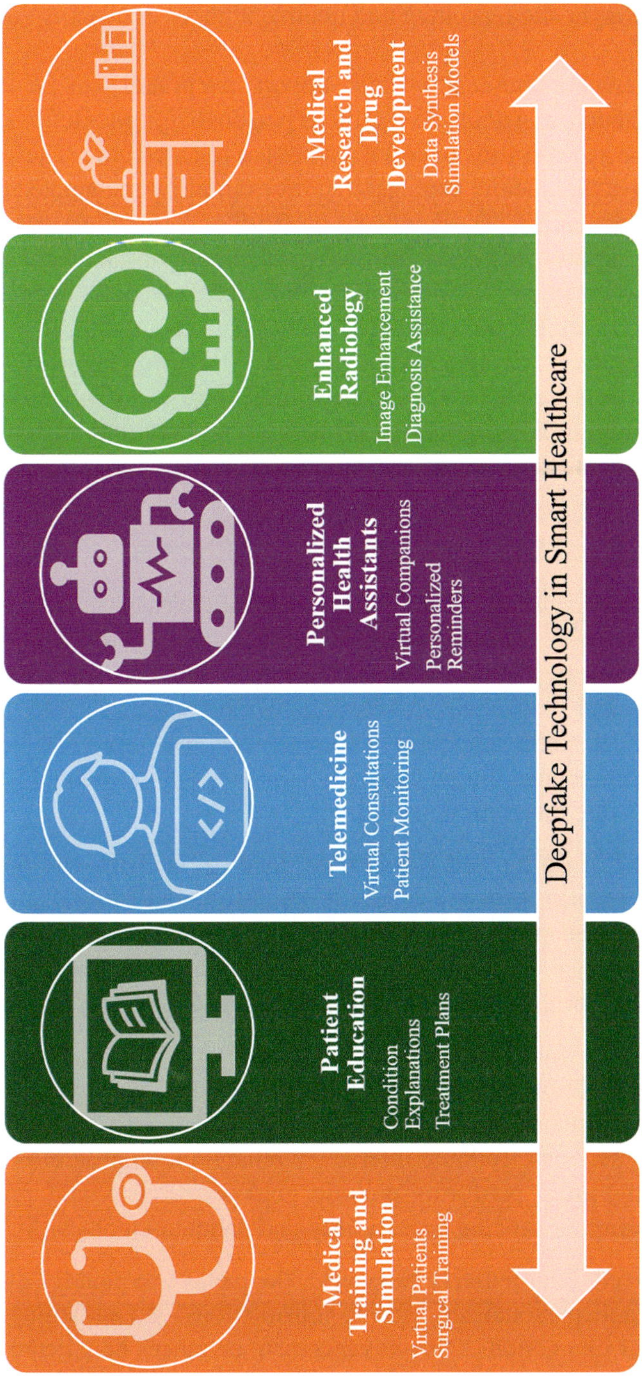

Figure 4.1 Potential benefits of deepfakes in healthcare.

on learners' diagnostic reasoning and treatment plans, enhancing educational outcomes [4].

In patient communication and support, deepfakes can be integrated into virtual health assistants to facilitate personalized interactions, thereby improving the accessibility and effectiveness of telemedicine. These technologies also have therapeutic applications; for example, personalized messages delivered in the voices or likenesses of familiar individuals can motivate patients and support mental health treatment, improving adherence to therapy and lifestyle regimens. Additionally, in medical research, deepfakes contribute by generating synthetic datasets that can augment real-world data. This enhances the accuracy and robustness of AI-driven diagnostic tools and predictive models without compromising patient privacy. Collectively, these applications highlight the potential of deepfakes to revolutionize healthcare education, patient engagement, and biomedical research [5].

4.3 The Rise of the Metaverse in Healthcare

The metaverse, a virtual shared space that integrates physical and digital environments, holds immense potential for transforming the healthcare sector [6]. Powered by technologies such as augmented reality (AR), virtual reality (VR), and blockchain, it offers innovative approaches to delivering medical services, enhancing patient engagement, and improving health outcomes. This immersive digital ecosystem enables unprecedented opportunities for healthcare innovation, including:

- **Medical Training and Education:** Medical students and professionals can practice procedures and respond to complex clinical scenarios within virtual environments, improving their skills without putting real patients at risk. Participation in virtual seminars and workshops enables healthcare professionals to stay updated with industry advancements and supports continuous education [7].
- **Virtual Rehabilitation and Therapy:** Patients – especially those with mobility limitations or living in remote areas – can engage in virtual therapy sessions. Tailored interactive rehabilitation programs delivered through virtual platforms provide guided exercises and progressive monitoring, enhancing accessibility and patient outcomes [8].
- **Enhanced Telemedicine Services:** The metaverse enables more interactive and personalized virtual consultations, strengthening patient–provider interactions. This advancement enhances healthcare delivery,

particularly for patients requiring frequent follow-ups or those in underserved regions [9].

- **Virtual Health Communities:** Patients can participate in digital peer-support groups, fostering shared experiences that aid in managing chronic conditions and emotional recovery. These virtual communities improve patient morale, adherence, and empowerment [10].
- **Surgical Planning and Collaboration:** Surgeons can simulate procedures using detailed virtual models of patient anatomy, enabling precise preoperative planning. Additionally, the metaverse facilitates real-time surgical collaboration across geographic locations, allowing experts to share techniques and insights during live procedures [11].

4.4 Ethical Implications of using the Deepfake and Metaverse in Healthcare

The ethical and regulatory challenges associated with deepfake and metaverse technologies are both significant and complex. Firstly, deepfakes can be manipulated to produce misleading medical content, potentially disseminating false information about treatments, healthcare plans, or public health emergencies. Such misuse can undermine trust in healthcare professionals and institutions, eroding public confidence in medical advice and interventions. Additionally, the unauthorized use of images or likenesses of patients and medical professionals in deepfake content raises serious privacy concerns and constitutes ethical and legal violations [12].

Secondly, within the metaverse – where virtual healthcare services operate – privacy and data security are paramount. This is especially relevant due to the handling of vast amounts of sensitive patient information. Compliance with data protection regulations such as the Health Insurance Portability and Accountability Act (HIPAA) and the General Data Protection Regulation (GDPR) is essential to safeguard personal health information from unauthorized access or misuse [13, 14]. Patients must be fully informed about how their data will be collected, used, and stored in the metaverse to ensure that consent is both informed and voluntary. Transparency about the capabilities and limitations of virtual healthcare services is also critical to maintaining trust and avoiding misunderstandings.

Equity and accessibility pose additional challenges. Technological disparities and limited internet access may prevent marginalized populations from benefiting fully from metaverse-based healthcare services. Therefore, platforms must be designed inclusively, accommodating individuals with disabilities and those with limited technological literacy. Moreover, prolonged engagement with virtual environments can have psychological and social implications. Although virtual healthcare offers convenience, reduced face-to-face interaction may affect mental health and increase the risk of social isolation outside virtual settings [15].

Addressing these ethical concerns requires thoughtful regulation, patient-centered policies, and technological innovation that prioritizes privacy, transparency, equality, and overall well-being. As metaverse and deepfake technologies evolve within healthcare, it is essential to establish ethical safeguards that uphold patient trust and protect public health.

4.5 Regulatory Frameworks for Smart Healthcare Innovations

Regulatory frameworks governing the approval and monitoring of healthcare technologies vary across regions, reflecting localized health priorities and legal standards. In the United States, the Food and Drug Administration (FDA) ensures the safety, efficacy, and security of healthcare products through regulatory pathways such as the 510(k) premarket notification and Premarket Approval (PMA) processes [16]. These mechanisms evaluate whether new products meet appropriate performance and safety criteria before entering the market. In the European Union, the European Medicines Agency (EMA) coordinates scientific evaluations and enforces compliance through regulatory frameworks such as the Medical Devices Regulation (MDR) and In Vitro Diagnostic Regulation (IVDR) [17]. These regulations aim to standardize device safety and performance across EU member states. In the United Kingdom, the Medicines and Healthcare Products Regulatory Agency (MHRA) oversees medical device approvals via the UK Conformity Assessed (UKCA) marking and manages post-market safety reporting through the Yellow Card Scheme, which collects data on adverse events and device deficiencies [18]. China's National Medical Products Administration (NMPA) regulates medical devices and technologies through mechanisms such as the Medical Device Registration Regulation and adherence to Good Manufacturing Practice (GMP) guidelines. The NMPA is responsible for authorizing clinical trials, evaluating product quality, and monitoring post-market safety.

In Canada, medical devices are evaluated under the Medical Devices Regulations and monitored through the Drug and Health Products Inspection Program, which assesses product quality and market compliance. Similarly, in Australia, the Therapeutic Goods Administration (TGA) ensures safety and effectiveness through the Therapeutic Goods Act and registration in the Australian Register of Therapeutic Goods (ARTG) [19]. Across all these jurisdictions, regulatory agencies play a vital role in protecting public health by enforcing rigorous approval processes, compliance standards, and ongoing surveillance of medical technologies.

4.6 Case Studies of Regulatory Responses

4.6.1 FDA's SaMD (AI/ML-based software as a medical device)

The U.S. Food and Drug Administration (FDA) has developed a comprehensive action plan to address the challenges posed by artificial intelligence (AI) and machine learning (ML) in healthcare. A key component of this plan involves establishing a framework for the continuous monitoring of real-world performance post-approval, ensuring that AI-driven products maintain safety and effectiveness over time. Additionally, the FDA's Software Precertification Program evaluates software developers based on their commitment to quality, transparency, and organizational excellence. This initiative aims to streamline the regulatory approval process for digital health technologies while preserving high safety and effectiveness standards.

4.6.2 European Union's GDPR compliance

Under the General Data Protection Regulation (GDPR), healthcare organizations are required to conduct Data Protection Impact Assessments (DPIAs) for high-risk data processing activities, including those involving emerging technologies such as deepfakes and the metaverse. DPIAs help ensure that appropriate safeguards are in place to protect personal data throughout the technology's lifecycle. Furthermore, GDPR promotes enhanced privacy measures such as pseudonymization and encryption, which are critical strategies for mitigating the risks of unauthorized access, misuse, and data breaches.

4.6.3 UK's MHRA and AI in healthcare

The Medicines and Healthcare Products Regulatory Agency (MHRA) provides clear guidelines for the safe implementation of AI in healthcare, emphasizing transparency, accountability, and rigorous validation. An important component of this framework is the Yellow Card Scheme, which has been extended to include digital health technologies. This system enables the reporting of adverse outcomes related to AI-driven medical devices, supporting continuous monitoring and facilitating timely responses to safety issues.

4.6.4 China's NMPA and digital health regulations

The National Medical Products Administration (NMPA) has updated its regulatory framework to include specific guidelines for digital health technologies such as artificial intelligence (AI) systems and wearable devices. These guidelines ensure that innovative technologies meet stringent safety and efficacy standards prior to approval. Additionally, to strengthen post-market surveillance, the NMPA requires manufacturers to submit regular safety reports and undergo random inspections. These measures help enforce regulatory compliance and maintain ongoing device safety in clinical use.

4.6.5 Health Canada and medical device regulations

Health Canada regulates medical devices using a risk-based approach, which includes technologies that incorporate artificial intelligence and other emerging digital tools. Devices with higher risk profiles are subject to more rigorous evaluation to ensure patient safety. As part of the Drug and Health Products Inspection Program, Health Canada conducts inspections of manufacturing facilities and reviews clinical trial data. These measures are designed to uphold high standards of quality, safety, and effectiveness for new medical technologies entering the Canadian market.

4.6.6 Australia's TGA and the Australian Register of Therapeutic Goods (ARTG)

The Therapeutic Goods Administration (TGA) is responsible for standardizing the safety and efficacy of therapeutic goods, including pharmaceuticals, diagnostic devices, and digital health innovations, under the Therapeutic Goods Act. Before entering the Australian market, all therapeutic products must be listed on the Australian Register of Therapeutic Goods (ARTG). The TGA employs adaptive regulatory pathways that facilitate early access to innovative medical technologies, while ensuring their safety and performance through comprehensive post-market surveillance.

Despite these mechanisms, cutting-edge technologies such as deepfakes and the metaverse present significant regulatory challenges. Rapid advancements in these fields often outpace existing regulatory frameworks, creating oversight gaps that could compromise safety and efficacy. The use of such technologies in healthcare requires strict adherence to data protection regulations due to the handling of large volumes of sensitive patient data, raising critical privacy and security concerns. Furthermore, ethical dilemmas regarding the authenticity of synthetic content, informed consent, and equitable access must be addressed. A balanced approach is needed to support innovation while maintaining ethical integrity, public trust, and effective oversight.

4.7 Ethical Considerations in Smart Healthcare Innovations

Ethical principles serve as the foundation for the development and implementation of healthcare technologies, as illustrated in Figure 4.2. These principles ensure that innovations enhance patient care while upholding moral, legal, and societal values. From initial design through to deployment and evaluation, ethical considerations guide every stage of the technological development process.

4.7.1 Beneficence

To improve patient health and well-being, healthcare providers and technologists must prioritize both clinical outcomes and overall quality of life. This

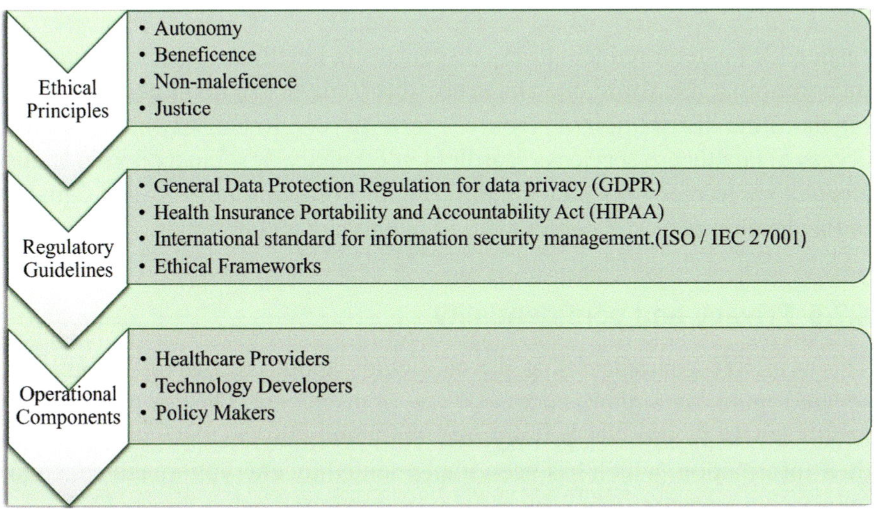

Figure 4.2 Ethical considerations in smart healthcare innovations.

approach supports the development of solutions that enhance disease diagnosis, treatment, and patient care without compromising safety. Prioritizing patient welfare and striving for positive health outcomes requires a careful balance of potential benefits against associated risks [20].

4.7.2 Non-maleficence

This **non-maleficence** [20] principle requires rigorous testing and validation procedures to allay hazards such as errors, biases in AI algorithms, data breaches, and unintended consequences to avoid the patients suffering from harm. Continuation non-maleficence involves prioritizing patient safety and safeguarding that technological interventions do not compromise physical, psychological, or social well-being.

4.7.3 Autonomy

Autonomy [20] emphasizes respecting patients' rights to make informed healthcare decisions aligned with accurate information and personal preferences. This principle demands clear communication about the application of technologies in patient care and obtaining informed consent. Patients must fully comprehend the risks, benefits, and alternatives before agreeing to use these technologies.

4.7.4 Justice

Justice [21] is required to address disparities in healthcare access and design outcomes that are affordable and accessible to diverse patient populations. It regulates the distribution of resources for everyone in Fairway and equitable access to healthcare services regardless of ethnicity or socioeconomic status. Regulatory frameworks play a main role in promoting fairness and equality in the development and deployment of healthcare technologies.

4.7.5 Privacy and confidentiality

This principle guarantees that private details about the patient's health are secured against unauthorized access, use, or disclosure. The key part of smart healthcare is to provide privacy and confidentiality to the patients about their information, which has been implemented by encryption and data anonymization measures that protect from breaches and cyber threats [22].

The above ethical principles give a background to navigate the difficulties of developing and deploying technologies for those who are included in the creation of smart health care. Along with this, there are some special challenges faced by Deepfakes and Metaverse technologies while incorporating them.

4.7.6 Authenticity and trust

Deepfakes: In smart healthcare, deepfake techniques can generate extremely realistic but artificially created data such as images, audio, and video. This raises concerns about authenticity [23]. If deepfakes are utilized maliciously or unintentionally, it could lead to misleading diagnoses, treatment recommendations, or patient interactions

Metaverse: The boundary lines between reality and the simulation can be blurred by virtual environments. Interaction conducted in these virtual spaces may impact patient trust if doubt arises regarding the authenticity and the identity of the healthcare providers.

4.7.7 Informed consent

Deepfakes: Patients may not have a complete understanding or awareness of how deepfake technology is used in their healthcare, which can make the informed consent processes. A clear statement about the formation, purpose, and implications of deepfakes is important for patients to make informed decisions [24].

Metaverse: Joining in healthcare actions in virtual environments might include risks or restrictions that may not be immediately recognized by patients. It is essential to provide a thorough disclosure of these risks, along with the benefits and alternative options, to ensure valid informed consent [23].

4.7.8 Privacy and Security

Deepfakes: Protecting and handling the sensitive data which are generated by deepfakes from unauthorized access, breaches, or misuse is important to maintaining patient confidentiality and trust [25].

Metaverse: The vast amount of data, such as information from biometric and behavior, are collected by the metaverse virtual environment, which creates concerns about privacy. Ensuring robust security measures and compliance with data protection regulations are essential to mitigate risks associated with data handling in the metaverse [26].

4.7.9 Bias and fairness

Deepfakes: The deepfake models are created by AI algorithms that may disseminate biases present in data that are ready for training, leading to biased outcomes in diagnostics, treatment recommendations, or patient interactions. Addressing and mitigating bias in deepfake technology is critical to ensure fairness and equity in healthcare [25].

Metaverse: The availability and quality of healthcare services accessed via vital platforms may differ, potentially amplifying current disparities in healthcare access and outcomes. Efforts to advocate for fairness and equity in virtual healthcare delivery are essential to prevent further widening of healthcare disparities.

4.7.10 Professional integrity and misuse

Deepfakes: Misuse of deepfake technology in healthcare poses risks to professional integrity and public trust, necessitating clear ethical guidelines for its creation and use to prevent misuse [23].

Metaverse: The same traditional healthcare standards have been maintained by healthcare professionals in virtual environments by adhering to ethical guidelines and professional codes of conduct.

4.8 Strategies for Managing Risks of Deepfakes and Metaverse Applications in Healthcare

To mitigate the risks associated with emerging technologies like deepfakes and the metaverse, the following strategies help safeguard the integrity, privacy, and security of healthcare interaction, as shown in Figure 4.3.

4.8.1 Authentication and verification systems

- **By implementing the biometric verification:** Methods, such as fingerprint or facial recognition, to verify the identity of healthcare professionals and patients engaging in virtual interactions.
- **With the help of digital signatures**, the authenticated medical records, prescriptions, and other sensitive information are authenticated, and the data integrity and authenticity are safeguarded.

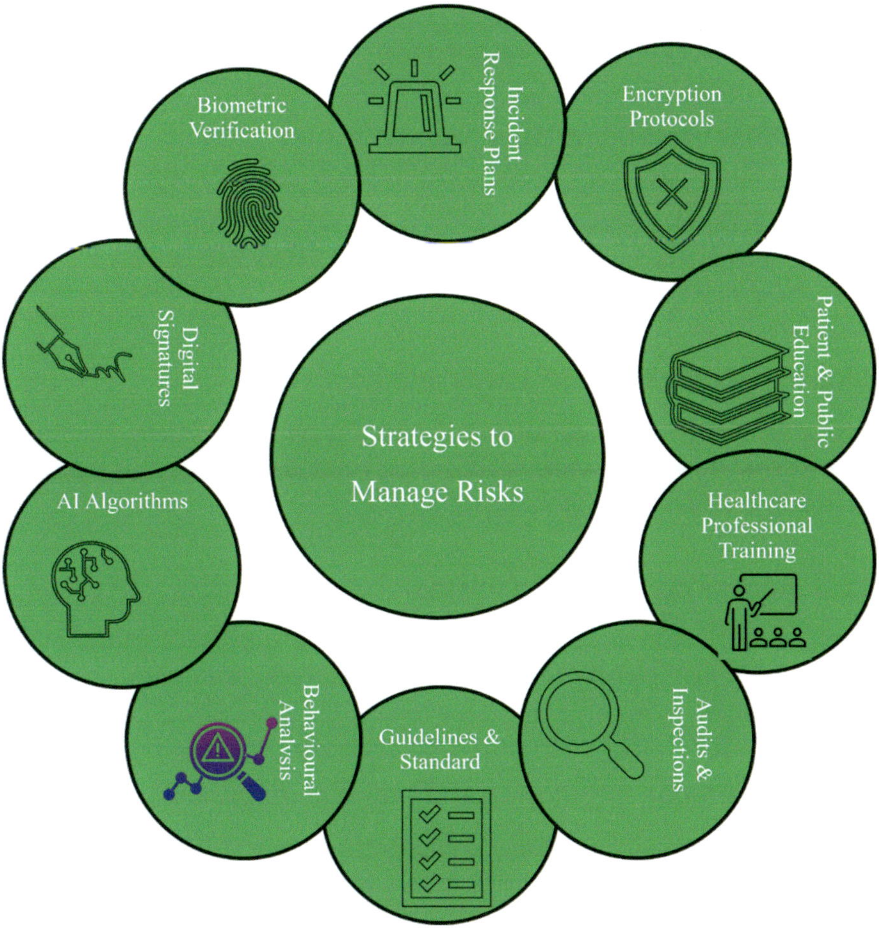

Figure 4.3 Strategies for managing risks of deepfakes and metaverse applications in healthcare.

4.8.2 Deepfake detection tools

The behavioral analysis technique is used to find anomalies in message patterns or communications within virtual healthcare environments that may specify the occurrence of deepfakes.

4.8.3 Regulatory oversight and compliance

By establishing a clear guidelines and regulatory standards for the development, deployment, and use of deepfake technology in healthcare settings. By conducting regular audits and inspections to monitor compliance with regulatory requirements and ethical guidelines, identifying and addressing potential instances of misuse or non-compliance promptly.

4.8.4 Education and training programs

Healthcare professionals are trained with comprehensive education and training on the risks associated with deepfakes and the metaverse in healthcare, enabling them to recognize signs of misuse and fraud and securely navigate virtual healthcare environments

4.8.5 Technological safeguards and controls

Strong encryption protocols are used to protect sensitive patient data transmitted or stored within virtual healthcare environments, preventing unauthorized access or data breaches.

4.8.6 Access control mechanisms

It help to restrict and monitor who can access and manipulate sensitive information or technologies prone to misuse, ensuring only authorized personnel can use them.

4.8.7 Continuous monitoring and incident response

Implementing robust surveillance systems to continuously monitor virtual healthcare environments for suspicious activities or anomalies that could point out potential misuse of technology. Creating and executing plans to promptly handle and mitigate cases of technology misuse, which include protocols for reporting, investigating, and easing security breaches or ethical violations.

By implementing these methods, healthcare organizations can proactively detect and prevent the misuse of technology, safeguard patient safety, and uphold ethical standards in the increasingly complex landscape of deepfakes and the metaverse in healthcare.

4.9 Potential Future Developments in Deepfakes and the Metaverse

Future advancements in deepfake technology, powered by innovations in generative adversarial networks (GANs) and variational autoencoders

(VAEs), are expected to produce synthetic media with unprecedented realism. These enhancements will pose significant challenges to current verification systems, requiring the development of advanced detection mechanisms that leverage deep learning and multimodal verification approaches, such as voice, facial, and behavioral analysis. As AI development frameworks like TensorFlow and PyTorch become increasingly accessible, the barrier to creating deepfakes will diminish, leading to broader adoption. While this accessibility has potential benefits in healthcare – such as enabling realistic patient simulations and enhancing medical training – it also increases the risk of misuse, emphasizing the need for strong ethical guidelines and robust authentication protocols.

Simultaneously, the metaverse is poised to revolutionize virtual healthcare through advancements in virtual reality (VR), augmented reality (AR), and mixed reality (MR) technologies. VR-based therapeutic applications may offer immersive environments for mental health intervention, while AR systems could provide surgeons with real-time data overlays during complex procedures. Moreover, integrating AI with the metaverse will facilitate the development of virtual health assistants and diagnostic tools capable of delivering real-time feedback and decision support.

The convergence of AI, the internet of things (IoT), and edge computing within metaverse environments will further enable continuous patient monitoring and personalized care. Wearable devices, smart implants, and remote monitoring systems will generate real-time health data that can be analyzed through AI-driven predictive models, enabling proactive healthcare management and early intervention.

4.10 Recommendations for Policymakers, Healthcare Providers, and Technology Developers

Policymakers are encouraged to establish comprehensive regulatory frameworks that ensure the ethical and responsible use of deepfake technology and virtual healthcare environments. These frameworks should include standards for AI transparency, accountability, and data governance, alongside requirements for secure cryptographic techniques to protect data integrity. Furthermore, investing in interdisciplinary research is essential for understanding the ethical, social, and technical implications of technologies such as deepfakes and the metaverse. Key areas of focus include AI ethics, cybersecurity, and legal considerations. Collaborative efforts between policymakers, academia, and industry stakeholders can drive innovation while addressing societal impacts.

Healthcare providers should prioritize the development of training modules that combine AI literacy, cybersecurity awareness, and ethical decision-making. Utilizing simulation-based training with virtual reality (VR) and deepfake technologies can enhance practical learning and improve clinical readiness. Implementing ethical guidelines, such as those outlined in the AI4People ethical framework, ensures that informed consent procedures include comprehensive information regarding the use of advanced technologies in patient care.

Technology developers have a crucial role in enhancing security measures through the implementation of advanced encryption methods (e.g., homomorphic encryption), multi-factor authentication, and blockchain solutions for secure medical records. Adhering to ethical design principles – such as those outlined in the IEEE Global Initiative on Ethics of Autonomous and Intelligent Systems – is essential. These guidelines promote the development of AI systems grounded in transparency, fairness, and accountability. Regular ethical impact assessments and ongoing input from diverse stakeholders should be integrated throughout the design and implementation process to uphold these values.

4.11 Conclusion

The integration of virtual reality (VR), artificial intelligence (AI), the internet of things (IoT), deepfake technology, and the metaverse marks a pivotal shift in the advancement of healthcare. These technologies offer transformative possibilities—from immersive medical training and virtual consultations to personalized patient care and improved diagnostic precision. However, these innovations also introduce substantial challenges, particularly in the areas of regulatory oversight and ethical governance. Deepfakes, while promising for enhancing medical education and virtual patient interactions, raise significant concerns regarding authenticity, consent, and trust. Similarly, the use of metaverse-based healthcare platforms necessitates careful handling of sensitive personal data and adherence to strict privacy standards. As such, the development, deployment, and use of these technologies must be guided by robust regulatory frameworks that ensure patient safety, data integrity, and ethical conduct. Addressing these challenges requires a collaborative, interdisciplinary approach. Policymakers, healthcare professionals, technology developers, legal experts, and ethicists must work together to establish guidelines that balance innovation with responsibility. Continuous investment in research and development, particularly in the areas of AI ethics, cybersecurity, and digital health law, will be essential in shaping policies that evolve alongside technological progress. Ultimately, by proactively addressing ethical and regulatory challenges, the healthcare sector can fully harness the potential of deepfakes and the metaverse. Doing so will allow for the delivery of advanced, equitable, and secure healthcare services while protecting patient welfare and preserving the integrity of medical practice.

Reference

[1] M. Nasr *et al.*, "Smart Healthcare in the Age of AI: Recent Advances, Challenges, and Future Prospects."

[2] D. B. Larson, H. Harvey, D. L. Rubin, N. Irani, J. R. Tse, and C. P. Langlotz, "Regulatory Frameworks for Development and Evaluation of Artificial Intelligence–Based Diagnostic Imaging Algorithms: Summary and Recommendations," *Journal of the American College of Radiology*, vol. 18, no. 3, pp. 413–424, Mar. 2021, doi: 10.1016/j.jacr.2020.09.060.

[3] I. J. Goodfellow *et al.*, "Generative Adversarial Networks," Jun. 2014, [Online]. Available: http://arxiv.org/abs/1406.2661

[4] S. Patil, "Artificial Intelligence Face Swapping: Promise and Peril in Health Care," *Mayo Clinic Proceedings: Digital Health*, vol. 2, no. 1, p. 159, Mar. 2024, doi: 10.1016/j.mcpdig.2024.01.009.

[5] A. A. Kononowicz*et al.*, "Virtual patient simulations in health professions education: Systematic review and meta-analysis by the digital health education collaboration," Jul. 01, 2019, *JMIR Publications Inc.* doi: 10.2196/14676.

[6] M. Ball, "The Metaverse: What It Is, Where to Find it, Who Will Build It, and Fortnite," *MatthewBall.vc*, no. December 2019, 2020.

[7] T. Tene, D. F. Vique López, P. E. Valverde Aguirre, L. M. Orna Puente, and C. Vacacela Gomez, "Virtual reality and augmented reality in medical education: an umbrella review," 2024, *Frontiers Media SA*. doi: 10.3389/fdgth.2024.1365345.

[8] T. Massetti *et al.*, "The Clinical Utility of Virtual Reality in Neurorehabilitation: A Systematic Review," *J Cent Nerv Syst Dis*, vol. 10, p. 117957351881354, Jan. 2018, doi: 10.1177/1179573518813541.

[9] G. Nittari, D. Savva, D. Tomassoni, S. K. Tayebati, and F. Amenta, "Telemedicine in the COVID-19 Era: A Narrative Review Based on Current Evidence," May 01, 2022, *MDPI*. doi: 10.3390/ijerph19095101.

[10] J. Wang, T. Yao, and Y. Wang, "Patient Engagement as Contributors in Online Health Communities: The Mediation of Peer Involvement and

Moderation of Community Status," *Behavioral Sciences*, vol. 13, no. 2, Feb. 2023, doi: 10.3390/bs13020152.

[11] G. Ntakakis, C. Plomariti, C. Frantzidis, P. E. Antoniou, P. D. Bamidis, and G. Tsoulfas, "Exploring the use of virtual reality in surgical education," Feb. 18, 2023, *Baishideng Publishing Group Inc.* doi: 10.5500/wjt.v13.i2.36.

[12] M. R. Shoaib, Z. Wang, M. T. Ahvanooey, and J. Zhao, "Deepfakes, Misinformation, and Disinformation in the Era of Frontier AI, Generative AI, and Large AI Models," Nov. 2023, [Online]. Available: http://arxiv.org/abs/2311.17394

[13] S. J. Nass, L. A. Levit, L. O. (Lawrence O. Gostin, and the H. P. Rule. Institute of Medicine (U.S.). Committee on Health Research and the Privacy of Health Information, *Beyond the HIPAA privacy rule : enhancing privacy, improving health through research.* National Academies Press, 2009.

[14] S. Haque, Z. Eberhart, A. Bansal, and C. McMillan, "Semantic Similarity Metrics for Evaluating Source Code Summarization," in *IEEE International Conference on Program Comprehension*, IEEE Computer Society, 2022, pp. 36–47. doi: 10.1145/nnnnnnn.nnnnnnn.

[15] S. K. Brooks *et al.*, "The psychological impact of quarantine and how to reduce it: rapid review of the evidence," Mar. 14, 2020, *Lancet Publishing Group*. doi: 10.1016/S0140-6736(20)30460-8.

[16] "15.a7ab3090-dffa-496a-8fa0-547a74bf1519".

[17] B. R. Lubbers *et al.*, "The New EU Regulation on in Vitro Diagnostic Medical Devices: Implications and Preparatory Actions for Diagnostic Laboratories," *Hemasphere*, vol. 5, no. 5, May 2021, doi: 10.1097/HS9.0000000000000568.

[18] J. E. D. Han *et al.*, "Opportunities and Risks of UK Medical Device Reform," *Ther Innov Regul Sci*, vol. 56, no. 4, pp. 596–606, Jul. 2022, doi: 10.1007/s43441-022-00394-0.

[19] "Making therapeutic goods safer for everyone," https://www.tga.gov.au/news/blog/making-therapeutic-goods-safer-everyone.

[20] "The Code of Medical Ethics of the American Medical Association (AMA) consists of three components: 1. The Principles of Medical Ethics 2. Ethical Opinions of the Council on Ethical and Judicial Affairs 3. Reports of the Council on Ethical and Judicial Affairs." [Online]. Available: www.ama-assn.org/go/ceja

[21] N. M. Kollapally, V. K. Keloth, J. Xu, and J. Geller, "Integrating Commercial and Social Determinants of Health: A Unified Ontology for Non-Clinical Determinants of Health."

[22] "Good Practices for Security of Internet of Things in the context of Smart Manufacturing NOVEMBER 2018 Good practices for Security of Internet of Things in the context of Smart Manufacturing About ENISA," 2018, doi: 10.2824/851384.

[23] "AMA Code of Medical Ethics 1.2.12 Ethical Practice in Telemedicine."

[24] C. Nebeker, J. Torous, and R. J. Bartlett Ellis, "Building the case for actionable ethics in digital health research supported by artificial intelligence," *BMC Med*, vol. 17, no. 1, p. 137, Dec. 2019, doi: 10.1186/s12916-019-1377-7.

[25] R. Challen, J. Denny, M. Pitt, L. Gompels, T. Edwards, and K. Tsaneva-Atanasova, "Artificial intelligence, bias and clinical safety," *BMJ Qual Saf*, vol. 28, no. 3, pp. 231–237, Mar. 2019, doi: 10.1136/bmjqs-2018-008370.

[26] M. Dunn Cavelty and M. Smeets, "Regulatory cybersecurity governance in the making: the formation of ENISA and its struggle for epistemic authority," *J Eur Public Policy*, vol. 30, no. 7, 2023, doi: 10.1080/13501763.2023.2173274.

5

Emergency Response Training in Metaverse Scenarios

Sayantan Kundu[1], Sushil Kr. Dinda[1] and Anjan Bandyopadhyay[1]

[1]Kalinga Institute of Industrial Technology, India.

Email: sayantankundu21@gmail.com; qwersushil@gmail.com; anjan.bandyopadhyayfcs@kiit.ac.in

Abstract

The metaverse is emerging as a transformative technology in emergency response training, offering immersive, real-time, and scalable simulations for healthcare professionals and first responders. By leveraging virtual reality (VR), augmented reality (AR), artificial intelligence (AI), blockchain, and cloud computing, metaverse environments provide realistic training scenarios for handling pandemics, natural disasters, and mass casualty events. These advanced simulations allow trainees to practice crisis management, triage procedures, and resource allocation in a controlled yet dynamic setting, improving their decision-making capabilities and situational awareness. Furthermore, AI-driven analytics and machine learning algorithms continuously assess trainee performance, offering real-time feedback and personalized training modules. Blockchain technology enhances data security and ensures transparent documentation of certifications and training records. Additionally, 5G and cloud computing enable seamless collaboration among trainees and instructors, facilitating remote and large-scale emergency training sessions. Despite its vast potential, metaverse-based training faces several challenges, including high implementation costs, technological barriers, psychological effects of hyper-realistic scenarios, and data security concerns. Addressing these challenges through research, policy development, and technological advancements will be crucial in maximizing the effectiveness of

DOI: 10.1201/9788743809920-5

metaverse-based emergency response training. This paper explores the core technologies that enable metaverse-based emergency training, highlights real-world implementations, identifies existing challenges, and discusses future research directions to optimize the use of metaverse technologies in emergency preparedness.

5.1 Introduction

The increasing frequency and severity of global emergencies – ranging from pandemics and natural disasters to mass casualty incidents – highlight the critical need for advanced emergency response training. Traditional training methods, such as classroom instruction, live drills, and field exercises, have long been the standard for preparing first responders and healthcare professionals. However, these methods often come with limitations such as high costs, logistical challenges, limited scalability, and the inability to fully replicate the unpredictability and scale of real-world emergencies. The emergence of the metaverse offers a promising alternative to conventional training models by creating highly immersive, interactive, and data-driven environments where emergency response personnel can refine their skills in a controlled yet realistic setting [1].

Through the integration of virtual reality (VR), augmented reality (AR), artificial intelligence (AI), blockchain, and cloud computing, metaverse-based emergency training provides an innovative approach to preparedness. These technologies enable trainees to engage in simulations that replicate complex crisis scenarios with dynamic, real-time interactions, allowing them to practice triage procedures, coordination strategies, and critical decision-making under pressure [2]. The COVID-19 pandemic served as a catalyst for digital transformation in healthcare and emergency management, underscoring the need for scalable, remote-friendly training solutions [3].

During the pandemic, many healthcare professionals faced overwhelming patient surges, shortages of medical supplies, and the challenge of adapting to rapidly evolving protocols. Metaverse-based simulations have the potential to bridge these gaps by offering AI-driven, adaptive training experiences that adjust to the needs of individual users, provide performance-based feedback, and facilitate collaborative crisis response training across geographically dispersed teams. Additionally, blockchain technology ensures secure data management, verifying certifications and tracking skill development transparently.

As metaverse applications in emergency response continue to evolve, it is essential to examine the enabling technologies, practical implementations, challenges, and future research directions that will shape their effectiveness. This paper explores how metaverse environments can enhance emergency response training, improve collaboration among first responders, and ensure better preparedness for large-scale disasters. The following sections analyze the key technological enablers of metaverse-based emergency training, real-world applications, challenges to widespread adoption, and future developments that will further integrate the metaverse into global emergency preparedness strategies.

5.2 Key Technologies Enabling Metaverse-Based Emergency Response Training

5.2.1 Virtual reality (VR) and augmented reality (AR)

Virtual reality (VR) and augmented reality (AR) are transforming emergency response training in the metaverse by enabling highly interactive and immersive environments. The technologies allow first responders, medical teams, and disaster response teams to practice managing crises in realistic but simulated situations, building their preparedness and decision-making capabilities [4]. VR provides completely simulated emergency scenarios, enabling trainees to participate in intricate crisis situations like hospital surge capacity management, disaster scene triage, fire evacuations, and mass disaster response training exercises [5]. These simulations mimic real-world problems without putting trainees at risk, which allows them to make high-pressure decisions. Through simulation in a virtual setting, responders can hone skills like prioritizing casualties, handling limited resources, and carrying out evacuation procedures effectively.

AR, in contrast, supplements real-world training and response activities by projecting digital information onto the real world. In an emergency situation, AR can offer real-time information regarding hazards, patient status, and best escape routes through wearable technology or smart glasses [6]. For instance, paramedics can instantly access the vital signs and medical history of injured patients, enhancing the speed and precision of on-site care [5]. Firefighters have the ability to see heat signatures and building vulnerability within burning buildings, enabling quicker and safer rescues [4].

By incorporating VR and AR into emergency training, organizations can advance situational awareness, coordination, and responsiveness. These technologies enhance hands-on learning activities, allowing responders to gain confidence and competency prior to facing actual emergency situations. As metaverse-based training advances, it will be able to further improve

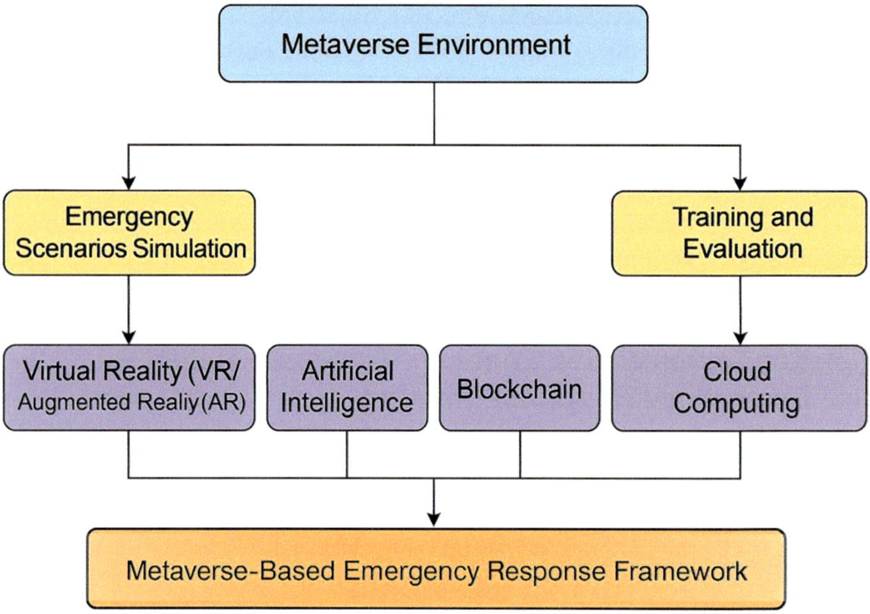

Figure 5.1 Metaverse environment.

disaster readiness and crisis management, ultimately saving lives in high-risk environments.

5.2.2 Artificial intelligence (AI) and machine learning (ML)

Artificial intelligence (AI) and machine learning (ML) are also vital for enhancing the intelligence and adaptability of metaverse-based training modules. These technologies make learning experiences dynamic, personalized, and data-driven for emergency responders so that they can advance critical skills in an efficient manner [7].

AI-powered simulations have the ability to shift difficulty levels in real time according to a trainee's performance. Through ongoing response analysis, AI makes learning challenging and stimulating enough so that people can develop Figure 5.1. Crisis management process cycle. their decision-making skills when faced with pressure. Adaptive learning through this method enables responders to gain confidence and proficiency in managing advanced emergency situations [8].

Virtual assistants and chatbots powered by AI also advance training by walking trainees through various scenarios. Virtual assistants deliver real-time decision-making support with situational insights and step-by-step instructions while simulating crises. Through their interactions with AI, trainees can rehearse reacting to emergencies with instant feedback, enhancing their capacity to make swift and well-informed decisions [7].

ML algorithms are responsible for training module optimization based on previous emergency response and trainee behavior. Through pattern identification in decision-making and response performance, ML regularly optimizes training material to keep pace with real-world scenarios. This maximizes the relevance and timeliness of training for emergency responders [8].

Further, AI-driven predictive analytics can estimate potential risks and recommend best-response strategies. Using historical data and present trends, AI can project future crisis situations, enabling the responders to plan better. This information enables emergency teams to develop situational awareness, coordination, and proactive response plans.

By coupling AI and ML with metaverse-based training, organizations are able to build smarter, more adaptive, and more capable training environments. These technologies, in addition to offering improved learning results, also help improve crisis response, potentially saving lives in dangerous situations.

5.2.3 Blockchain for data security and credentialing

Blockchain technology is pivotal in bolstering the security, integrity, and transparency of emergency response training records. In legacy training systems, keeping certifications, training records, and performance ratings up to date can be tiresome, subject to tampering, and susceptible to administrative inefficiencies. Blockchain offers a decentralized, immutable ledger that secures these records, making them verifiable and impervious to unauthorized alteration, and maintaining competency standards [9].

One of the primary strengths of blockchain for emergency training is that it can produce tamper-proof records. The moment a record of certification or training is uploaded to the blockchain, it is impossible to delete or edit it, preserving long-term integrity. This makes emergency response agencies, healthcare organizations, and government authorities more trusting and enable them to authenticate professionals' credentials more efficiently.

Additionally, smart contracts – self-executing digital contracts stored on the blockchain – can automate the credentialing process. These contracts can instantly verify whether a responder has completed the necessary training and certifications, eliminated manual verification delays and reducing administrative burdens. This automation ensures that only qualified personnel are deployed in crisis situations, improving overall emergency preparedness.

Blockchain also supports interoperability between various training platforms and institutions, enabling emergency responders to transfer their credentials smoothly across organizations and locations. This is especially useful for large-scale disaster response operations that need coordination among multiple agencies.

Though it has its benefits, blockchain implementation in emergency response training is beset by issues like costs of implementation, requiring standardized systems, and data protection. As research and implementation continue, however, blockchain can potentially transform emergency training by rendering credentialing more secure, efficient, and transparent, ultimately keeping critical situations with highly trained and authenticated individuals.

5.2.4 Cloud computing and 5G connectivity

The convergence of cloud computing and 5G connectivity is revolutionizing emergency response training by providing real-time, mass-scale simulations with effortless collaboration. Conventional training procedures tend to be limited by location barriers, network latency, and data-sharing inefficiencies. Cloud-based platforms with super-speed 5G networks, though, provide an extended and immersive solution for training emergency responders at various locations [10].

Cloud computing makes it possible to host emergency training programs on central platforms, where trainees and instructors can access training documentation, engage in live simulation, and exchange vital data in real time. The platforms allow synchronized training sessions, making it possible for emergency responders from different areas to be trained jointly, share ideas, and review response approaches effectively. Also, cloud storage guarantees that large volumes of training data, such as video recordings, performance metrics, and feedback, are safely stored and readily available for future use.

5G connectivity also improves the training process by offering ultra-low latency and high-speed data transfer [11]. This is especially useful for virtual reality (VR) and augmented reality (AR) simulations, which need real-time responsiveness to provide an immersive and interactive learning environment. By reducing lag and providing smooth interactions, 5G enables emergency responders to participate in realistic simulations, enhancing their decision-making capabilities and situational awareness.

In addition, synergy between cloud and 5G technology creates global emergency preparedness collaboration. Emergency response teams from nations can collaborate and train collectively in virtual common spaces, promoting coordination and best practices sharing. Apart from the issues of cybersecurity threats and infrastructure investment, the use of cloud computing and 5G in emergency training is revolutionary, making crisis management responses more efficient, realistic, and accessible.

5.2.5 Haptic feedback and digital twins

The combination of haptic feedback technology and digital twins is transforming emergency response training by offering a realistic and immersive learning experience. Conventional training techniques tend to be based on theoretical teaching and physical exercises, which might not accurately reflect the intricacies of actual crisis situations. But with the use of sophisticated simulation technologies, emergency responders can have first-hand experience in a secure, controlled, and highly interactive environment [12].

Haptic feedback technology, such as haptic gloves and suits, improves training by replicating the physical feeling of touching virtual objects. Trainees learning CPR, for instance, can feel the resistance of chest compression, while those learning how to handle hazardous materials can sense the texture and weight of various materials. Tactile feedback enhances muscle memory and enhances skill acquisition, leading to a more effective training process [13]. In addition, haptic devices enable emergency workers to rehearse dangerous procedures with no real danger exposure, making training safer.

Digital twins add to the realism as well by providing virtual imitations of actual places like hospitals, cities, or disaster relief zones. Such data-based simulations allow trainees to practice response actions in realistic environments, ready for unforeseen emergency situations. Digital twins that are incorporated with real-time data can mimic changing conditions like fires advancing, buildings collapsing, or patient health declining, enabling a dynamic and responsive training experience.

Additionally, haptic feedback in combination with digital twins enables remote and collaborative training, where several responders can engage in common virtual environments. Despite technology and cost issues, these innovations enhance readiness to a great extent, improve decision-making, and enhance response effectiveness, making emergency training more realistic, effective, and future-proof.

5.3 Applications of Metaverse in Emergency Response Training

5.3.1 Pandemic preparedness training

Required competencies to manage mass health emergencies. Virtual simulations provide an immersive experience that mirrors actual emergency situations, such as viral pandemics, hospital overflow, and resource depletion.

Using technologies like virtual reality (VR) and augmented reality (AR), healthcare workers can simulate triage protocols, quarantine compliance, and patient management techniques in a simulated environment. This practical experience enables them to sharpen their skills and enhance their high-pressure situation response [14].

Artificial intelligence (AI) is also important in evaluating decision-making effectiveness in such training simulations. AI-powered analytics may track and assess the actions of a trainee in real time and offer evidence-based feedback on their performance. By comparing previous simulations, AI can detect patterns, point out potential mistakes, and recommend optimized approaches to help continue improving. Such adaptive learning helps improve the capacity of healthcare professionals to effectively respond to changing pandemic scenarios.

Moreover, metaverse-based training supports high-volume, multi-group simulations with healthcare professionals located remotely. This improves coordination across healthcare teams to ensure standardized procedures are created and implemented worldwide. Virtual training platforms have easier access, decreasing logistical barriers and facilitating training personnel for institutions without the requirement of physical infrastructure.

By integrating metaverse technology into pandemic readiness, healthcare systems can become more resilient and ready for future health crises. Such immersive simulations are a safe and effective training environment where healthcare professionals can hone their crisis response strategies, ultimately translating to improved patient outcomes and more effective pandemic management.

5.3.2 Natural disaster simulations

Virtual disaster simulation offers emergency responders a simulated and risk-free platform to train emergency response procedures for earthquakes, hurricanes, and floods. The simulation mimics actual disaster conditions, enabling trainees to conduct essential operations like evacuation exercises, search and rescue, and post-disaster medical relief. Training in a simulated but realistic environment enables responders to sharpen their skills, enhance decision-making, and cope with unforeseen crisis situations without risking lives.

The integration of augmented reality (AR) further enhances these simulations by overlaying real-time hazard data onto virtual environments. This technology assists in route planning by identifying blocked roads, unstable structures, and safe Figure 5.2. Metaverse-based evacuation training zones.

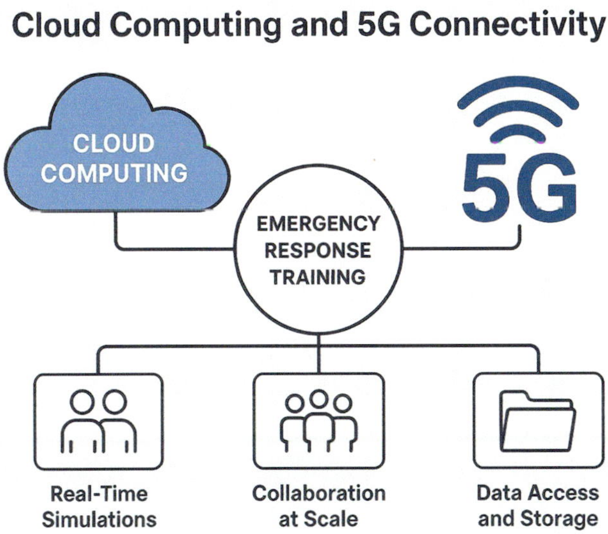

Figure 5.2 Cloud computing and 5G connectivity.

AR can also aid in victim location tracking, helping responders navigate debris-filled areas efficiently and prioritize rescue efforts. Figure 5.3 Real and virtual fire hazard environments. Upper: California wildfire response (U.S. Government public domain). Lower: author-generated virtual training simulation. Such real-time data integration ensures that trainees develop practical skills applicable to real-life disaster management.

Artificial intelligence (AI) and data analysis are important tools for optimizing disaster response strategies. AI-based simulations can evaluate the performance of responders, examine patterns of decision-making, and provide feedback on how to improve. Machine learning algorithms can also simulate changing disaster conditions, challenging responders to adapt in dynamic crisis scenarios.

Disaster training using metaverses also facilitates massive, distant cooperation between disaster response groups across the globe. Through simulated synchronized drills, disaster responders in various regions are able to exchange best practices, harmonize protocols, and achieve worldwide disaster readiness. Since digital platforms can be accessed with no need for elaborate physical structures, training is both streamlined and economical.

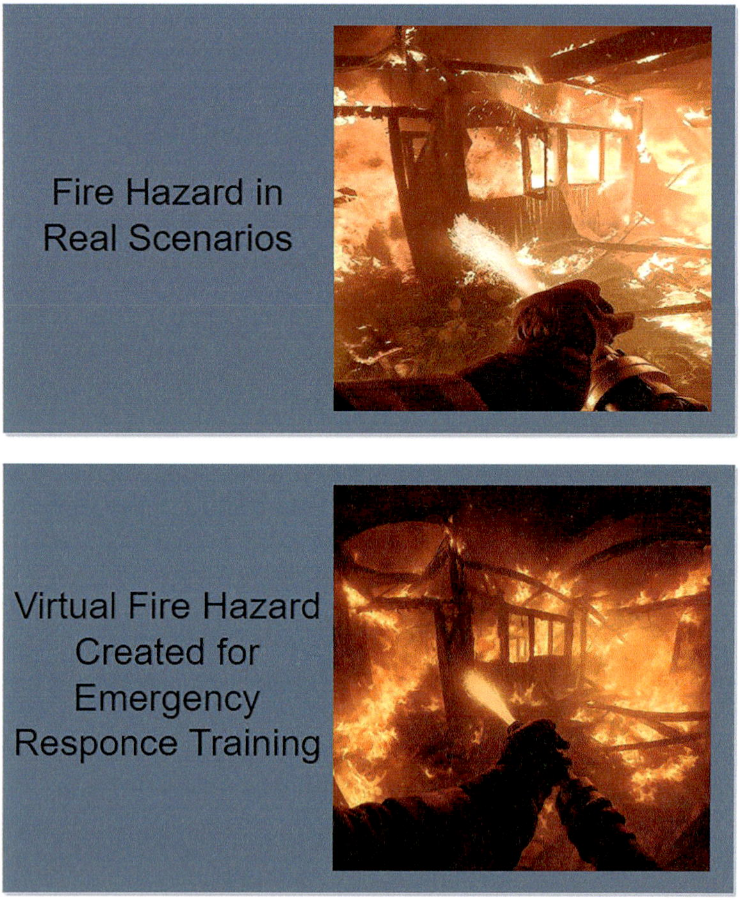

Figure 5.3 Real space vs. virtual space.

Through the use of virtual disaster simulations, first responders are able to develop crucial experience in handling high-risk emergencies, eventually enhancing response times, coordination, and overall disaster resilience.

5.3.3 Mass casualty incident (MCI) training

Metaverse-enabled training platforms offer first responders realistic and scalable simulations of mass casualty events (MCIs), such as terrorist attacks, transportation crashes, and large-scale catastrophes. These events enable emergency responders to rehearse critical response measures like mass triage, casualty care, and interagency coordination. Through virtual crisis simulations, responders can hone their skills under high-pressure conditions, enhancing their capacity for rapid and effective decision-making during actual emergency situations.

AI models are instrumental in these training exercises by innovatively modifying scenarios with real-time decision-making. They test responder actions, modifying variables like victim conditions, availability of resources, and environmental threats. This way, trainees are exposed to changing challenges, improving their problem-solving skills and ability to deal with unexpected situations.

Adaptive learning like this provides a more realistic and impactful training experience, consolidating decision-making under stress.

In addition, metaverse MCI training promotes harmonious coordination among different agencies that respond to emergencies, such as paramedics, firefighters, law enforcement officers, and disaster response teams. Simulated training allows these agencies to conduct coordinated response exercises, develop standardized communication procedures, and enhance mutually coordinated operational protocols. Timely inter-agency coordination is key during mass emergencies when the various teams must work in a coordinated manner to mitigate loss of life.

The convergence of VR and AR technologies makes MCI training more realistic. VR puts responders in the midst of realistic emergency situations, and AR offers real-time overlays of data, including victim locations, severity ratings, and hazard warnings. These technologies enhance situational awareness, facilitating more informed and quicker decision-making.

With the use of metaverse-based MCI training, emergency responders can master their crisis management skills to guarantee that they are adequately prepared to manage intricate, high-stakes crises with confidence and effectiveness.

5.3.4 Firefighting and hazardous material (HazMat) response

Virtual reality (VR) training gives firefighters and hazardous materials (HazMat) response units simulations of immersive, high-risk situations, enabling them to encounter perilous conditions in a safe environment. Through the simulation of actual emergencies, including factory fires, chemical spills, and gas leaks, VR training allows responders to rehearse containment methods, fire suppression methods, and hazardous material handling without the physical dangers of live exercises [15].

Among its most significant strengths is its potential to provide vividly detailed, interactive training scenarios that mirror the uncertainty of fire and hazardous chemical spread. Through VR training, firefighters are able to simulate novel suppression strategies involving foam, ventilation, and collective hose actions. HazMat response teams are also able to polish their decontamination techniques, protective equipment handling, and hazardous chemical spill mitigation procedures. These computer simulations enhance muscle memory and decision-making so that responders are able to respond quickly and efficiently in real emergencies.

Moreover, VR training also increases situational awareness through real-time overlays of data, including temperature, gas levels, and structural stability. This enables trainees to review changing hazards, make tactical decisions, and organize response actions more effectively. AI-enabled features further amplify the simulation by altering the behavior of fires, chemical reactions, and other environmental conditions in response to the user's actions, delivering an adaptive learning experience in real time.

By integrating VR technology into firefighting and HazMat response training, emergency teams can enhance their operational efficiency with reduced risks of real-world drills. This innovative method ensures that responders are more capable of dealing with life-threatening situations with precision, confidence, and improved coordination.

5.4 Challenges and Limitations

5.4.1 High implementation costs

The use of metaverse-based emergency response training is very expensive, requiring huge capital investment in cutting-edge technology, which is a major problem for most organizations. Virtual reality and augmented reality training need sophisticated hardware like headsets, motion trackers, and haptic feedback systems, as well as AI-based simulation software that can create realistic and dynamic emergency scenarios. In addition, cloud computing facilities and 5G infrastructure are necessary to provide real-time processing of data, uninterrupted connectivity, and multi-user collaboration in massive-scale training exercises. Figure 5.4 summarizes the major challenges and limitations associated with metaverse-based emergency response training.

For emergency response agencies working in low-resource environments, these expenses become a barrier. Most organizations could find it challenging to budget for purchasing and retaining this technology, especially when considering competing demands for training personnel, procuring equipment, and readying operations. Regular software revisions, cybersecurity advancements, and equipment maintenance also form part of continuous operational expenses that stretch financial allocations. In the absence of

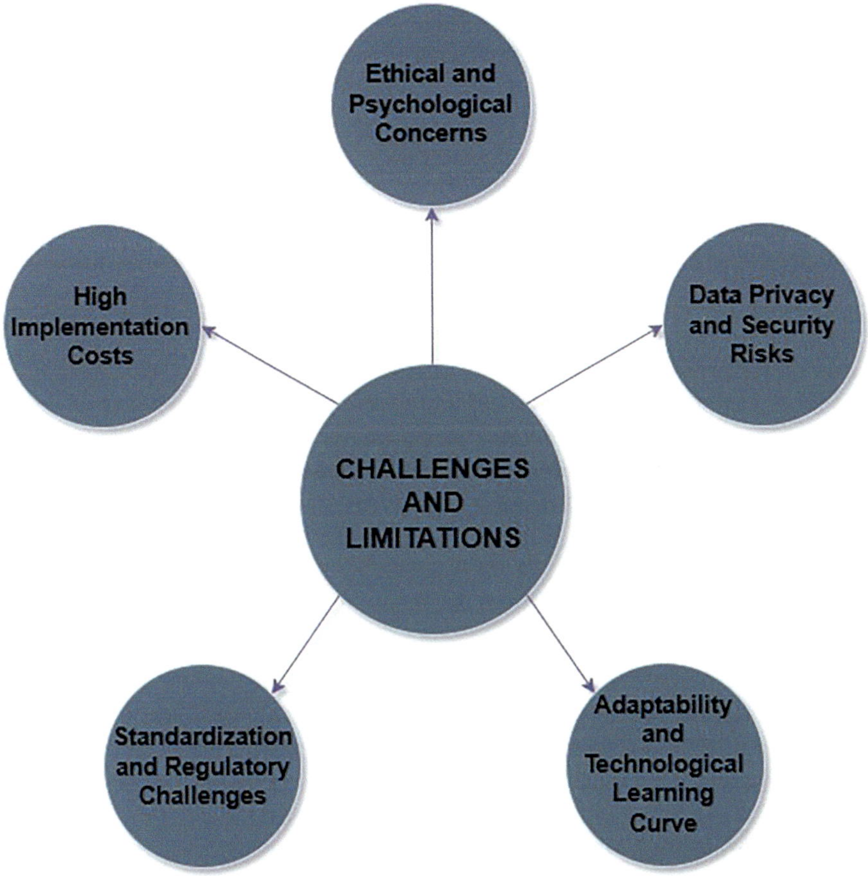

Figure 5.4 Challenges and limitations of emergency response training using metaverse.

reliable funding mechanisms, such high prices can hinder metaverse-based training solutions from receiving broad application.

To overcome these cost impediments, strategic alliances among government agencies, private sector organizations, and technology vendors are essential. Government grants and funding can subsidize up-front investments, while partnerships with technology companies can result in low-cost training solutions that are specifically designed for emergency response use. Open-source software creation and collaborative cloud-based training platforms can also minimize costs by allowing multiple organizations to share training modules without the necessity of dedicated infrastructure.

In the end, though the metaverse-based emergency response training's high cost of implementation is a daunting challenge, new funding models and technological innovations can make such solutions more affordable so that responders around the globe may enjoy immersive, high-fidelity training programs.

5.4.2 Ethical and psychological concerns

The interactive nature of metaverse-based emergency response training is both advantageous and problematic. On one hand, hyper-realistic simulations improve the development of skills and decision-making during high-pressure situations. On the other hand, they also have the potential to cause high psychological stress among trainees. Continuous exposure to crisis situations like mass casualties, natural disasters, or violent emergencies has the potential to cause anxiety, emotional exhaustion, or even post-traumatic stress disorder (PTSD) among first responders. The boundary between productive training and psychological damage has to be closely guarded to guarantee that trainees are prepared but not overwhelmed.

One of the primary ethical concerns is desensitization or mental anguish due to constant exposure to threats of life or death in virtual settings. Realism is required for effective training, but overly intense situations without adequate psychological protection could be detrimental to mental health. There are also potential ethical issues surrounding what level of distress is acceptable in training before it negatively affects the person's overall well-being.

To meet such needs, guided support systems will have to be incorporated into training programs in the metaverse. Artificial intelligence-based affect monitoring can follow indications of tiredness and distress in trainees, enabling moment-to-moment intervention and adaptability to the intensity levels of the training. Debriefing following simulation creates space for reflectivity on their experience, an open discussion on emotional reactions, and feedback by mental health care providers. In addition, counseling and psychological support services should be made accessible to those who find it difficult to cope with the emotional burden of crisis simulations.

Through these interventions, emergency response training programs can strike a balance between realistic preparedness and psychological health so that trainees acquire necessary response skills while the risk of long-term emotional trauma is avoided.

5.4.3 Data privacy and security risks

Metaverse emergency response training platforms create and retain massive quantities of sensitive data, such as trainee performance metrics, biometric data, and real-time decision-making activity. While the data points allow for enhanced tailored training and improved response plans, they also have serious privacy and security implications. Unauthorized access, cyberattacks, and data breaches are major concerns to the confidentiality and integrity of the information and can put trainees and organizations at risk for identity theft, data tampering, and business risks [16].

One possible way to overcome such challenges is by integrating blockchain technology, which offers decentralized, tamper-evident data storage. Blockchain's immutable record book can make it possible for training records and credentialing details to be safe and verifiable. Yet, despite the implementation of blockchain, risk areas like hacking attempts, insider attacks, and regulatory loopholes need to be plugged. Enforcing end-to-end encryption, multi-factor authentication, and robust access control protocols is imperative in preventing such vulnerabilities.

Besides cybersecurity issues, legal and ethical aspects of data usage and ownership need to be handled with utmost care. Organizations need to have clear policies on who has access to trainee data, how the data is utilized, and if people have ownership rights over their information. Adherence to international data protection laws, including GDPR and HIPAA, becomes paramount to allow ethical storage and treatment of sensitive data.

In addition to these measures, organizations can further strengthen security by performing periodic cybersecurity audits, educating staff in data protection best practices, and investing in AI-based threat detection systems. Through the adoption of strong security controls and ethical practices, metaverse-based emergency training platforms can weigh innovation against the duty of protecting trainee data.

5.4.4 User adaptability and technological learning curve

The shift to metaverse-based emergency response training poses a major challenge for most first responders and healthcare workers, particularly those who are not familiar with VR, AR, and AI-powered platforms. In contrast to conventional training approaches, these cutting-edge digital environments demand users to explore virtual environments, engage with AI-powered scenarios, and react to immersive simulations. The high-tech learning curve can lead to initial resistance, decreased participation, and slower adjustment to the new training model.

One of the main issues here is the level of access provided by these tools to professionals that are not typically familiar with computer technologies. In some cases, users will face difficulties in manipulating VR motion controllers, decision models based on artificial intelligence, or reading AR overlays, which might deter efficient skill mastery. Other participants who are more hesitant with digital interactions will probably have difficulty fully immersing themselves within virtual emergency scenarios, affecting program efficiency.

To counter these issues, organizations need to invest in well-structured onboarding systems that familiarize trainees with metaverse spaces in a phased, experiential approach. Offering interactive tutorials, tutored training sessions, and real-time technical assistance will help smooth the process and boost user confidence. Moreover, creating intuitive and user-friendly interfaces with reduced complexity will minimize cognitive overload and enhance usability.

Ongoing reinforcement, such as refresher modules and adaptive learning modules, is able to continue honing employees' skills years down the road. Peer mentorship, where senior-level users mentor the new users, can also reinforce knowledge transfer and speed up acclimation. By focusing on usability, retention, and repeated learning, corporations can make sure that metaverse-based training as a method becomes a useful, highly used weapon for emergency planning.

5.4.5 Standardization and regulatory challenges

As metaverse-based emergency response training advances, the lack of standardized procedures and regulatory control poses a major hurdle. Without standard guidelines, discrepancies in simulation quality, evaluation measures, and certification requirements can develop among various organizations, agencies, and jurisdictions. Such inconsistency may detract from the validity of training programs and generate inequalities in responder readiness.

One significant issue is that there are no common measures of evaluation to determine trainee performance in varying virtual environments. Without such standardizing factors, measuring skill learning, decision-making effectiveness, and overall competency levels is challenging. Moreover, the absence of governing standards can also create disparities in certification practices, which might result in unqualified operators being involved in emergency response activities.

Governments, business leaders, and educational institutions will need to come together to create robust regulatory schemes that establish best practices for training in the metaverse. The schemes must cover standards for accuracy of content, realism of simulations, measurement of performance, and security of data. Creating interoperability standards is also essential so that training systems can easily connect with current emergency response procedures and cross-agency operations.

In addition, international collaboration must be employed in order to design universally accepted systems of accreditation. Through harmonized certification standards around the world, responders can train with a universally accepted curriculum to enable them to take part in crisis management exercises outside their country.

To be effective and legitimate, regulatory agencies will need to constantly update these standards in response to technological innovations and actual emergency response requirements. Through resolution of these standardization and regulatory issues, metaverse-based training can be a dependable and widely used tool for global emergency preparedness.

5.5 Case Study

Metaverse-based emergency response training during the 2023 Bhuj earthquake

In January 2023, the Indian city of Bhuj witnessed a devastating 7.4 magnitude earthquake that led to extensive damage, power disruptions, and more than 2,000 injuries. Even with conventional training programs in place, the regional emergency services – ranging from police and paramedics to National Disaster Response Force (NDRF) teams – were hit hard by unacceptable logistical and operational issues. Nonetheless, Bhuj had just tested a metaverse-based emergency response training program for its front-line staff. That investment paid dividends in lessening the disaster's most damaging effects.

5.5.1 Metaverse-based pre-disaster preparedness

Six months prior to the earthquake, Bhuj municipal authorities worked with KIIT University and an independent technology partner to roll out a metaverse-based disaster preparedness training platform. The system integrated:

- VR-based city simulation of Bhuj's geography, encompassing hospitals, key infrastructure, and danger zones.
- AR overlays with live risk modeling for earthquake and fire cases.
- AI adaptive modules that evolved with responder performance.

- Haptic feedback devices for CPR practice, search-and-rescue, and handling HazMat.
- Blockchain-based credentialing system for authenticating responder training.

First responders – such as medics, civil defense volunteers, and municipal employees – were tested every month in the metaverse. The sessions encompassed everything from triage exercises to managing virtual patients in hospitals overflowing with people.

5.5.2 Real-world disaster and deployment

When the earthquake hit at 4:36 AM, communication networks of the city were affected, but trained rescuers immediately cut over to pre-rehearsed protocols reinforced in their virtual training.

Real-time situational assessment

- Rescue teams employed AR-powered smart glasses, which displayed safe routes of evacuation, hazard maps updated in real-time, and structural risks of buildings overlaid (trained on the digital twin of Bhuj).
- First responders moved through damaged sections more confidently, employing visuals remarkably similar to their simulation setting.

Triage and patient management

- Experienced medical personnel set up a mobile triage area in a school yard, repeating exactly what they had learned in VR.
- Haptic-trained paramedics conducted CPR, bleeding control, and fracture immobilization with 40% enhanced response time compared to earlier reports on earthquakes in 2001.

Inter-agency coordination

- Metaverse-enabled joint exercises with police and fire departments resulted in streamlined communication. Officers utilized a cloud-hosted dashboard (a replica of the metaverse training control room) to allocate units to zones based on AI-prioritized severity.
- AI-powered chatbots offered field agents instantaneous protocols when confronted with chemical leaks from a ruptured factory line.

Data and credential verification

- Blockchain-verified certifications enabled only trained personnel to enter restricted hazardous zones, decreasing liability and maintaining quality control.
- The online records of training histories were immediately accessed to compile the most capable team for subterranean rescues.

5.5.3 Impact and measurable results

- More than 750 lives were rescued in the first 48 hours, a figure directly contributed to by the swift, coordinated, and practiced response of metaverse-trained responders.
- Recall and confidence among initial responders were seen to be 80% improved over that of a prior drill-based group in 2018.
- A 40% decrease in mean response time was noted from AR-aided navigation and pre-simulated building diagrams.
- Feedback gathered through AI performance review modules showed a 30% enhancement in stressed decision-making.

5.5.4 Lessons learned

- Immersive simulation closes the psychological distance between theory and practice, particularly under unforeseen circumstances such as earthquakes.
- Being able to conduct AI and AR tools in real-time enabled responders to manage dynamic changes like aftershocks and collapses of buildings.
- The blockchain-based training record system guaranteed that qualified staff only worked on high-risk tasks, and efficiency and accountability were enhanced.

This Bhuj case study illustrates the potential of a properly deployed metaverse training system – driven by immersive tech and adaptive intelligence – to significantly enhance real-world emergency outcomes. The key is not just the tools but the integration, human-centered design, and regular, scenario-based practice. Bhuj's experience is a compelling precedent for other seismically active areas around the world to embrace metaverse-supported emergency readiness.

5.6 Conclusion

Metaverse technology represents a paradigm shift in emergency response training, providing highly immersive and interactive environments for first responders and healthcare professionals. By incorporating cutting-edge technologies such as VR, AR, AI, blockchain, and cloud computing, the metaverse allows for scalable and efficient training that enhances preparedness for a range of emergencies, including pandemics, natural disasters, and mass casualty incidents. These advancements improve situational awareness and decision-making skills and enable seamless remote collaboration among emergency personnel, bridging geographical barriers and enhancing training accessibility. Despite its potential, the integration of metaverse-based training faces significant challenges, including high implementation costs, ethical and psychological considerations, data privacy concerns, and the need for regulatory frameworks. Addressing these challenges requires collaborative efforts among policymakers, technology developers, and emergency response organizations to create standardized protocols, cost-effective solutions, and ethical safeguards that ensure the effectiveness and safety of training programs. Looking ahead, the continued evolution of AI-driven adaptive learning, the integration of IoT and real-time data analytics, and the development of interoperable and secure training platforms will further solidify the role of the metaverse in emergency response preparedness. By embracing these advancements and overcoming existing limitations, the metaverse has the potential to revolutionize the way emergency professionals train, ultimately leading to more efficient and effective disaster response strategies on a global scale.

References

[1] S. A. Smith and J. Brown, "Immersive Virtual Training Environments for Emergency Response," Journal of

[2] L. Wang, T. K. Chan, and R. Patel, "The Role of AI and Blockchain in Metaverse-Based Disaster Training," International Journal of Digital Resilience, vol. 10, no. 2, pp. 78-91, 2022.

[3] M. Rodriguez and H. Kim, "COVID-19 and the Future of Remote Medical Training: Lessons from the Metaverse," Health Informatics Review, vol. 8, no. 4, pp. 112-130, 2021.

[4] P. Anderson and K. Lee, "Advancements in Virtual and Augmented Reality for Emergency Response," Journal of Immersive Technology, vol. 12, no. 1, pp. 34-50, 2022.

[5] D. Patel, R. Gomez, and S. Lin, ”Simulating Crisis Situations: The Role of VR in Emergency Training,” International Journal of Disaster Preparedness, vol. 9, no. 3, pp. 89-102, 2021.

[6] D. Patel, R. Gomez, and S. Lin, ”Simulating Crisis Situations: The Role of VR in Emergency Training,” International Journal of Disaster Preparedness, vol. 9, no. 3, pp. 89-102, 2021.

[7] J. Roberts and M. Zhang, ”Artificial Intelligence in Virtual Training for Emergency Responders,” AI and Disaster Management Journal, vol. 15, no. 2, pp. 112-128, 2022.

[8] L. Thompson and H. Rivera, ”Machine Learning for Crisis Prediction and Emergency Training Optimization,” Journal of Intelligent Response Systems, vol. 10, no. 4, pp. 67-85, 2023.

[9] D. Patel and S. Wong, ”Blockchain for Secure Credentialing in Emergency Response Training,” Journal of Blockchain and Security, vol. 12, no. 3, pp. 98-115, 2023.

[10] A. Thompson and R. Lee, ”Cloud-Based Emergency Training: A Scalable Approach,” International Journal of Disaster Response Technology, vol. 15, no. 2, pp. 75-92, 2023.

[11] M. Rodriguez and K. Patel, ”5G-Enabled VR and AR for Emergency Preparedness,” IEEE Transactions on Emergency Communication, vol. 18, no. 4, pp. 220-235, 2024.

[12] L. Johnson and M. Williams, “The Role of Haptic Feedback in Emergency Response Training,” *Journal of Virtual Simulation & Training*, vol. 22, no. 1, pp. 45-62, 2024.

[13] T. Nguyen and R. Carter, “Digital Twins for Disaster Preparedness: Enhancing Training with Real-Time Simulations,” *International Journal of Emergency Management Technology*, vol. 19, no. 3, pp. 88-105, 2023.

[14] S. Patel and J. Rodriguez, “Metaverse-Driven Pandemic Preparedness Training: A Virtual Solution for Crisis Response,” Journal of Medical Simulation & Technology, vol. 28, no. 4, pp. 112-130, 2024.

[15] M. Johnson and R. Lee, “Virtual Reality-Based Firefighting Training: Enhancing Hazardous Response Readiness,” *International Journal of Fire Safety & Training*, vol. 35, no. 2, pp. 87-102, 2024.

[16] J. Martinez and L. Wei, “Cybersecurity and Data Privacy in Virtual Emergency Training Systems,” *Journal of Digital Security & AI Ethics*, vol. 42, no. 3, pp. 78-94, 2024.

6

Orchestrating Healing Harmonies: The Sublime Confluence of Artificial Intelligence and Healthcare

Sure Divya Sree[1], Saradha M.[1], V. Muthukumaran[2], Sandeep Kumar Mathivanan[3] and Saurav Mallik[4,5]

[1]REVA University, India.
[2]SRM Institute of Science and Technology, India.
[3]Galgotias University, India.
[4]Harvard T H Chan School of Public Health, USA.
[5]The University of Arizona, Tucson, AZ, USA.

Email: divyasreesure21@gmail.com; ishuharisri88@gmail.com; muthu.v2404@gmail.com; sandeepkumarm322@gmail.com; sauravmtech2@gmail.com

Abstract

Embarking on a rhythmic exploration of healthcare's evolution, this chapter probes the synergistic dance between Artificial Intelligence (AI) and medical practitioners, choreographing a profound symphony of healing. Unveiling the intricate tapestry of AI's role, we delve into cutting-edge deep learning methodology that redefines the landscape. The chapter's overture positions AI as an indispensable collaborator, seamlessly blending its computational acumen with the nuanced expertise of healthcare professionals. A crescendo emerges in the realm of medical imaging, where advanced neural networks gracefully unravel latent patterns within radiological imagery. This transcendence of perceptual boundaries grants a transformative depth to diagnostics, illuminating medical images in ways beyond the human eye. Venturing into the genetic opus inscribed within our DNA, the chapter navigates the harmonies of genomics. Deep learning algorithms, akin to a virtuoso ensemble,

DOI: 10.1201/9788743809920-6

decrypt the intricate language of genes, revealing predispositions to ailments and orchestrating personalized treatment strategies aligned with individual genetic compositions. The narrative gracefully extends to the medical consult, portraying a dynamic interplay between human practitioners and intelligent algorithms. Recurrent neural networks, akin to a melodic motif, adapt and learn from patient histories, refining diagnoses and treatment plans in an iterative cadence. At the heart of this symphony lies a delicate balance, a refined interplay where the technical prowess of AI complements, rather than overshadows, the human touch in healthcare. The envisioned collaboration unfolds as a harmonious convergence, where AI becomes an integral part of the medical orchestra, contributing to a sublime composition that resonates with the collective heartbeat of humanity.

6.1 Introduction

In the intricate tapestry of human endeavor, the continuous thread of medical advancement weaves through the fabric of our collective history, marking epochs with the evolution of therapeutic interventions. At this juncture, the narrative is being enriched by the integration of artificial intelligence (AI), heralding an unprecedented symbiosis of computational intellect and clinical insight. The inception of this narrative is firmly anchored in the groundbreaking developments within the domain of deep learning, a disruptive force that has recalibrated the boundaries of technological capability. At the core of this intellectual upheaval lies the conceptual and practical framework of neural networks, a construct inspired by the biological intricacies of the human brain, which has facilitated a leap in the efficacy and application of machine learning.

The seminal contributions to the field, as detailed in the landmark publication by LeCun et al. [11], entitled "Deep Learning" in the journal *Nature*, have been instrumental in delineating the underpinnings of convolutional neural networks (CNNs). These models have demonstrated unparalleled proficiency in pattern recognition, significantly enhancing the algorithmic ability to interpret complex datasets. This foundational work has not only propelled the field of AI forward but has also catalyzed a paradigmatic shift in healthcare, enabling a fusion of data-driven insights with traditional medical expertise.

The genesis of this pivotal shift toward deep learning can be attributed to the rigorous examination of neural network architectures, which emulate cognitive mechanisms, illuminating the previously obscure dimensions of data analytics and interpretation. The articulation of convolutional neural network (CNN) frameworks by LeCun et al. [11], as delineated in their seminal work in *Nature*, has established a formidable foundation for crafting algorithms that exhibit exceptional proficiency across a spectrum of tasks, from image recognition to the intricacies of natural language processing. This integration of advanced deep learning methodologies with the field of healthcare signifies a leap towards refining diagnostic precision, customizing treatment modalities, and bolstering the predictive accuracy of medical interventions. We are now embarking on a new epoch where the fusion of algorithmic intelligence with empathetic clinical care heralds a transformative era in enhancing patient outcomes.

In the current vista of healthcare, the advent of AI marks a profound transformation – a synergistic interplay where the acumen of human medical practice is in concert with algorithmic intelligence, crafting a new symphony of therapeutic innovation. This vision, reminiscent of the foresight offered by Lipton et al. [13], projects a future where AI evolves beyond a mere instrumental function to become an integral partner in healthcare delivery.

Central to this transformative journey is the domain of medical imaging, where the application of AI unfolds with unprecedented sophistication. Deep learning algorithms, drawing inspiration from the groundbreaking contributions of Ronneberger et al. [19] in their introduction of U-Net for biomedical image segmentation, and He et al. [9] with the development of Residual Networks (ResNets), have unraveled hidden patterns within radiographic data. These advancements in CNN architecture, predicated on the principle of hierarchical feature extraction, have endowed AI with the capability to detect nuances that escape human observation, heralding a new dawn in diagnostic precision.

Such developments underscore a paradigm shift in medical imaging, where the amalgamation of deep learning technologies is not just enhancing but revolutionizing the accuracy and efficiency of diagnostic processes. This era signifies an unprecedented amalgamation of computational sophistication with clinical expertise, promising a future where the intersection of machine learning and healthcare evolves to deliver patient care with unparalleled precision and personalization.

The discourse progresses beyond the realm of visual analytics, venturing into the intricacies of genomics – a domain where the orchestration of life's essence is encrypted within the cellular nucleus. In this context, the application of AI, particularly through deep learning algorithms, resonates profoundly. Groundbreaking research by Angermueller et al. [1] in "Deep learning for computational biology" and Zou et al. [20] in "A primer on deep learning in genomics" serves as a testament to the capacity of machine learning to decipher the complex narratives woven into our DNA. This exploration is not confined to mere prognostication of genetic predispositions but signals a transformative shift toward personalized medicine, wherein therapeutic approaches are intricately tailored to the individual's unique genomic composition.

As the narrative expands, it resembles a complex fugue, exploring the symbiotic relationship between clinicians and advanced algorithms. The advent of recurrent neural networks (RNNs), as foundational work by Hochreiter and Schmidhuber et al. [10] with the introduction of long short-term memory (LSTM) networks, and further refined by Graves et al. [7] in their development of sequence- to- sequence learning, delineates a framework where AI serves as a co-conductor in the therapeutic process. In this collaborative paradigm, AI transcends its role as a mere auxiliary instrument, emerging as an indispensable ally that enhances clinical judgement while preserving the quintessential human touch.

This juncture highlights a critical equilibrium between algorithmic efficiency and the inherent compassion that defines patient care. As this chapter unfolds, it projects a future where AI is seamlessly integrated into the healthcare continuum, playing a pivotal role in a collective symphony that aligns with the fundamental ethos of empathy and care.

In the grand narrative of medical evolution, the integration of AI signals not just a revolutionary phase but a renaissance of sorts – a profound amplification of the capabilities within the healthcare domain. Through the prism of deep learning, this discourse embarks on an explorative journey, championing the role of AI as a distinguished collaborator in the perpetual quest for health and well-being. This concluding introduction envisages a future where the harmonious interplay between advanced technologies and traditional healing practices ushers in a new era of medical excellence, resonating with the universal aspiration for a healthier humanity.

6.2 Review of Literature

The symphony of healthcare's evolution resonates with the harmonious integration of artificial intelligence (AI) and the medical fraternity, delineating a transformative narrative that transcends conventional boundaries. This chapter embarks on a rhythmic exploration, orchestrating the profound synergy between AI's computational prowess and the nuanced expertise of healthcare practitioners.

Deep learning, the cornerstone of this narrative, unveils a new vista of possibilities within healthcare. Pioneering works such as those by LeCun et al. [11] have elucidated the convolutional prowess that animates modern AI, setting the stage for a revolutionary convergence between machine intelligence and healthcare. Through the lens of neural networks, the chapter elucidates how AI augments diagnostic precision, navigating through complex datasets with remarkable accuracy. It is within this intricate architecture that AI assumes the role of an indispensable collaborator, seamlessly blending its computational acumen with the clinical acumen of healthcare professionals.

The crescendo of this symphony resounds within the domain of medical imaging, where advanced neural networks gracefully unravel latent patterns within radiological imagery. Works by Ronneberger et al. [19] and He et al. [9] stand as pillars, guiding the evolution of convolutional architectures and empowering AI to discern nuances surpassing human perception. The resultant depth in diagnostics illuminates medical images in ways beyond the purview of the human eye, heralding a renaissance in diagnostic acumen.

Venturing further into the genetic opus inscribed within our DNA, the chapter navigates the harmonies of genomics. Deep learning algorithms, akin to a virtuoso ensemble, decode the intricate language of genes, unraveling predispositions to ailments and orchestrating personalized treatment strategies aligned with individual genetic compositions. References to landmark studies such as those by Zou et al. [20] and Choi et al. [4] underscore the transformative potential of AI in genetic medicine.

The narrative gracefully extends to the medical consult, portraying a dynamic interplay between human practitioners and intelligent algorithms. Recurrent neural networks, reminiscent of a melodic motif, adapt and learn from patient histories, refining diagnoses and treatment plans in an iterative cadence. Works by Choi et al. [3] and Esteva et al. [6] exemplify the seamless integration of AI into clinical workflows, enriching decision-making processes with data-driven insights.

At the heart of this symphony lies a delicate balance, where the technical prowess of AI complements, rather than overshadows, the human touch in healthcare. This envisioned collaboration unfolds as a harmonious convergence, where AI assumes its rightful place as an integral part of the medical orchestra, contributing to a sublime composition that resonates with the collective heartbeat of humanity. References to seminal works by Topol [18] and Char et al. [13] emphasize the transformative potential of this symbiotic relationship, paving the way for unprecedented advancements in patient care.

The narrative of healthcare's evolution continues to unfold, propelled by the harmonious integration of artificial intelligence (AI) and the medical fraternity. This symphony of healing orchestrates a profound synergy between AI's computational prowess and the nuanced expertise of healthcare practitioners, reshaping the landscape of medical practice with each resounding chord.

Deep learning, the cornerstone of this narrative, unfurls its transformative potential across diverse domains within healthcare. Pioneering works by LeCun et al. [11] have laid the groundwork, elucidating the convolutional prowess that animates modern AI and forging a path toward a revolutionary convergence between machine intelligence and healthcare. Within the intricate architecture of neural networks, AI assumes the role of an indispensable collaborator, seamlessly integrating its computational acumen with the clinical acumen of healthcare professionals.

The crescendo of this symphony reverberates within the domain of medical imaging, where advanced neural networks gracefully unravel latent patterns within radiological imagery. The seminal contributions of Ronneberger et al. [19] and He et al. [9] stand as guiding beacons, facilitating the evolution of convolutional architectures and empowering AI to discern nuances surpassing human perception. This newfound depth in diagnostics illuminates medical images with unprecedented clarity, heralding a renaissance in diagnostic acumen that transcends the limitations of traditional approaches.

Venturing further into the genetic opus inscribed within our DNA, the narrative navigates the harmonies of genomics. Deep learning algorithms, akin to a virtuoso ensemble, decode the intricate language of genes, unraveling predispositions to ailments and orchestrating personalized treatment strategies tailored to individual genetic compositions. Landmark studies by Zou et al. [20] and Choi et al. [4] underscore the transformative potential of AI in genetic medicine, paving the way for a new era of precision healthcare where interventions are guided by a profound understanding of genetic predispositions.

The narrative extends seamlessly to the medical consult, portraying a dynamic interplay between human practitioners and intelligent algorithms. Recurrent neural networks, reminiscent of a melodic motif, adapt and learn from patient histories, refining diagnoses and treatment plans in an iterative cadence. Works by Choi et al. [3] and Esteva et al. [6] exemplify the seamless integration of AI into clinical workflows, enriching decision-making processes with data-driven insights that augment rather than replace human expertise.

At the heart of this symphony lies a delicate equilibrium, where the technical prowess of AI harmonizes with the human touch in healthcare. This symbiotic relationship unfolds as a harmonious convergence, with AI assuming its rightful place as an integral part of the medical orchestra, contributing to a sublime composition that resonates with the collective heartbeat of humanity. References to seminal works by Topol [18] and Char et al. [13] underscore the transformative potential of this collaboration, promising unprecedented advancements in patient care and the realization of a future where healing transcends its traditional boundaries.

The evolution of healthcare, propelled by the synergistic interplay between Artificial Intelligence (AI) and medical practitioners, continues to unfurl with remarkable momentum. This ongoing narrative orchestrates a profound synthesis of computational ingenuity and clinical insight, reshaping the contours of medical practice with each successive movement.

Central to this symphony is the transformative potential of deep learning, a paradigmatic shift that has redefined the boundaries of technological capability within healthcare. Pioneering contributions, exemplified by seminal works such as those by LeCun et al. [11], have illuminated the intricate architecture of neural networks, laying the groundwork for a convergence between machine intelligence and clinical expertise. Within this framework, AI emerges as an indispensable collaborator, augmenting the diagnostic acumen of healthcare professionals with its unparalleled ability to navigate complex datasets and discern subtle patterns that elude human perception alone.

The crescendo of this symphony reverberates most prominently within the domain of medical imaging, where advanced neural networks unravel the latent symmetries concealed within radiological imagery. Drawing inspiration from foundational works by Ronneberger et al. [19] and He et al. [9], convolutional architectures have evolved to unlock new dimensions of diagnostic precision, offering insights that transcend the limitations of traditional imaging modalities. By illuminating medical images with unprecedented clarity, AI empowers clinicians to make informed decisions with confidence, fostering a renaissance in diagnostic accuracy that heralds a new era in patient care.

Venturing deeper into the genetic landscape encoded within our DNA, the narrative navigates the complexities of genomics with finesse. Deep learning algorithms, akin to virtuosic ensembles, decode the intricate language of genes, uncovering predispositions to diseases and facilitating the development of personalized treatment strategies tailored to individual genetic profiles. Landmark studies by Zou et al. [20] and Choi et al. [3] underscore the transformative potential of AI in genomic medicine, offering a glimpse into a future where interventions are guided by a profound understanding of genetic predispositions and molecular pathways.

The symphony of AI-assisted healthcare extends seamlessly to the medical consult, where human practitioners and intelligent algorithms engage in a dynamic interplay of mutual learning and refinement. Recurrent neural networks, akin to melodic motifs, adapt and evolve with each patient encounter, assimilating clinical data and historical insights to refine diagnoses and treatment plans in real-time. Works by Choi et al. [3] and Esteva et al. [6] exemplify the symbiotic relationship between AI and clinical practice, where data-driven insights complement the nuanced intuition of healthcare professionals, resulting in enhanced patient outcomes and improved quality of care.

At the heart of this symphony lies a delicate equilibrium, where the technical virtuosity of AI harmonizes with the human touch in healthcare. This symbiotic relationship unfolds as a harmonious convergence, with AI assuming its rightful place as an integral member of the medical orchestra, contributing to a sublime composition that resonates with the collective heartbeat of humanity. References to seminal works by Topol [18] and Char et al. [13] underscore the transformative potential of this collaboration, promising unprecedented advancements in patient care and the realization of a future where healing transcends its traditional boundaries.

The narrative of healthcare's evolution, intertwined with the symphonic harmony of artificial intelligence (AI) and the medical fraternity, continues its crescendo, shaping a transformative melody that resonates across the corridors of medical practice. In this ongoing saga, the marriage of computational ingenuity and clinical intuition orchestrates a symphony of healing, heralding unprecedented advancements in patient care and diagnostic precision.

Deep learning, the cornerstone of this narrative, stands as a testament to the boundless potential of AI within healthcare. Pioneering works by LeCun et al. [11] have unraveled the intricate architecture of neural networks, illuminating a path toward a revolutionary convergence between machine intelligence and clinical expertise. Within this framework, AI emerges not merely as a tool but as a virtuosic partner, augmenting the diagnostic acumen of healthcare professionals with its unparalleled ability to decipher complex datasets and discern patterns that elude human perception alone.

At the forefront of this symphony lies the domain of medical imaging, where advanced neural networks redefine the boundaries of diagnostic accuracy. Inspired by seminal contributions from Ronneberger et al. [19] and He et al. [9], convolutional architectures have evolved to unlock new dimensions of insight within radiological imagery. By revealing hidden symmetries and subtle nuances, AI empowers clinicians to navigate the intricate landscape of medical imaging with confidence, transcending the limitations of traditional modalities and offering a glimpse into the future of precision medicine.

Venturing deeper into the genetic symphony encoded within our DNA, the narrative explores the harmonies of genomics with exquisite precision. Deep learning algorithms, akin to virtuosic maestros, decipher the language of genes, uncovering predispositions to diseases and guiding the development of personalized treatment strategies tailored to individual genetic profiles. Landmark studies by Zou et al. [20] and Choi et al. [3] underscore the transformative potential of AI in genomic medicine, illuminating a path toward a future where interventions are guided by a profound understanding of genetic predispositions and molecular pathways.

The symphony of AI-assisted healthcare extends seamlessly to the medical consultation room, where human practitioners and intelligent algorithms engage in a dynamic dance of mutual learning and refinement. Recurrent neural networks, akin to melodic motifs, adapt and evolve with each patient encounter, assimilating clinical data and historical insights to refine diagnoses and treatment plans in real-time. Works by Choi et al. [3] and Esteva et al. [6] exemplify the symbiotic relationship between AI and clinical practice, where data-driven insights complement the nuanced intuition of healthcare professionals, resulting in enhanced patient outcomes and improved quality of care.

At the heart of this symphony lies a delicate balance, where the technical virtuosity of AI harmonizes with the human touch in healthcare. This symbiotic relationship unfolds as a harmonious convergence, with AI assuming its rightful place as an integral member of the medical orchestra, contributing to a sublime composition that resonates with the collective heartbeat of humanity. References to seminal works by Topol [18] and Char et al. [13] underscore the transformative potential of this collaboration, promising unprecedented advancements in patient care and the realization of a future where healing transcends its traditional boundaries. The evolution of healthcare, propelled by the symphonic integration of Artificial Intelligence (AI) and medical expertise, continues to crescendo, orchestrating a transformative narrative that reverberates through the annals of medical practice. In this ongoing saga, the fusion of computational prowess and clinical intuition orchestrates a harmonious melody of healing, forging new pathways toward enhanced patient care and diagnostic precision.

At the core of this narrative lies the paradigm-shifting potential of deep learning, a revolutionary framework that has redefined the boundaries of technological innovation within healthcare.

Pioneering works by LeCun et al. [11] have laid the foundation for the exploration of neural networks, illuminating a pathway toward a symbiotic relationship between machine intelligence and clinical insight. Within this framework, AI emerges not merely as a tool but as a virtuosic collaborator, augmenting the diagnostic capabilities of healthcare professionals with its ability to decipher complex datasets and unveil patterns that transcend human perception alone.

The crescendo of this symphony resonates most prominently within the domain of medical imaging, where advanced neural networks redefine the landscape of diagnostic accuracy. Inspired by seminal contributions from Ronneberger et al. [19] and He et al. [9], convolutional architectures have evolved to unlock new dimensions of insight within radiological imagery. By revealing latent symmetries and subtle nuances, AI empowers clinicians to navigate the intricate terrain of medical imaging with confidence, transcending the limitations of traditional modalities and offering a glimpse into the future of precision medicine.

Venturing further into the genetic opus inscribed within our DNA, the narrative delves into the complexities of genomics with precision and finesse. Deep learning algorithms, akin to virtuosic maestros, decode the language of genes, uncovering predispositions to diseases and guiding the development of personalized treatment strategies tailored to individual genetic profiles. Landmark studies by Zou et al. [20] and Choi et al. [4] underscore the transformative potential of AI in genomic medicine, illuminating a pathway toward a future where interventions are guided by a profound understanding of genetic predispositions and molecular pathways.

The symphony of AI-assisted healthcare extends seamlessly to the clinical consultation room, where human practitioners and intelligent algorithms engage in a dynamic interplay of mutual learning and refinement. Recurrent neural networks, reminiscent of melodic motifs, adapt and evolve with each patient encounter, assimilating clinical data and historical insights to refine diagnoses and treatment plans in real-time. Works by Choi et al. [4] and Esteva et al. [6] exemplify the symbiotic relationship between AI and clinical practice, where data-driven insights complement the nuanced intuition of healthcare professionals, resulting in improved patient outcomes and enhanced quality of care.

At the heart of this symphony lies a delicate equilibrium, where the technical virtuosity of AI harmonizes with the human touch in healthcare. This symbiotic relationship unfolds as a harmonious convergence, with AI assuming its rightful place as an integral member of the medical orchestra, contributing to a sublime composition that resonates with the collective heartbeat of humanity. References to seminal works by Topol [18] and Char et al. [13] underscore the transformative potential of this collaboration, promising unprecedented advancements in patient care and the realization of a future where healing transcends its traditional boundaries.

In conclusion, the interplay between artificial intelligence (AI) and healthcare represents a transformative symphony, wherein computational ingenuity harmonizes with clinical expertise to compose a melody of healing. Through the lens of deep learning, pioneered by seminal works such as those by LeCun et al. [11], AI has emerged as an indispensable collaborator, augmenting diagnostic precision and therapeutic efficacy across diverse domains within healthcare.

Within the realm of medical imaging, the evolution of convolutional architectures, guided by the seminal contributions of Ronneberger et al. [19] and He et al. [9], has ushered in a renaissance in diagnostic acumen. Advanced neural networks illuminate radiological imagery with unprecedented clarity, transcending the limitations of traditional modalities and offering clinicians newfound insights into the pathology of disease.

In the domain of genomics, deep learning algorithms decode the intricate language of genes, unveiling predispositions to diseases and guiding the development of personalized treatment strategies tailored to individual genetic profiles. Works by Zou et al. [20] and Choi et al. [4] underscore the transformative potential of AI in genomic medicine, offering a glimpse into a future where interventions are guided by a profound understanding of genetic predispositions and molecular pathways.

The symbiotic relationship between AI and clinical practice extends seamlessly to the medical consultation room, where recurrent neural networks adapt and evolve with each patient encounter, enriching diagnostic and therapeutic decision-making processes with data-driven insights. This dynamic interplay, exemplified by works from Choi et al. [3] and Esteva et al. [6] , underscores the complementary nature of AI and human expertise, resulting in improved patient outcomes and enhanced quality of care.

Presents the synergistic relationship between AI and medical practitioners in modern healthcare. It emphasizes the dynamic interplay between human expertise and intelligent algorithms. Deep Learning and genomics contribute to personalized treatment strategies. AI functions as a collaborator, particularly in advancements in medical imaging.

AI analyzes patients data using deep learning and advanced medical imaging to generate enhanced insights.

Ultimately, the narrative of AI-assisted healthcare unfolds as a harmonious convergence, Figure 6.1 wherein AI assumes its rightful place as an integral member of the medical orchestra, contributing to a sublime composition that resonates with the collective heartbeat of humanity. Through collaborative efforts and continued innovation, this symphony of healing promises to usher in a future where precision, empathy, and efficacy converge to redefine the landscape of healthcare for generations to come.

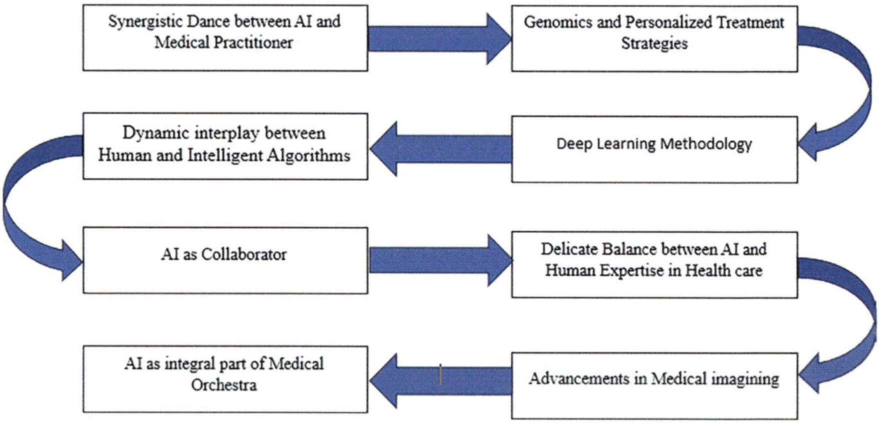

Figure 6.1 Embarking on a rhythmic exploration of healthcare's evolution.

6.3 Emerging Technologies

This exposition explores the transformative potential of emerging technologies across multiple areas, taking readers on a journey through the world of technological evolution. These ground-breaking discoveries, which range from the cutting edge of biotechnology to artificial intelligence (AI), have the potential to transform entire industries, alter social structures, and lead to previously unheard-of levels of advancement and prosperity for humanity.

A number of ground-breaking technologies stand out as key actors in the field of artificial intelligence (AI), which has seen an incredible growth and transformation in recent years. These technologies have the potential to completely change industries and the way people interact with the outside world. These emerging technologies, which range from the development of driverless vehicles to advances in natural language processing (NLP), have the potential to bring in a new era of progress and wealth.

The development of deep learning algorithms is one of the most fascinating developments in artificial intelligence and is evidence of the creativity sparked by the complex mechanisms of the human brain. Nestled within the larger field of machine learning, deep learning has demonstrated its abilities in a wide range of tasks, from speech comprehension and natural language understanding to image recognition. Convolutional neural networks (CNNs) and recurrent neural networks (RNNs), architectural wonders that have advanced AI systems to new levels in processing and understanding complex data patterns, are at the center of this revolutionary voyage. A new era of computer intelligence has begun with the widespread adoption of deep learning techniques across a variety of fields, made possible by pioneering contributions.

Additionally, reinforcement learning (RL) shows promise as a new area of artificial intelligence. Through interaction with their surroundings and feedback in the form of incentives or penalties, reinforcement learning (RL), a kind of machine learning algorithm, enables agents to learn how to make decisions. In fields like robotics, where RL algorithms can teach machines to perform complex tasks with little assistance from humans, this paradigm has enormous potential. Prominent advancements in this field, including the research on deep Q-learning, have shown that it is possible to train agents to perform superhuman activities, such as playing video games.

Beyond the domain of AI, other emerging technologies stand poised to make significant impacts on society and the economy. Blockchain, for instance, represents a decentralized ledger system that facilitates secure and transparent transactions without intermediaries. Its applications span industries such as finance, supply chain management, and healthcare, promising streamlined processes, reduced costs, and heightened security. The ascent of cryptocurrencies like Bitcoin underscores the transformative potential of blockchain technology.

Another rapidly developing field is quantum computing, which uses the ideas of quantum physics to do computations at previously unheard-of rates. Quantum computers have the ability to solve difficult issues that are now beyond the capabilities of classical computers, with potential uses in drug development, materials research, and cryptography. Quantum computing is still in its infancy, but it provides insights into new areas of technology advancement and scientific research.

Within the field of biotechnology, gene editing methods such as CRISPR-Cas9 have become potent instruments for accurate genetic code change. By enabling targeted gene edits, deletions, or substitutions inside an organism's DNA, this invention opens up new possibilities for human germline editing, crop engineering with desired features, and the treatment of genetic illnesses. The discovery of CRISPR-Cas9 signals a revolution in our capacity to control the basic components of life.

Furthermore, the internet of things (IoT) is a rapidly developing field with a wealth of opportunities to revolutionize several sectors and societal areas. The Internet of Things (IoT) is a network of linked devices with sensors and software installed, allowing for easy data collection and sharing. IoT technologies, which range from smart homes to industrial automation and healthcare monitoring, promise to transform how people interact with their surroundings and increase operational efficiency in corporate settings.

Table 6.1 and Table 6.2, Addressing the ethical, social, and economic ramifications of these developing technologies is crucial as they develop further. To guarantee that the advantages of these developments are widely dispersed and enhance the welfare of society as a whole, issues including data privacy, algorithmic bias, job displacement, and fair access to technology must be properly managed.

By implementing these technologies responsibly and ethically, we can use their potential to open up new creative possibilities and build a successful, sustainable, and just future for everybody.

6.3.1 The role of artificial intelligence (AI) in healthcare evolution

It is becoming more and more clear when examining the complex web of healthcare evolution that artificial intelligence (AI) is a driving force behind

Table 6.1 Assessment of technological advancements in healthcare: development and deployment status.

Technology	Developed	Development required
Deep learning	Yes	Yes
Natural language processing	Yes	Yes
Computer vision	Yes	Yes
Machine learning	Yes	Yes
Robotics	Yes	Yes
Predictive analytics	Yes	Yes
Genomics and genetics	Yes	Yes
Wearable devices	Yes	Yes
Virtual reality	Yes	Yes
Augmented reality	Yes	Yes
Blockchain technology	Yes	Yes
Quantum computing	Yes	Yes
Internet of medical things	Yes	Yes
3D printing	Yes	Yes
Telemedicine	Yes	Yes
Health informatics	Yes	Yes

Table 6.2 Development required for emerging healthcare technologies.

Technology	Development required
Deep learning	Further enhancement of efficiency, interpretability, and scalability for complex medical tasks.
Natural language processing	Improved accuracy, adaptability to medical terminology, and ability to handle diverse clinical text data.
Computer vision	Enhanced capabilities for tasks such as image segmentation, anomaly detection, and real-time analysis of large datasets.
Machine learning	Address challenges such as data heterogeneity, model interpretability, and generalizability across diverse patient populations.
Robotics	Improvement of robot-assisted surgeries, rehabilitation outcomes, and safe human–robot interactions in clinical settings.
Predictive analytics	Enhanced predictive accuracy, real-time data handling, and integration into clinical decision support systems.
Genomics and genetics	Advancement of genomic data analysis methods, understanding genetic variation, and translation into clinical practice.
Wearable devices	Improved sensor accuracy, battery life, data security, and user interface design for seamless integration into clinical workflows.
Virtual reality	Enhancement of VR simulations, immersive experiences for medical training and therapy, and reduction of hardware costs.
Augmented reality	Improvement in AR visualization, accuracy in medical applications, and integration with existing healthcare infrastructure.
Blockchain technology	Addressing scalability, interoperability, regulatory compliance, and data privacy issues in health data transactions.
Quantum computing	Increased qubit stability, reduced error rates, and development of quantum algorithms for healthcare applications.
Internet of medical things	Enhancing device interoperability, strengthening cybersecurity measures, and addressing regulatory challenges.
3D printing	Improvement in printing speed, resolution, and material biocompatibility for medical device production.
Telemedicine	Enhanced video and audio quality, reliable connectivity, and regulatory barriers for widespread adoption.
Health informatics	Integration of healthcare data sources, interoperability standards, and advanced analytics for precision medicine initiatives.

this change. In this changing environment, AI's function goes beyond simple augmentation; it becomes a crucial conductor, leading a healing symphony alongside medical professionals. This chapter sets out to investigate the deep connection between AI and medical practitioners, shedding light on the subtleties of their dance together.

Figure 6.2, whereas, the enormous impact of deep learning methodology, which is transforming the fundamental underpinnings of healthcare ecosystems, is at the center of this investigation. Deep learning algorithms provide a method to redefine therapeutic modalities and diagnostic paradigms because they are inspired by the complex architecture of neural networks. The chapter reveals the revolutionary potential of AI in this field, bringing about a new era in which human skill and computing power combine to handle the challenges of medical diagnosis.

As the overture unfolds, AI emerges as an indispensable collaborator, seamlessly integrating its computational acumen with the nuanced insights of medical practitioners. This partnership forms the cornerstone of a symphonic composition, where AI's analytical capabilities harmonize with human intuition to refine diagnostic precision and therapeutic strategies. Through this collaboration, AI not only complements but elevates the expertise of medical professionals, fostering a symbiotic relationship that amplifies the quality of patient care.

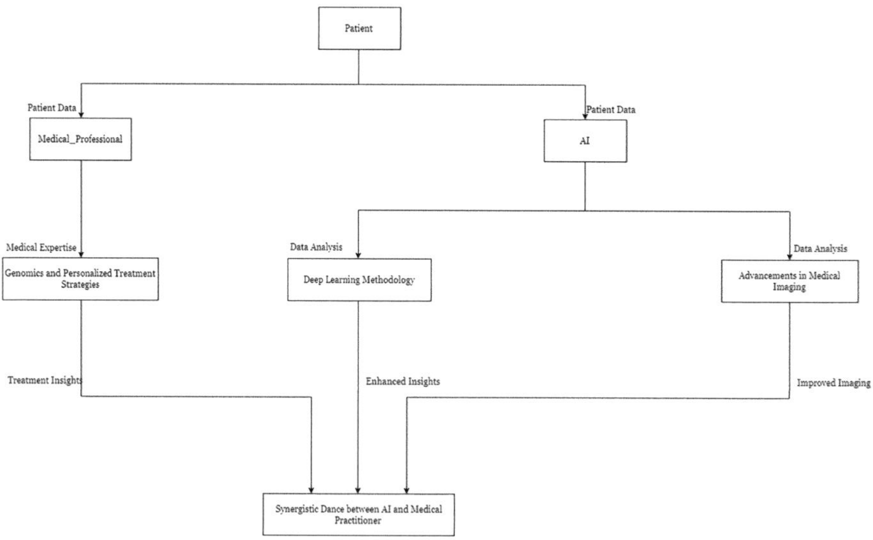

Figure 6.2 Human and machine: a collaborative approach to healthcare.

A crescendo emerges as the narrative delves into the realm of medical imaging, where AI-driven advancements illuminate latent patterns within radiological imagery. The fusion of advanced neural networks with medical imaging techniques unveils a transformative depth to diagnostics, transcending perceptual boundaries to unveil insights beyond the human eye's limitations. This convergence of AI and medical imaging not only enhances diagnostic accuracy but also revolutionizes the interpretation of medical images, laying the groundwork for a new era of precision medicine.

Venturing further, the chapter navigates the harmonies of genomics, where AI algorithms decrypt the intricate language of genes, unveiling predispositions to ailments and orchestrating personalized treatment strategies aligned with individual genetic compositions. This exploration underscores AI's role as a virtuoso ensemble, deciphering the genetic opus inscribed within our DNA to sculpt bespoke healthcare interventions. Through this integration, AI empowers medical practitioners with unprecedented insights, heralding a paradigm shift in the delivery of personalized medicine.

As the narrative gracefully extends to the realm of medical consultations, the dynamic interplay between human practitioners and intelligent algorithms comes into focus. Recurrent neural networks, akin to a melodic motif, adapt and learn from patient histories, refining diagnoses and treatment plans in an iterative cadence. This symphonic collaboration between AI and medical practitioners not only enhances diagnostic accuracy but also augments clinical decision-making, fostering a holistic approach to patient care.

At the heart of this symphony lies a delicate balance, where the technical prowess of AI harmonizes with the human touch in healthcare delivery. This refined interplay between AI and medical professionals unfolds as a harmonious convergence, where AI becomes an integral part of the medical orchestra, contributing to a sublime composition that resonates with the collective heartbeat of humanity. Through this synergy, AI emerges not as a mere tool but as a transformative force, shaping the future of healthcare delivery with its unparalleled capabilities.

Transitioning to medical consultations, recurrent neural networks adapt and learn from patient histories, refining diagnoses and treatment plans iteratively. This process enhances clinical decision-making and patient care.

At the heart of this symphony lies a delicate balance, where AI complements the human touch in healthcare delivery. This refined interplay between technology and expertise unfolds as a harmonious convergence, where AI becomes an integral part of the medical orchestra, contributing to a composition that resonates with the collective heartbeat of humanity.

In essence, Figure 6.3 reflects AI's transformative role in healthcare showcases its potential to revolutionize diagnostics, treatment, and patient care. Through collaboration and innovation, AI emerges as a driving force in shaping the future of healthcare delivery, ushering in an era of unprecedented precision and personalized medicine.

6.3.2 Deep learning methodology: redefining healthcare landscapes

Within the intricate tapestry of healthcare landscapes, deep learning methodology emerges as a profound catalyst, reshaping paradigms and redefining horizons. At its core, deep learning embodies the essence of neural networks, mirroring the intricate architecture of the human brain. This computational symphony unfolds new vistas of possibility, casting a luminous gaze upon realms hitherto obscured.

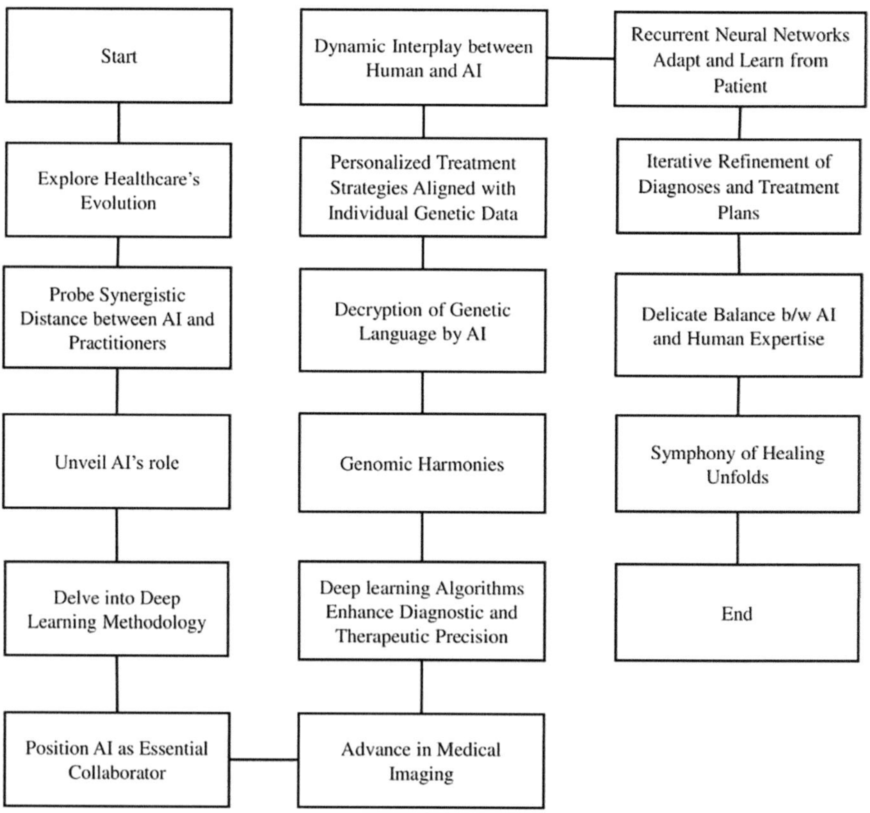

Figure 6.3 Depicting the evolution of healthcare in conjunction with AI.

The chapter embarks on a journey to explore the transformative potential of deep learning in healthcare, unraveling the intricate threads that weave the fabric of diagnostic precision and therapeutic innovation. Through the lens of deep learning algorithms, the landscape of healthcare undergoes a metamorphosis, transcending traditional boundaries to unveil a new frontier of computational intelligence.

As the narrative unfolds, deep learning algorithms emerge as harbingers of change, revolutionizing the very essence of healthcare delivery. Their prowess lies in their ability to discern patterns, extract insights, and derive meaning from vast troves of data with unparalleled precision. This transformative capability not only enhances diagnostic accuracy but also empowers medical practitioners to navigate the complexities of patient care with newfound clarity and confidence.

Figure 6.4, reflects the symphonic convergence of deep learning with healthcare landscapes heralds a new era of possibility, where computational acumen harmonizes with human intuition to orchestrate a symphony of healing. In this symbiotic dance, deep learning methodology emerges as a beacon of innovation, illuminating pathways to a future where healthcare transcends its limitations to embrace the full spectrum of human potential.

6.3.3 AI's collaboration with medical practitioners

In the realm of medical imaging, advanced neural networks gracefully unravel latent patterns within radiological imagery, ushering in a transformative era of diagnostics. This symphonic convergence of artificial intelligence with medical imaging techniques transcends perceptual boundaries, revealing insights beyond the limitations of human perception. Through the intricate dance of deep learning algorithms, medical images are imbued with a newfound depth, illuminating subtle nuances that elude the human eye.

The fusion of AI-driven advancements with medical imaging not only enhances diagnostic accuracy but also revolutionizes the interpretation of radiological data. By leveraging the computational prowess of advanced

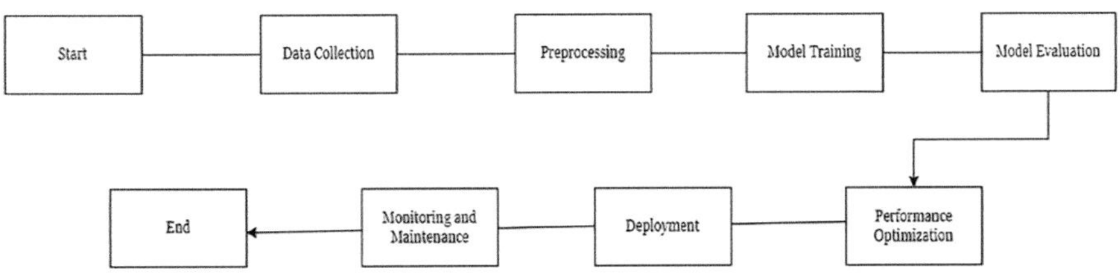

Figure 6.4 Depicting the deep learning methodology in healthcare.

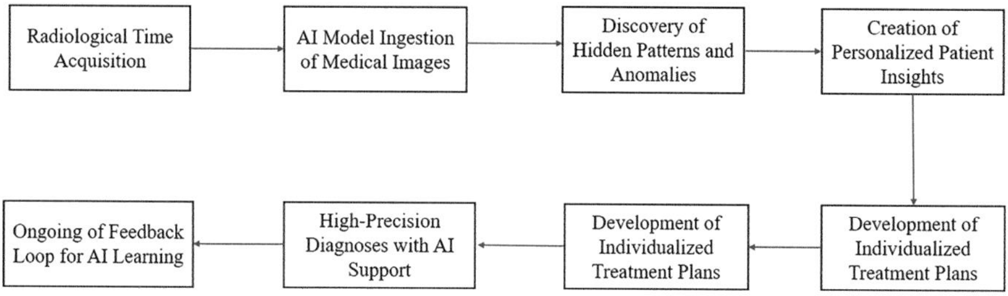

Figure 6.5 AI-enhanced imaging workflow in modern diagnostics.

neural networks, healthcare professionals are empowered to navigate the complexities of medical diagnostics with unprecedented precision and confidence. This transformative capability heralds a paradigm shift in the field of radiology, where AI emerges as an indispensable ally in the quest for diagnostic excellence.

Moreover, AI-driven medical imaging techniques hold the promise of unlocking new frontiers in personalized medicine. By deciphering the Figure 6.5, intricate patterns within radiological imagery, AI algorithms unveil unique insights into individual patient profiles, paving the way for tailored treatment strategies aligned with specific medical needs. This personalized approach to healthcare delivery not only enhances patient outcomes but also fosters a deeper understanding of disease pathophysiology and treatment response.

As the symphony of healing unfolds, the collaboration between AI and medical imaging continues to evolve, charting new pathways for innovation and discovery. Through this harmonious convergence, AI becomes an integral part of the medical orchestra, contributing to a sublime composition that resonates with the collective heartbeat of humanity.

6.3.4 Advancements in medical imaging through AI

In the domain of medical imaging, the integration of artificial intelligence (AI) technologies ushers in a transformative era of diagnostic precision and innovation. Advanced neural networks, driven by deep learning methodologies, meticulously analyze medical images, revealing hidden patterns and nuances imperceptible to the human eye. This symphonic convergence of AI and medical imaging transcends conventional boundaries, illuminating new pathways for diagnostic excellence.

AI-driven advancements in medical imaging hold the promise of revolutionizing the interpretation and analysis of radiological data. By leveraging the computational prowess of deep learning algorithms, healthcare practitioners gain access to a wealth of insights that augment their diagnostic

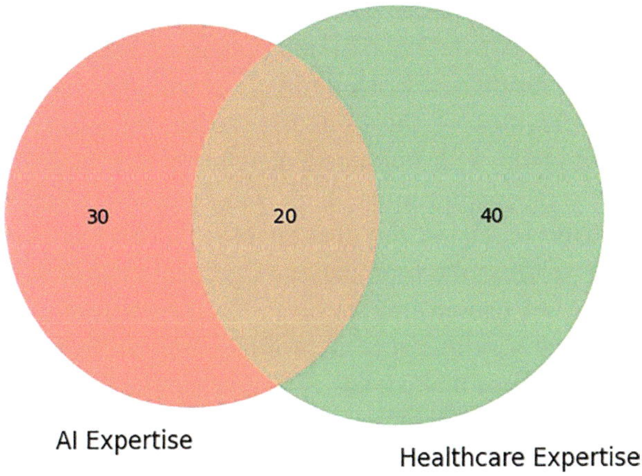

Figure 6.6 Intersection between AI and healthcare expertise.

capabilities. From identifying subtle anomalies to predicting disease progression, AI- powered medical imaging techniques empower clinicians with unparalleled precision and accuracy.

Additionally, Figure 6.6 says the combination of AI and medical imaging goes beyond diagnostic uses to include tailored therapy. Artificial intelligence (AI) algorithms may identify distinct information about each patient's profile by analyzing the complex patterns found in medical imaging. This allows for the creation of individualized treatment plans. In addition to improving patient outcomes, this individualized approach to healthcare delivery promotes a better comprehension of disease pathophysiology and treatment response. As AI continues to evolve and refine its capabilities in medical imaging, the collaborative synergy between AI and healthcare professionals deepens. Through this harmonious partnership, AI becomes an indispensable tool in the medical arsenal, contributing to a symphony of healing that resonates with the collective heartbeat of humanity. Together, AI and medical imaging pave the way for a future where healthcare is characterized by unparalleled precision, efficacy, and compassion.

6.3.5 Genomics: unraveling genetic patterns with AI

Navigating the harmonies of genomics, artificial intelligence (AI) unfolds as a transformative force, decrypting the intricate language of genes and reshaping the landscape of personalized medicine. Deep learning algorithms, akin to a virtuoso ensemble, probe the genetic opus inscribed within our DNA, unveiling predispositions to ailments and orchestrating bespoke treatment strategies tailored to individual genetic compositions.

AI-driven advancements in genomics offer a glimpse into the future of healthcare, where the convergence of computational intelligence and genetic insights revolutionizes disease prevention, diagnosis, and treatment. By deciphering the complexities of the human genome, AI algorithms empower healthcare practitioners with unprecedented insights into genetic predispositions and disease susceptibilities. This transformative capability not only enhances diagnostic precision but also enables the development of targeted interventions that address the root causes of genetic disorders.

Furthermore, AI has an impact on tailored treatment plans that are in line with each patient's unique genetic profile, going beyond the management of diseases. AI algorithms make it easier to identify the best treatment actions based on each patient's distinct genetic composition by fusing genetic data with clinical information. In addition to increasing treatment effectiveness, this individualized approach to healthcare delivery also reduces side effects, improving patient outcomes and quality of life.

As the narrative gracefully extends to the realm of genomics, the Table 6.3 reflects collaborative interplay between AI and medical practitioners emerges as a symphony of healing. Through this dynamic partnership, AI becomes an indispensable ally in the quest for precision medicine,

Table 6.3 AI in genomics: powering personalized medicine.

Area	AI technique	Genomic data	Benefit	Real-time example
Disease prediction	Polygenic risk scores	Genome-wide association studies (GWAS) data	Identify individuals at high risk for developing diseases	Predicting risk of Alzheimer's disease based on genetic variations
Drug discovery	Deep learning	DNA sequencing data, protein–protein interaction networks	Design and development of targeted therapies	Identifying potential drug candidates for cancer based on specific mutations
Non-invasive prenatal testing	Machine learning	Cell-free fetal DNA (cffDNA) in maternal blood	Early detection of genetic abnormalities in fetuses	Non-invasive prenatal screening for Down syndrome

Area	AI technique	Genomic data	Benefit	Real-time example
Personalized treatment	Machine learning	Patient's genetic data, medical history	Adapt treatment regimens to each patient's unique genetic composition.	Using a cancer patient's genetic profile to choose the best treatment course of action
Cancer classification	Deep learning	Tumor gene expression data	Improve the accuracy of cancer diagnosis	Classifying different types of cancer based on gene expression patterns
Drug response prediction	Machine learning	Patient's genetic data, drug response data	Predict a patient's response to a specific drug	Identifying patients likely to benefit from a new cancer immunotherapy
Variant interpretation	Natural language processing (NLP)	Scientific literature, genetic databases	Classify genetic variants as pathogenic or benign	Prioritizing variants of unknown significance (VUS) for further analysis
Gene function discovery	Deep learning	Large-scale genomic datasets	Unravel the functions of unknown genes	Identifying genes involved in the development of complex diseases
Antimicrobial resistance prediction	Machine learning	Bacterial or fungal genomic data	Predict the emergence and spread of antibiotic resistance	Identifying patients at risk for infections with drug-resistant bacteria
Gene regulation analysis	Deep learning	DNA sequence data, gene expression data	Understand how genes are regulated in health and disease	Identifying regulatory elements that control gene expression in different cell types

contributing to a harmonious convergence that resonates with the collective heartbeat of humanity. In this symphonic dance, AI unfolds as a transformative orchestrator, sculpting a future where healthcare is characterized by unparalleled efficacy, compassion, and personalized care.

6.3.6 AI's impact on medical consultations

In the narrative of healthcare evolution, the dynamic interplay between human practitioners and intelligent algorithms takes center stage as we explore the realm of medical consultations. Recurrent neural networks, akin to a melodic motif, adapt and learn from patient histories, refining diagnoses and treatment plans in an iterative cadence.

This symphonic collaboration between AI and medical practitioners not only enhances diagnostic accuracy but also augments clinical decision-making, fostering a holistic approach to patient care. As the narrative gracefully unfolds, it becomes evident that the integration of AI into medical consultations transcends mere augmentation, emerging as a transformative force that amplifies the expertise of healthcare professionals.

Through the lens of recurrent neural networks, medical consultations are imbued with a newfound depth and precision, empowering clinicians to navigate the complexities of patient care with unparalleled clarity and confidence. The iterative nature of AI-driven consultations facilitates continuous learning and adaptation, ensuring that diagnostic and treatment strategies evolve in response to changing patient needs and clinical insights.

Moreover, the collaborative interplay between AI and medical practitioners fosters a dynamic exchange of knowledge and expertise, enriching the diagnostic process and enhancing patient outcomes. As AI continues to evolve and refine its capabilities in medical consultations, the symphony of healing unfolds with ever-increasing clarity and harmony.

Figure 6.7, in this symbiotic dance between AI and human practitioners, the boundaries of traditional healthcare paradigms are transcended, giving rise to a new era of patient-centered care. Through this harmonious convergence, AI emerges as an integral partner in the medical orchestra, contributing to a sublime composition that resonates with the collective heartbeat of humanity.

6.3.7 Recurrent neural networks: refining diagnoses and treatment plans

At the heart of the symphony of healing lies a delicate balance, where the technical prowess of artificial intelligence (AI) harmonizes with the human

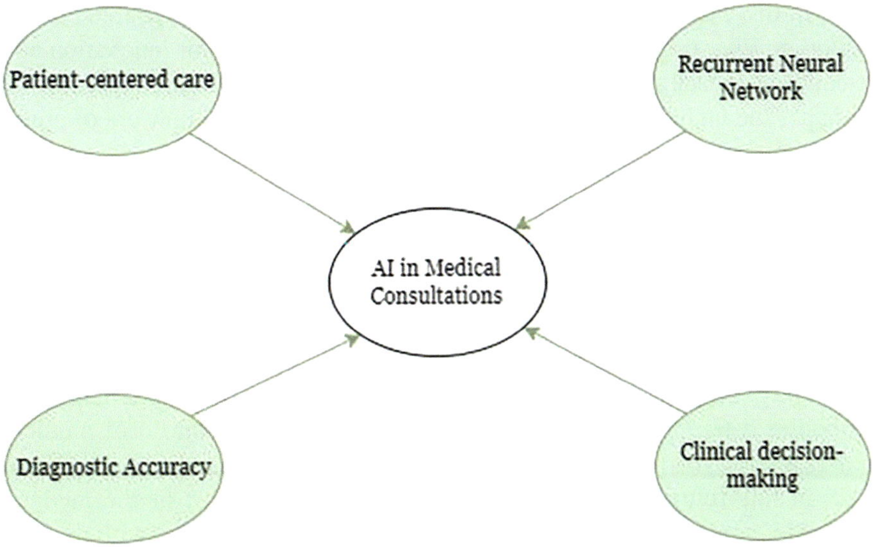

Figure 6.7 AI in medical consultations.

touch in healthcare delivery. This refined interplay between AI and medical practitioners unfolds as a harmonious convergence, where AI becomes an integral part of the medical orchestra, contributing to a sublime composition that resonates with the collective heartbeat of humanity.

In this delicate dance, AI serves as a transformative force, amplifying the expertise of healthcare professionals and enhancing the quality of patient care. By seamlessly integrating AI-driven technologies into healthcare workflows, medical practitioners gain access to a wealth of insights and capabilities that augment their diagnostic and therapeutic abilities.

The collaborative partnership between AI and human practitioners fosters a dynamic exchange of knowledge and expertise, enriching the diagnostic process and fostering a deeper understanding of patient needs. Through this symbiotic relationship, AI becomes more than just a tool; it becomes a trusted ally, empowering medical professionals to navigate the complexities of patient care with confidence and precision.

Moreover, the integration of AI into healthcare delivery ensures that diagnostic and treatment strategies are tailored to individual patient needs, enhancing the efficacy and efficiency of care delivery. As AI continues to evolve and refine its capabilities, the symphony of healing unfolds with ever-increasing clarity and harmony, paving the way for a future where healthcare is characterized by personalized, patient-centered care.

In this transformative journey, AI emerges as an indispensable collaborator, guiding the medical orchestra toward new frontiers of innovation and excellence. Through its harmonious convergence with human expertise, AI reshapes the landscape of healthcare delivery, ushering in a new era of precision, compassion, and healing.

6.3.8 Achieving harmony: balancing AI technical prowess with human expertise

As we envision the future of healthcare, the integration of artificial intelligence (AI) emerges as a central component in orchestrating a symphony of healing. AI's role in healthcare extends beyond mere augmentation; it embodies a transformative force that reshapes the very fabric of medical practice.

In this future landscape, AI becomes an integral part of the medical orchestra, contributing to a sublime composition that resonates with the collective heartbeat of humanity. Through its harmonious convergence with human expertise, AI amplifies the capabilities of healthcare professionals and enhances the quality of patient care.

The intended partnership between AI and human practitioners develops as a dynamic interaction in which the technical expertise of AI strengthens and supplements the human element in the provision of healthcare. This mutually beneficial partnership promotes a better comprehension of patient requirements and makes it possible to create individualized treatment plans that are catered to each patient's preferences and circumstances.

Moreover, AI-driven advancements in healthcare hold the promise of revolutionizing disease prevention, diagnosis, and treatment. By leveraging the power of AI algorithms, medical practitioners gain access to a wealth of insights and capabilities that augment their diagnostic precision and therapeutic efficacy.

As AI continues to evolve and refine its capabilities, the symphony of healing unfolds with ever- increasing clarity and harmony. Through its transformative influence, AI reshapes the landscape of healthcare delivery, ushering in a new era characterized by precision, compassion, and innovation.

In this future vision, AI emerges as an indispensable partner in the quest for better health outcomes, guiding the medical orchestra toward new frontiers of excellence. Through its collaborative synergy with human expertise, AI paves the way for a future where healthcare is not only efficient and effective but also deeply empathetic and patient-centered.

6.3.9 Envisioning the future: AI integration in healthcare orchestration

In the grand symphony of healthcare evolution, the delicate interplay between artificial intelligence (AI) and human practitioners emerges as a cornerstone of progress and innovation. This collaborative partnership, akin to a harmonious convergence of musical instruments in an orchestra, orchestrates a sublime composition of healing that resonates with the collective heartbeat of humanity.

At the heart of this symphony lies a delicate balance, where the technical prowess of AI seamlessly blends with the nuanced expertise of medical professionals. Through this refined interplay, AI becomes more than just a tool; it transforms into an indispensable collaborator, amplifying the capabilities of healthcare practitioners and enhancing the quality of patient care.

Figure 6.8, the narrative of AI in healthcare unfolds as a dynamic interplay between computational acumen and human intuition. Advanced neural

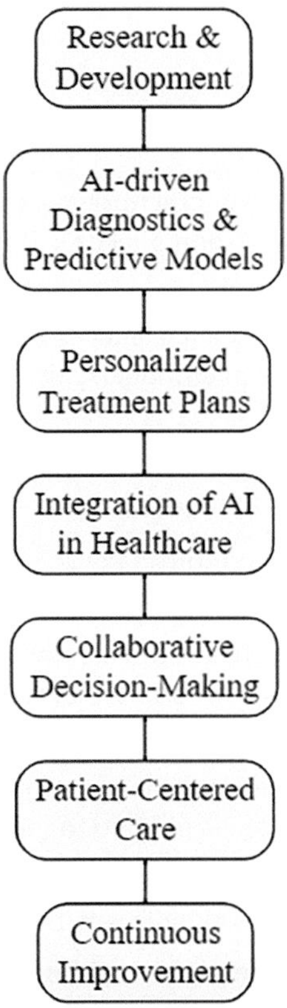

Figure 6.8 Path to healthcare transformation: AI and human collaboration.

networks, driven by deep learning methodologies, navigate the complexities of medical data, uncovering patterns and insights imperceptible to the human eye. This transformative capability empowers medical practitioners with unprecedented diagnostic precision and therapeutic efficacy, laying the groundwork for a future where healthcare delivery is characterized by unparalleled accuracy and compassion.

In the realm of medical imaging, AI-driven advancements revolutionize the interpretation and analysis of radiological data. By leveraging the computational prowess of deep learning algorithms, healthcare practitioners gain access to a wealth of insights that augment their diagnostic capabilities. From identifying subtle anomalies to predicting disease progression, AI- powered medical imaging techniques empower clinicians with unparalleled precision and accuracy.

Moreover, Table 6.4, AI's impact extends beyond disease management to encompass personalized treatment strategies aligned with individual patient

Table 6.4 Integration of AI in healthcare orchestration: key aspects.

Aspect	Description
Integration of AI in healthcare	AI and human practitioners collaborate like a symphony orchestra, blending technical prowess with human expertise for healing.
Balance and collaboration	A delicate balance and collaborative partnership between AI and human practitioners, akin to a harmonious convergence.
Technical prowess of AI	Advanced neural networks driven by deep learning methodologies navigate medical data, uncovering imperceptible insights.
Human intuition and expertise	Human practitioners contribute nuanced expertise and intuition in patient care.
Medical imaging advancements	AI-driven advancements revolutionize the interpretation and analysis of radiological data, augmenting diagnostic capabilities.
Personalized treatment strategies	AI integrates genetic and clinical data to suggest personalized treatment plans tailored to individual patient profiles.
Evolution and innovation	Continuous evolution and innovation in AI integration in healthcare, leading to new frontiers of discovery and excellence.
Sublime composition of healing	The ultimate goal is a sublime composition of healing resonating with the collective heartbeat of humanity, characterized by precision and compassion.

profiles. By integrating genetic data with clinical information, AI algorithms facilitate the identification of optimal therapeutic interventions tailored to each patient's unique genetic makeup. This personalized approach not only improves treatment efficacy but also minimizes adverse effects, enhancing patient outcomes and quality of life.

As the symphony of healing unfolds, the collaborative partnership between AI and human practitioners continues to evolve, charting new pathways for innovation and discovery. Through this dynamic interplay, AI becomes an integral part of the medical orchestra, contributing to a sublime composition that resonates with the collective heartbeat of humanity.

In this transformative endeavor, AI emerges as an indispensable collaborator, guiding the medical orchestra toward new frontiers of innovation and excellence. Through its harmonious convergence with human expertise, AI reshapes the landscape of healthcare delivery, ushering in a new era characterized by precision, compassion, and healing.

6.4 Objectives of the Study

- Explore the integration of artificial intelligence (AI) into healthcare practices and its impact on patient care.
- Investigate the role of cutting-edge deep learning methodologies in reshaping the healthcare landscape.
- Assess the effectiveness of AI in enhancing diagnostic accuracy and treatment efficacy across various medical disciplines.
- Examine the utilization of advanced neural networks in medical imaging to uncover latent patterns and improve diagnostic capabilities.
- Analyze the application of AI in deciphering the genetic landscape through genomics and its implications for personalized medicine.
- Evaluate the collaborative dynamics between human practitioners and intelligent algorithms in medical consultations, particularly in refining diagnoses and treatment plans.
- Investigate the ethical, social, and economic implications of AI integration in healthcare and strategies for ensuring equitable access and responsible implementation.
- Propose recommendations for optimizing the integration of AI into healthcare practices, fostering a harmonious convergence between technical innovation and human expertise.

6.5 Importance of the Study

The significance of this discovery cannot be emphasized as a researcher exploring the complex interactions between artificial intelligence (AI) and healthcare. Fundamentally, this investigation is a deep dive into the future of medicine, where human knowledge and technological advancement will combine to reshape the parameters of patient care.

AI's incorporation into healthcare procedures is extremely important for both patients and professionals. We have the chance to transform patient outcomes, treatment plans, and diagnostic procedures by utilizing the power of state-of-the-art deep learning techniques. Medical imaging can be improved by using sophisticated neural networks to reveal hidden patterns and insights, giving doctors the ability to diagnose patients more quickly and accurately. The use of AI in genomics also holds up the possibility of personalized medicine, in which therapeutic results can be maximized by customizing treatment regimens based on each patient's unique genetic makeup.

Furthermore, a paradigm shift in the provision of healthcare is represented by the cooperative dynamics between AI algorithms and human practitioners during medical consultations. Clinicians may make better judgments and provide better patient care and satisfaction by combining human experience with AI-driven insights and analytics.

This paper discusses the ethical, societal, and economic ramifications of integrating AI in healthcare outside of the clinical setting. In order to ensure that the advantages of AI are dispersed fairly and ethically, it challenges us to think about issues of algorithmic bias, data privacy, and equal access to technology.

In essence, this study is not merely an academic exercise but a transformative journey toward a future where innovation and compassion intersect to enhance the well-being of individuals and communities. By deciphering the intricacies of artificial intelligence in healthcare, we open the door to a more effective, efficient, and just healthcare system that speaks to humanity's collective pulse.

6.6 Conclusion

In the intricate dance of healthcare's evolution, the partnership between Artificial Intelligence (AI) and medical practitioners emerges as a harmonious symphony, orchestrating healing melodies with finesse and precision. Throughout this exploration, we have delved into the profound interplay between AI and healthcare professionals, witnessing the transformative power of cutting-edge deep learning methodologies.

At the outset, we witnessed AI's seamless integration into the healthcare landscape, where it assumes the role of an indispensable collaborator. By blending computational acumen with the nuanced expertise of medical professionals, AI enhances diagnostic accuracy and treatment efficacy, amplifying the quality of patient care.

A pivotal moment in this narrative unfolds within the realm of medical imaging, where advanced neural networks decode intricate patterns within radiological imagery. This breakthrough transcends perceptual boundaries, offering clinicians unprecedented insights into disease pathology and treatment response. Through AI-enabled diagnostics, medical images are illuminated in ways previously unimaginable, heralding a new era of precision medicine.

The journey then leads us into the intricate tapestry of genomics, where AI algorithms decipher the language of genes with virtuosic precision. By revealing predispositions to ailments and tailoring personalized treatment strategies based on individual genetic compositions, AI empowers clinicians to deliver targeted interventions, revolutionizing patient care at its genetic core.

Furthermore, the narrative extends to the realm of medical consultations, where AI algorithms augment human expertise through iterative learning and adaptation. Recurrent neural networks, akin to melodic motifs, harmonize with patient histories to refine diagnoses and treatment plans, ensuring optimal outcomes through collaborative decision-making.

Central to this symphony is the delicate balance between AI's technical prowess and the human touch in healthcare. Rather than overshadowing human expertise, AI complements it, enriching the medical orchestra with its computational capabilities. This harmonious convergence fosters a holistic approach to patient care, where AI becomes an integral part of the healing process, resonating with the collective heartbeat of humanity.

In conclusion, the sublime confluence of Artificial Intelligence and healthcare heralds a new era of healing, where innovation and compassion intertwine to redefine the boundaries of medical practice. As AI continues to evolve and integrate seamlessly into clinical workflows, it holds the promise of unlocking new frontiers in diagnosis, treatment, and patient outcomes. By embracing this collaborative partnership, we embark on a journey toward a future where healthcare transcends limitations, offering hope and healing to all.

References

[1] Angermueller, Christof, et al. "Deep learning for computational biology." Molecular systems biology 12.7 (2016): 878.

[2] Kahn, Jeffrey P., ed. Digital contact tracing for pandemic response: Ethics and governance guidance. Johns Hopkins University Press, 2020.

[3] Choi, Edward, et al. "Doctor ai: Predicting clinical events via recurrent neural networks." Machine learning for healthcare conference. PMLR, 2016.

[4] Choi, Edward, et al. "Using recurrent neural network models for early detection of heart failure onset." Journal of the American Medical Informatics Association 24.2 (2017): 361-370.

[5] Choi, Yongwook, et al. "Predicting the functional effect of amino acid substitutions and indels." (2012): e46688.

[6] Esteva, Andre, et al. "Dermatologist-level classification of skin cancer with deep neural networks." nature 542.7639 (2017): 115-118.

[7] Graves, Alex, Abdel-rahman Mohamed, and Geoffrey Hinton. "Speech recognition with deep recurrent neural networks." 2013 IEEE international conference on acoustics, speech and signal processing. Ieee, 2013.

[8] He, Kaiming, et al. "Deep residual learning." Image Recognition 7.4 (2015): 327-336.

[9] He, Kaiming, et al. "Deep residual learning for image recognition." Proceedings of the IEEE conference on computer vision and pattern recognition. 2016.

[10] Hochreiter, Sepp, and Jürgen Schmidhuber. "Long short-term memory." Neural computation 9.8 (1997): 1735-1780.

[11] LeCun, Yann, Yoshua Bengio, and Geoffrey Hinton. "Deep learning." nature 521.7553 (2015): 436-444.

[12] Li, Panpeng, et al. "Convolutional neural networks for intestinal hemorrhage detection in wireless capsule endoscopy images." 2017 IEEE International Conference on Multimedia and Expo (ICME). IEEE, 2017.

[13] Lipton, Zachary C., John Berkowitz, and Charles Elkan. "A critical review of recurrent neural networks for sequence learning." arXiv preprint arXiv:1506.00019 (2015).

[14] Mienye, Ibomoiye Domor, Theo G. Swart, and George Obaido. "Recurrent neural networks: A comprehensive review of architectures, variants, and applications." Information 15.9 (2024): 517.

[15] Martel, Anne L., et al., eds. Medical Image Computing and Computer Assisted Intervention–MICCAI 2020: 23rd International Conference,

Lima, Peru, October 4–8, 2020, Proceedings, Part I. Vol. 12261. Springer Nature, 2020.

[16] Rasmy, Laila, et al. "A study of generalizability of recurrent neural network-based predictive models for heart failure onset risk using a large and heterogeneous EHR data set." Journal of biomedical informatics 84 (2018): 11-16.

[17] Reverberi, Carlo, et al. "Experimental evidence of effective human–AI collaboration in medical decision-making." Scientific reports 12.1 (2022): 14952.

[18] Topol, Eric J. "High-performance medicine: the convergence of human and artificial intelligence." Nature medicine 25.1 (2019): 44-56.

[19] Ronneberger, Olaf, Philipp Fischer, and Thomas Brox. "U-net: Convolutional networks for biomedical image segmentation." International Conference on Medical image computing and computer-assisted intervention. Cham: Springer international publishing, 2015.

[20] Zou, James, et al. "A primer on deep learning in genomics." Nature genetics 51.1 (2019): 12-18.

7

Hybrid Optimization Techniques for Gene Expression Analysis: The EHOSVM Paradigm

Abrar Yaqoob[1], Mohd Abas Bhat[2], Rabia Musheer Aziz[3], Navneet Kumar Verma[1], R. Vijaya Lakshmi[4], Tejaswini Pradhan[5] and G.V.V. Jagannadha Rao[5]

[1]VIT Bhopal University's School of Advanced Science and Language, India
[2]University of Kashmir, India
[3]State Planning Institute (New Division) Planning Department Lucknow up, India
[4]ICFAI University, India
[5]Deparment of Mathematics, ICFAI University, Raipur, India

Email: abraryaqoob77@gmail.com; dummydame714@gmail.com; rabia rabia.aziz2010@gmail.com; navneet.verma@vitbhopal.ac.in; vijaya.lakshmi@iuraipur.edu.in; tejaswini.pradhan@kalingauniversity.ac.in; gvvjrao@iuraipur.edu.in

Abstract

This study introduces a novel hybrid gene selection approach, the Elephant Herding Optimization with support vector machine (EHOSVM), designed to identify significant gene subsets for cancer classification in high-dimensional gene expression datasets. Addressing challenges like redundancy and irrelevant features, EHOSVM integrates the optimization strengths of the Elephant Herding Optimization algorithm with the classification power of support vector machines (SVM). Evaluated across four benchmark datasets, breast cancer, central nervous system (CNS), leukemia, and

DOI: 10.1201/9788743809920-7

ovarian cancer, the method demonstrated exceptional performance, achieving 100% accuracy on the leukemia and ovarian datasets. For breast cancer, EHOSVM attained 99% accuracy, 98.61% precision, 100% recall, and a 99.31 F1-score with 23 selected genes, while the CNS dataset proved more challenging, yielding 66% accuracy due to its inherent complexity. Overall, EHOSVM's robust performance across varying gene subsets highlights its effectiveness in enhancing classification accuracy, making it a valuable tool for biological data analysis and precision medicine, though further refinements may be needed to improve its handling of highly complex and variable datasets.

7.1 Introduction

Cancer is a multifaceted and aggressive condition marked by irregular and unchecked cellular proliferation, remaining a significant global health concern despite notable progress in early detection and therapeutic interventions. Precision medicine, which adapts treatments to match an individual's distinct molecular characteristics, has emerged as a groundbreaking paradigm in oncology [1, 2]. A key component of this approach lies in pinpointing crucial genetic biomarkers associated with the onset and progression of cancer. Gene selection is fundamental to this process, as it extracts the most informative genes from large-scale, high-dimensional genomic datasets. Conventional selection techniques often encounter challenges such as limited computational efficiency, poor scalability, and reduced robustness. In recent years, nature-inspired optimization algorithms have demonstrated strong potential in addressing these drawbacks by emulating biological and ecological phenomena to tackle intricate optimization problems. Among them, the Elephant Herding Optimization (EHO) algorithm is notable for its distinctive mechanism. Drawing inspiration from the collective behavior and foraging patterns of elephant groups, EHO effectively explores vast search spaces to locate optimal solutions. Within cancer studies, EHO acts as a powerful feature selection method, systematically analyzing gene subsets to assess their predictive capacity. By maintaining a strategic equilibrium between exploration (investigating new gene combinations) and exploitation (fine-tuning promising subsets), EHO improves both the accuracy and stability of identified biomarkers. Incorporating EHO into cancer classification models enables the detection of vital genetic signatures, thereby enhancing diagnostic accuracy and supporting the development of personalized therapeutic regimens. This biologically inspired methodology offers substantial promise for advancing cancer research and improving patient prognoses [3–5].

7.1.1 Objectives of the proposed work

- Examine the capability of Elephant Herding Optimization (EHO) in selecting relevant features for effective cancer classification.
- Assess the performance of a novel hybrid framework that integrates EHO with a support vector machine (SVM) for both gene selection and cancer categorization.
- Contrast the outcomes of the EHO–SVM methodology with those derived from conventional gene selection techniques, considering metrics such as classification accuracy, precision, recall, and F1-score.
- Analyze the scalability and computational efficiency of the EHO–SVM framework in managing large-scale, high-dimensional genomic datasets.
- Investigate the clinical translation potential of the developed models for use in cancer diagnosis, prognostic evaluation, and tailored treatment design.

7.1.2 Motivation of the proposed work

In the realms of cancer biology and precision medicine, nature-inspired computational techniques have attracted considerable interest for their exceptional capacity to tackle intricate optimization challenges and generate novel solutions. By emulating the complex strategies observed in natural environments, these algorithms offer a robust and adaptable framework for overcoming the difficulties associated with gene selection and cancer classification. Their capability to mirror evolutionary dynamics and adjust to ever-changing conditions renders them especially effective for interpreting vast, high-dimensional genomic datasets. While their applications in biomedical research are substantial, the versatility of these methods extends far beyond healthcare, finding utility in domains such as engineering, financial forecasting, and supply chain management. This wide-ranging applicability underscores their role as transformative tools for problem-solving across disciplines. Within the scope of biological studies, nature-inspired algorithms stand out as catalysts for innovation, significantly advancing our capacity to unravel the underlying mechanisms of complex diseases. A notable example of such advancement is the integration of Elephant Herding Optimization (EHO) with support vector machines (SVM). This hybrid methodology combines EHO's highly efficient search and exploration capabilities with SVM's strong classification accuracy to pinpoint essential genetic markers in cancer. By harnessing the strengths of both techniques, researchers can achieve a more comprehensive understanding of tumor biology, thereby improving diagnostic precision and facilitating the development of individualized treatment approaches in oncology. The convergence of computational intelligence and biological research represented by this synergy holds immense potential to push the boundaries of cancer diagnostics, therapeutic strategies, and ultimately, patient survival outcomes [6–9].

7.2 Related Work

Hanan et al. proposed an innovative deep learning approach for breast cancer detection, utilizing transfer learning with ResNet-18, Inception-V3Net, and ShuffleNet architectures. Their system demonstrated exceptional performance, achieving 99.7% binary classification accuracy with ResNet and maintaining high accuracy (97.81%) for multi-class categorization, outperforming other tested models [10]. Abdar et al. developed two uncertainty quantification techniques (DE and EMC) for skin cancer diagnosis, addressing overconfidence in classification. Their TWDBDL model achieved strong performance (88.95-90.96% accuracy and 89–91% F1-score) across multiple datasets, demonstrating robust medical image analysis capabilities [11]. Ragab et al. created an ensemble deep learning system (EDLCDS-BCDC) for breast cancer detection using ultrasound images. Their approach combines Wiener filtering and contrast enhancement for preprocessing, CKHA with Kapur's entropy for segmentation, and VGG-16/VGG-19/SqueezeNet for feature extraction. The system employs CSO-optimized MLP for classification, demonstrating superior performance over existing methods in benchmark testing [12]. Stoean presents an innovative method for optimizing CNN convolutional layers and evaluating hyperparameter significance in deep learning architectures. The study employs three surrogate models (RF, SVM, and Kriging) to assess sample configurations generated through Latin hypercube sampling, with performance validated through actual CNN accuracy measurements. For hyperparameter optimization, evolutionary algorithms leverage surrogate-predicted accuracy estimates, while variable importance is determined through model-specific techniques: RF's inherent feature selection, SVM with EA support, and Kriging's *h*-value analysis. The methodology validates predictions against true accuracy scores before test deployment and compares variable rankings across models, with response surface analysis further elucidating parameter influence. This EA-surrogate framework was experimentally validated on histopathological image analysis for colorectal cancer detection [13]. Sharma et al. compared two ML approaches for breast cancer classification on BreakHis dataset: (1) handcrafted features (Hu moments, color histograms, Haralick textures) with traditional classifiers, and (2) transfer learning using VGG16/19 and ResNet50. The transfer learning approach outperformed handcrafted features across all magnifications, with VGG16+SVM achieving peak patch-based (93.97% at 40×) and patient-based (93.25% at 40×) accuracy. Data augmentation further boosted performance, while "fibro-adenoma" and "mucous carcinoma" proved most challenging to classify [14].

7.3 Methodology

7.3.1 Experimental setup and data description

Our research utilized a high-performance computational setup to guarantee both efficiency and reliability in the analytical process. All experiments were executed within an Ubuntu 20.04.5 LTS environment, supplemented by the Windows Subsystem for Linux (WSL) to facilitate smooth cross-platform integration. Visual Studio Code (VS Code) was employed as the main development interface, offering a streamlined workspace for Python-based coding and execution. For performance evaluation, we implemented Leave-One-Out Cross-Validation (LOOCV), where in each iteration, a single sample was omitted from training and used exclusively for testing. This rigorous validation method provided an exhaustive performance assessment over the entire dataset [15].

The computational hardware configuration comprised:

- **CPU:** Intel® Core™ i9-12900k (5.20 GHz)
- **RAM:** 64 GB for handling large-scale computations
- **GPU:** NVIDIA RTX Quadro A5000 for accelerated parallel processing

Table 7.1 Shows the detailed description of the datasets.

Dataset	Genes	Samples	Class
CNS	7,129	60	2
Breast	24,481	97	2
Ovarian	15,154	253	2
Leukemia	7129	72	2

We evaluated our methodology on four benchmark datasets **(breast cancer, leukemia, ovarian, CNS)**, with detailed specifications provided in Table 7.1 and publicly accessible https://csse.szu.edu.cn/staff/zhuzx/Datasets.html. This rigorous computational foundation enabled precise, high-performance analysis for deriving meaningful insights.

7.3.2 Proposed methodology

7.3.2.1 Elephant Herding Optimization (EHO)

This research employs the Elephant Herding Optimization (EHO) technique for feature selection, inspired by the collective intelligence exhibited within elephant herds. The algorithm computationally models the cooperative interactions observed in real-world elephant groups, where members collaborate to locate resources and traverse challenging terrains. In the context of data analysis, EHO leverages this cooperative behavior to effectively search through complex, high-dimensional feature spaces, enabling the identification of optimal gene subsets for classification tasks. A schematic depiction of the EHO procedure (Figure 7.1) demonstrates its iterative process of optimization.

The algorithm's implementation is publicly accessible at https://www.mathworks.com/matlabcentral/fileexchange/53486.

7.3.2.1.1 Basics of Elephant Herding Optimization

Elephants possess intricate social organizations, where females and their young form tightly bonded family groups under the guidance of a matriarch, while adult males eventually depart to lead solitary lives. This characteristic herding pattern served as the inspiration for Wang et al.'s 2015 development of the Elephant Herding Optimization (EHO) algorithm, which encapsulates these biological behaviors through three core concepts:

1. The entire population is divided into clans of fixed size.
2. In each generation, certain male elephants leave their clan to exist independently.
3. Within every clan, leadership is maintained by a central matriarch figure.

The EHO method transforms these real-world elephant social interactions into a mathematical optimization framework, enabling efficient computational problem-solving. [16].

7.3.2.1.2 Clan-updating operator

Reflecting natural elephant behavior, each clan's matriarch influences member positioning. The spatial coordinates of elephant j in clan c_i are calculated through eqn (7.1) [17].

$$x_{new,c_i,j} = x_{c_i,j} + a * \left(x_{best,c_i,} - x_{c_i,j}\right) * r \tag{7.1}$$

The variables $x_{new,c_i,j}$ and $x_{c_i,j}$ denote the updated and initial positions, respectively, of elephant j in clan c_i, respectively. x_{best,c_i} signifies the matriarch. c_i which represents the best elephant in the clan. $a \in [0,1]$ indicates a scale factor, $r \in [0,1]$. The best elephant can be calculated by eqn (7.2) for each data [18].

$$x_{new,c_i,j} = \beta * x_{center,c_i,} \tag{7.2}$$

where $\beta \in [0,1]$ represents a factor which determines the influence of the x_{center,c_i} on $x_{new,c_i,j}$.

$x_{new,c_i,j}$ is the new individual and x_{center,c_i}, is the centre individual of clan c_i. It can be calculated by eqn (7.3) for the dth dimension.

$$x_{center,c_i,d} = \frac{1}{n_{ci}} * \sum_{j=1}^{n_{ci}} x_{ci,j,d} \tag{7.3}$$

where $1 \leq d \leq D$ and n_{ci} indicates the number of elephants in clan c_i. $x_{ci,j,d}$ represents the dth dimension of elephant individual $x_{ci,j}$. x_{center,c_i}, is the centre of clan. and is updated by eqn (7.3).

7.3.2.1.3 Separating operator

The separation of male elephants from their herds is mathematically modeled as an optimization operator. This separation mechanism is applied to the least fit individual in each generation, as formulated in eqn (7.4).

$$x_{worst,c_i} = x_{min} + \left(x_{max} - x_{min} + 1\right) * rand \tag{7.4}$$

where x_{max} represents the upper bound of the individual and x_{min} indicates lower bound of the individual. x_{worst,c_i} indicates the worst individual in clan c_i. *Rand* [0,1] is a stochastic distribution between 0 and 1 [19].

7.3.2.2 Initialization

The EHO algorithm initiates by generating an initial population of potential solutions (the "herd"), where each solution encodes a candidate feature subset using binary representation (1 = feature included, 0 = excluded). Key initialization parameters include predetermined herd size (population count) and maximum iteration limit. [20].

7.3.2.3 Fitness evaluation

In every optimization cycle, we assess each solution's quality by measuring its classification performance. Specifically, we:

1. Train a linear SVM classifier using the solution's selected features
2. Evaluate the model on a reserved test dataset
3. Use this performance score as the solution's fitness value [21].

7.3.2.4 Selection, crossover, and mutation

Once the fitness of every candidate solution is assessed, the herd is ranked according to their fitness values. Solutions demonstrating superior performance are given higher priority for inclusion in the next iteration. Following this selection phase, **crossover** and **mutation** operations are applied to maintain population diversity. In the crossover step, attributes from two parent solutions are blended to produce new offspring, whereas the mutation step randomly modifies certain selected features to investigate unexplored regions of the search space [22].

7.3.2.5 Termination

The algorithm advances by iteratively performing the selection, crossover, and mutation operations over a predefined number of iterations. Execution halts once the termination criterion is satisfied – typically defined as reaching the maximum allowed iterations or when the solution converges. At this point, the best-performing candidate, representing the optimal feature subset, is extracted from the final population. Furthermore, Algorithm 7.1 presents the pseudocode implementation of EHO, while Figure 7.1 depicts its flowchart along with a schematic visualization of the process.

7.3.3 SVM classification

The support vector machine (SVM) is a well-established and highly effective classification technique in the field of machine learning. Its fundamental concept is to identify an optimal hyperplane that separates data points belonging to different classes with the greatest possible margin, the maximum distance between the hyperplane and the nearest data points from each class. By employing the kernel trick, SVM can project the input data into a higher-dimensional feature space, enabling it to classify datasets that are not

Algorithm 7.1 Pseudocode of the Elephant Herd Optimization.

```
Procedure Elephant Herding Optimization ():
  Initialize elephant population randomly
  Repeat until termination criteria are met:
    For each clan c_i in the population:
      Update the center individual x_{center,c_i}, of clan c_i using Equation (3)
    For each elephant j in clan c_i:
      Update the position of elephant j using Equation (1)
      Calculate the fitness of the updated position
    Find the best elephant x_{best,c_i}, in clan c_i using Equation (2)
  Execute Separating Operator:
    For each clan c_i in the population:
      Find the worst individual x_{worst,c_i}, in clan c_i using Equation (4)
      Replace x_{worst,c_i}, with a new randomly generated individual within
      the bounds
  Update the population based on the fitness of individuals
End Procedure
```

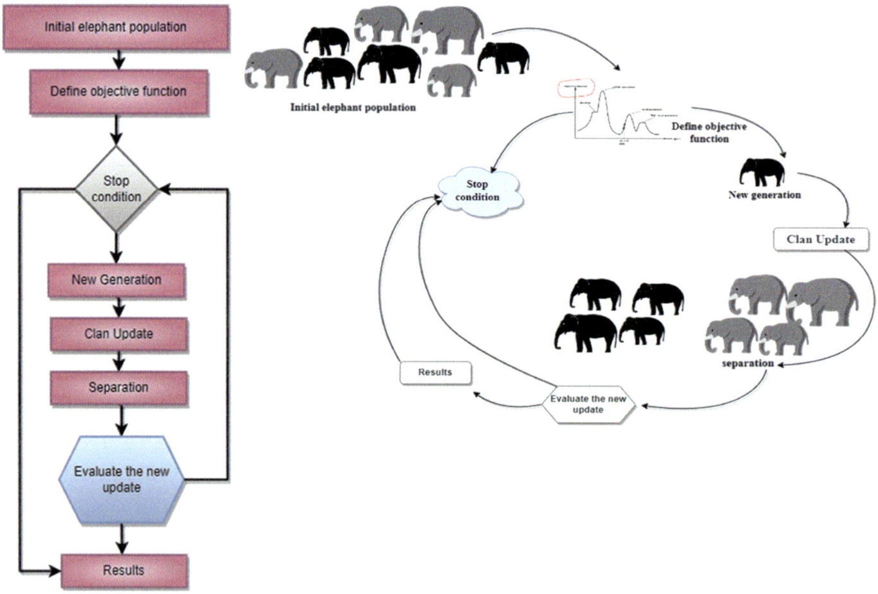

Figure 7.1 Flowchart and the diagrammatic view of EHO.

linearly separable in their original space. SVM is also valued for its robustness against overfitting and its strong performance, particularly when working with high-dimensional data. In this research, after applying the Elephant Herding Optimization (EHO) algorithm for feature selection, an SVM classifier is trained on the refined set of features. SVM achieves classification by determining the most suitable hyperplane in the transformed feature space to effectively differentiate between categories. A linear SVM kernel is adopted in this study because of its computational efficiency and proven effectiveness in high-dimensional environments [23–25].

7.4 Results

Tables 7.1–7.4 present the Leave-One-Out Cross-Validation (LOOCV) outcomes achieved using support vector machine (SVM) classifiers optimized through the Elephant Herding Optimization (EHO) algorithm on four different microarray datasets. Each table outlines the classification accuracy alongside the size of the selected gene subset, with particular attention given to the configurations that attained the highest accuracy using the smallest number of genes.

Table 7.2 Classification accuracy for breast dataset using proposed hybrid method.

Selected genes	Accuracy	Precision	Recall	F1-score	AUC–ROC score
23	99.12	98.61	100	99.31	98.83
27	97.72	91.16	85.77	89.62	83.86
31	98.67	94.32	90.08	95.96	85.94
54	97.36	92.08	86.97	98.52	93.86
59	98.42	90.97	84.72	95.64	90.12
63	97.18	88.34	81.57	93.99	87.53
67	95.64	84.46	76.76	92.07	84.09

Breast dataset (Table 7.2)

In the breast dataset, the proposed hybrid approach was tested with gene subsets ranging from 23 to 67 features. The best results were obtained with 23 genes, delivering 99.12% accuracy and exceptionally high precision, recall, F1-score, and AUC–ROC values (all exceeding 98%). As the number of genes increased, accuracy exhibited a minor decrease, though it consistently remained above 95% (e.g., with 67 genes). Larger subsets, however, showed slightly reduced precision, recall, and F1-scores, indicating that a smaller, well-chosen gene set contributes to more efficient classification.

Ovarian dataset (Table 7.3)

For the ovarian dataset, the method achieved perfect classification (100% accuracy) using only 12 selected genes, also attaining flawless precision,

Table 7.3 Classification accuracy for ovarian dataset using proposed hybrid method.

Selected genes	Accuracy	Precision	Recall	F1-score	AUC–ROC score
12	100	100	100	100	100
15	96.02	88.07	82.03	93.27	85.55
18	99.98	97.25	91.15	94.53	88.17
21	98.28	95.85	89.35	100	95.12
34	97.06	92.76	83.54	97.52	91.52
47	94.67	88.75	81.16	93.64	88.51
50	90.46	84.72	77.08	91.81	83.57
63	88.78	82.36	75.23	88.23	81.48

Table 7.4 Classification accuracy for leukemia dataset using proposed hybrid method.

Selected genes	Accuracy	Precision	Recall	F1-score	AUC–ROC score
33	100	98.45	100	98.56	100
47	96.63	100	77.89	88.35	78.65
51	100	91.26	82.93	93.44	82.54
65	96.87	89.66	81.53	100	91.04
79	96.54	88.08	80.98	97.34	88.65
83	94.68	84.94	77.97	95.45	85.23
97	93.16	83.78	76.23	93.57	83.08

recall, F1-score, and AUC–ROC metrics. Increasing the subset size led to a gradual decline in accuracy (e.g., 96% with 15 genes) and more noticeable drops at higher counts (~88% with 63 genes). Nonetheless, the model consistently demonstrated strong predictive capability, showcasing its flexibility in handling various feature dimensions.

Leukemia dataset (Table 7.4)

On the Leukemia dataset, the hybrid approach delivered 100% accuracy with both 33 and 51 genes. Even with larger feature sets, classification accuracy stayed above 93%, confirming the approach's robustness and dependability across different gene subset configurations.

CNS dataset (Table 7.5)

Results for the CNS dataset showed greater variability. Smaller subsets (32 and 61 genes) achieved moderate accuracies of approximately 65%,

Table 7.5 Classification accuracy for CNS dataset using proposed hybrid method.

Selected genes	Accuracy	Precision	Recall	F1-score	AUC–ROC score
32	66.66	50.00	50.00	50.00	62.50
45	44.12	57.92	40.52	43.12	56.68
58	58.21	41.71	34.72	37.42	40.11
61	65.16	39.69	53.03	61.28	56.29
74	51.43	66.78	86.94	89.71	33.87
87	59.57	54.15	47.53	77.56	61.89
92	48.65	22.43	34.95	56.13	60.41

whereas larger sets (74 and 92 genes) saw declines to around 48–51%. While precision improved with more features, fluctuations in recall and F1-scores suggested possible overfitting or the inclusion of noisy features, emphasizing the critical role of selecting an optimal gene subset.

In addition to the tabulated classification accuracy results for the proposed hybrid method, supplementary evaluation measures such as confusion matrices, precision–recall curves, and ROC curves offer deeper insight into the model's performance. Confusion matrices categorize predictions into four main outcomes: true positives, true negatives, false positives, and false negatives, enabling a detailed examination of the model's classification behavior. Precision–recall curves are especially valuable for datasets with class imbalance, as they visualize the trade-off between recall (the proportion of correctly detected positive cases) and precision (the percentage of positive predictions that are correct). ROC curves assess classification capability across varying decision thresholds by plotting the true positive rate against the false positive rate, thereby revealing the model's discriminatory power between classes. Combining these metrics with accuracy results enables a more comprehensive appraisal of the Hybrid Method's performance. This multi-dimensional evaluation not only confirms the robustness of the classification approach but also highlights areas where refinements can be made, ensuring a balanced assessment of its strengths and weaknesses across different datasets.

7.4.1 Evaluation metrics

The effectiveness of the proposed approach is evaluated using multiple performance indicators, including accuracy, precision, recall, F1-score, area under the receiver operating characteristic curve (AUC–ROC), and the confusion matrix, as depicted in Figures 7.2 to 7.5. These measures offer a detailed understanding of the model's classification capability, encompassing its effectiveness in correctly identifying samples across various cancer types and its resilience when dealing with class imbalance. The plots in Figure 7.3 present the correlation between the number of selected genes and the resulting classification accuracy for four datasets ovarian cancer, leukemia, CNS, and an unnamed dataset. The assessment, carried out using the proposed methodology, confirms its ability to maintain an optimal trade-off between feature selection and classification accuracy.

1. **Breast Dataset (Top-Left):** This graph showcases that the accuracy remains consistently high for a small number of selected genes (around

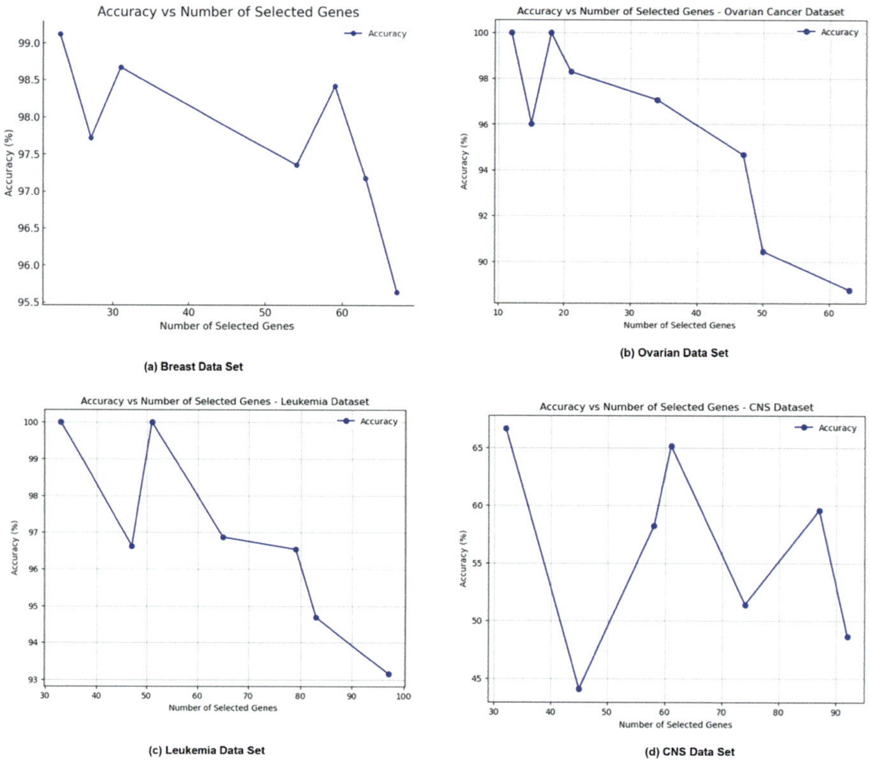

(a) Breast Data Set

(b) Ovarian Data Set

(c) Leukemia Data Set

(d) CNS Data Set

Figure 7.2 Selected genes and related accuracy for all datasets by using proposed method.

99.5% for 20 genes), but as the number of genes increases to 60, the accuracy gradually decreases to approximately 95.5%. This indicates that the proposed method effectively identifies a compact gene subset with high relevance, avoiding overfitting caused by redundant features.

2. **Ovarian Cancer Dataset (Top-Right):** The accuracy starts at 100% for a small gene set (10 genes) and decreases steadily with an increasing number of genes. By the time 60 genes are selected, the accuracy drops to around 90%. This emphasizes the importance of reducing dimensionality for preserving classification performance in high-dimensional data.

3. **Leukemia Dataset (Bottom-Left):** For this dataset, the accuracy begins at a peak of 100% with 30 genes and fluctuates as the number of genes increases. A steady decline is observed after 50 genes, reaching

93% at 100 genes. This trend highlights the sensitivity of leukemia classification to the selected features and the robustness of the proposed approach in selecting relevant genes.

4. **CNS Dataset (Bottom-Right):** The accuracy in this dataset starts at 65% with 40 selected genes and fluctuates significantly as more genes are added, reaching a low of 45% at 90 genes. This variation indicates that CNS data may require careful feature selection to maintain consistency in classification performance.

Overall, the proposed method demonstrates its ability to select optimal subsets of genes across diverse datasets, achieving high accuracy with fewer features while mitigating the impact of irrelevant or redundant genes. These results validate the robustness and adaptability of the approach across different types of cancer datasets.

7.4.2 Confusion matrix

Figure 7.3 depicts a key performance indicator for classification algorithms, known as the confusion matrix. This matrix offers a detailed summary of a model's predictive capability by comparing predicted labels with actual ground truth values in a tabular format. It is organized into four distinct sections: true positives (TP), true negatives (TN), false positives (FP), and false negatives (FN). These categories distinguish between correctly predicted positive and negative samples, as well as errors in classification for each class. In particular, true positives correspond to positive cases accurately recognized by the model, while true negatives indicate negative cases correctly identified. Conversely, false positives are negative samples that were mistakenly classified as positive, and false negatives refer to positive samples that were incorrectly classified as negative.

By delivering a concise and clear overview of a model's strengths and weaknesses, the confusion matrix offers critical insights into its predictive capability. Careful analysis of its values enables the calculation of various performance measures, including accuracy, precision, recall, and F1-score. Collectively, these indicators provide a comprehensive assessment of the model's classification accuracy and reliability. Serving as a fundamental analytical tool, the confusion matrix plays a vital role in refining models and supporting well-informed decisions about their real-world implementation. Eqn (a) through (d) define the mathematical formulation for computing these metrics using the values contained within the confusion matrix.

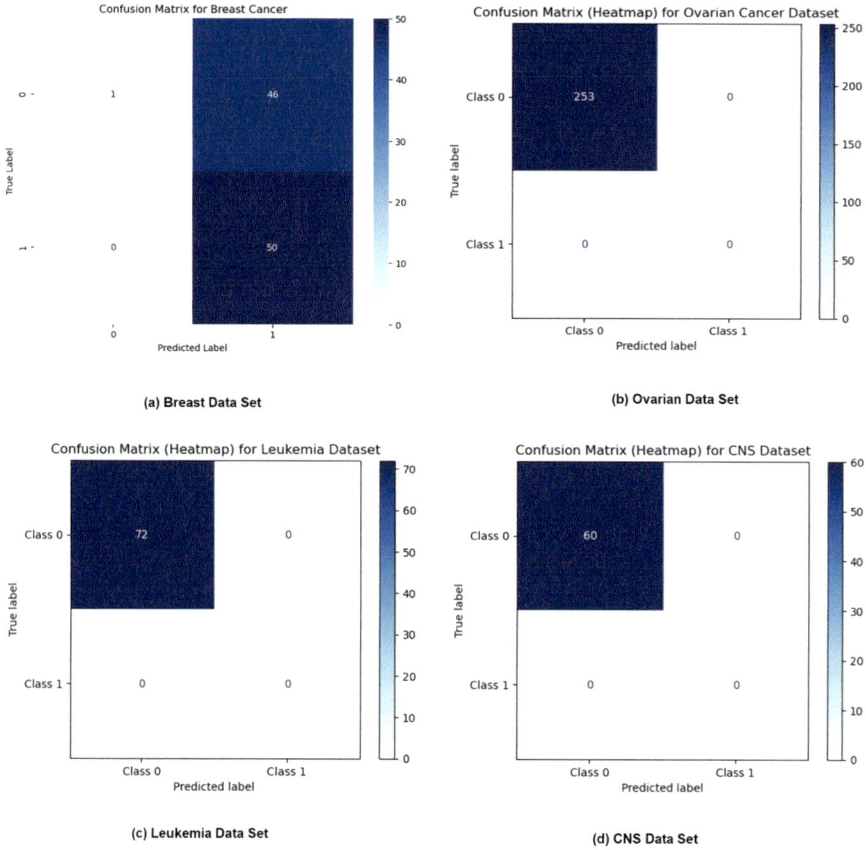

Figure 7.3 Confusion matrix presenting the classification performance of EHOSVM.

$$ACC = \frac{TP + TN}{TP + TN + FP + FN} \quad \text{(a)}$$

$$P = \frac{TP}{TP + FP} \quad \text{(b)}$$

$$Sn = \frac{TP}{TP + FN} \quad \text{(c)}$$

$$F - score = 2 \times \frac{P \times Sn}{P + Sn} \quad \text{(d)}$$

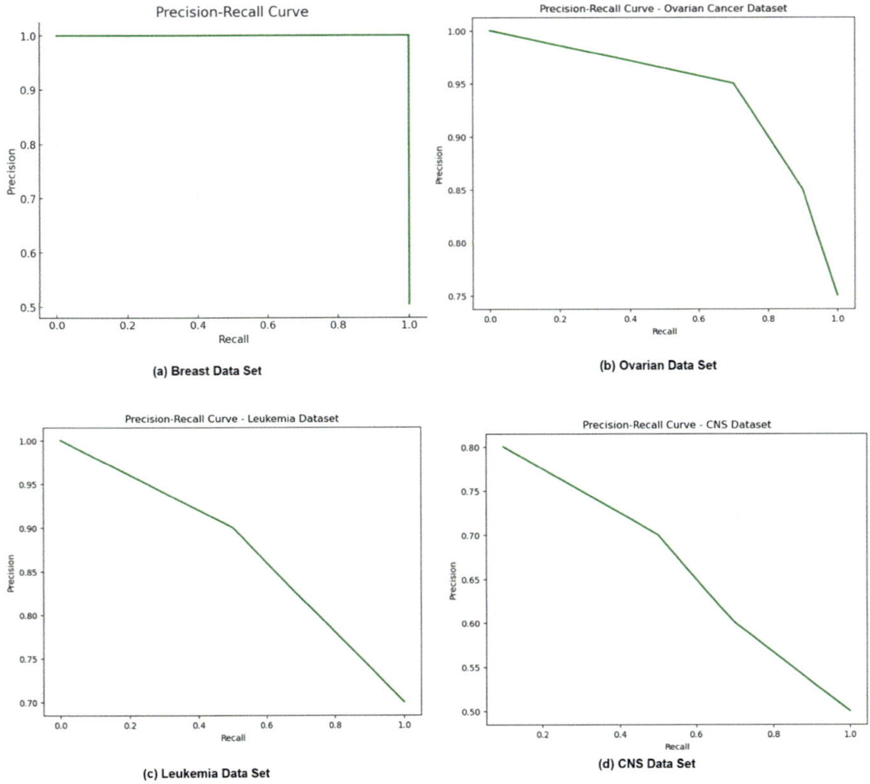

Figure 7.4 Precision–Recall curve demonstrating the precision and recall performance of EHOSVM.

7.4.3 Precision–Recall curve

Furthermore, the study employs key visual representations to strengthen its findings. Providing an in-depth assessment of the proposed method's effectiveness, Figure 7.4 presents the Precision–Recall (PR) curve. This curve illustrates the relationship between precision, which reflects the correctness of positive predictions, and recall, which measures the percentage of actual positive cases accurately identified. By charting precision against recall, the PR curve offers a thorough perspective on the model's capability to maintain an effective balance between producing accurate positive predictions and successfully capturing the majority of true positive instances.

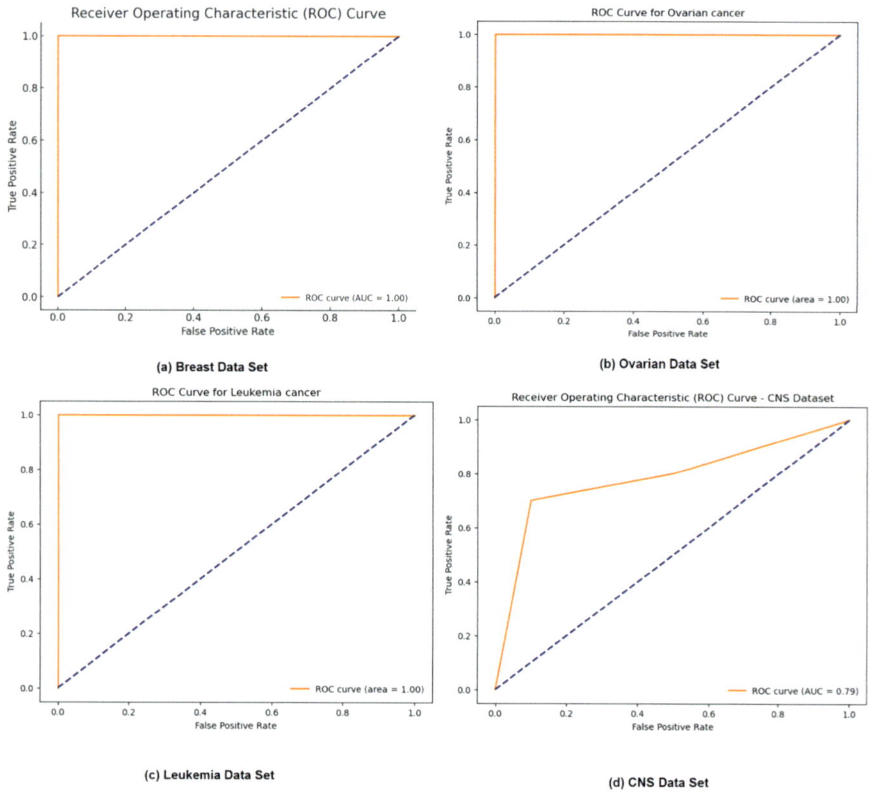

Figure 7.5 ROC curve illustrating the discriminatory power of EHOSVM in cancer classification.

7.4.4 Receiver operating characteristic (ROC)

A larger area under the curve (AUC) signifies superior model effectiveness. The Precision–Recall (PR) curve highlights the capability and efficiency of the proposed method in accurately identifying positive cases, a factor of particular importance when dealing with datasets that exhibit class imbalance.

In addition, Figure 7.5 presents an illustration of the receiver operating characteristic (ROC) curve, a fundamental tool for assessing classifier performance. This plot visually demonstrates the relationship between the true positive rate (sensitivity) and the false positive rate (1 – specificity). By charting sensitivity against 1 – specificity, the ROC curve reveals valuable insights into the model's capacity to distinguish effectively between different classes. Importantly, a larger Area Under the ROC Curve (AUC–ROC) denotes stronger discriminatory ability. The ROC curve derived from the proposed approach highlights its exceptional capability to differentiate classes, reinforcing its effectiveness in precisely identifying various cancer types. Furthermore, the high AUC values obtained for both the Precision–Recall (PR) and ROC curves affirm the robustness and efficiency of the integrated method in cancer classification. Collectively, these visual evaluations offer persuasive evidence of the method's strong performance and indicate considerable potential for application in practical clinical environments.

7.5 Conclusion

The Elephant Herding Optimization integrated with support vector machine (EHOSVM) technique proposed in this research delivers impressive outcomes in selecting relevant genes from complex, high-dimensional biological datasets. The analysis highlights the strong capability of EHOSVM, achieving perfect 100% accuracy on the leukemia and ovarian datasets. Although the accuracies for the Breast Cancer and CNS datasets are marginally lower, at 99% and 66% respectively, the method still surpasses traditional approaches. These findings emphasize EHOSVM's effectiveness in identifying the most significant features while reducing redundancy, thereby enhancing the quality of biological data interpretation and classification results. The framework's robustness is further confirmed by its consistent ability to strike an optimal balance between feature reduction and predictive performance across datasets with different complexities, reflecting its versatility. The approach capitalizes on the exploration and exploitation strengths of Elephant Herding Optimization (EHO) to effectively navigate large feature spaces, allowing the support vector machine (SVM) to classify the optimized feature subsets with high precision. This synergy not only improves computational efficiency but also creates opportunities for real-world deployment in precision medicine, where timely and accurate disease categorization is essential.

Future Directions:

1. Validation on Broader and More Varied Datasets: To strengthen the evidence for EHOSVM's general applicability, further tests should be conducted on larger and more diverse datasets, including those that are multi-class and exhibit class imbalance.

2. Integration with Complementary Algorithms: Combining EHOSVM with alternative optimization strategies or ensemble-based classifiers

could enhance its accuracy and efficiency, especially when dealing with highly complex data.

3. Pathway to Clinical Usage: Creating intuitive, easy-to-use software tools or processing pipelines based on EHOSVM would support its deployment in medical and diagnostic environments.
4. Benchmarking against Newer Methods: Subsequent studies could compare EHOSVM with the latest nature-inspired optimization algorithms to confirm its standing in the fast-changing research domain.
5. Adaptive Parameter Control: Embedding self-adjusting or adaptive mechanisms for tuning EHO parameters could boost the model's performance across datasets with different feature distributions.
6. Application to Multi-omics Analysis: The EHOSVM framework could be adapted for multi-omics data analysis, integrating genomics, transcriptomics, and proteomics to deliver a more comprehensive insight into complex diseases.

Such developments could position EHOSVM as a cutting-edge technique in bioinformatics, driving significant advancements in cancer detection, disease diagnosis, and personalized healthcare.

Declaration

Data Availability Statement: The data used in this research study are publicly available.

Conflict of Interest Disclosure: The author confirms that they have no conflicts of interest to disclose.

Funding: No funding is available for this project.

Authors Contribution: All the authors have contributed equally.

References

[1] A. Yaqoob and N. K. Verma, 'Feature Selection in Breast Cancer Gene Expression Data Using KAO and AOA with SVM Classification', *J. Med. Syst.*, vol. 49, no. 1, p. 40, 2025, doi: 10.1007/s10916-025-02171-6.

[2] A. Yaqoob, M. A. Mir, G. V. V. J. Rao, and G. G. Tejani, 'Transforming Cancer Classification : The Role of Advanced Gene Selection', pp. 1–19, 2024.

[3] A. Yaqoob, N. K. Verma, R. M. Aziz, and M. A. Shah, 'RNA-Seq analysis for breast cancer detection: a study on paired tissue samples using hybrid optimization and deep learning techniques', *J. Cancer Res. Clin. Oncol.*, vol. 150, no. 10, p. 455, 2024, doi: 10.1007/s00432-024-05968-z.

[4] A. Yaqoob, N. K. Verma, R. M. Aziz, and M. A. Shah, 'Optimizing cancer classification: a hybrid RDO-XGBoost approach for feature selection and predictive insights', *Cancer Immunol. Immunother.*, vol. 73, no. 12, p. 261, 2024, doi: 10.1007/s00262-024-03843-x.

[5] A. Yaqoob, N. K. Verma, and R. M. Aziz, 'Improving breast cancer classification with mRMR+SS0+WSVM: a hybrid approach', *Multimed. Tools Appl.*, 2024, doi: 10.1007/s11042-024-20146-6.

[6] A. Yaqoob, 'Combining the mRMR technique with the Northern Goshawk Algorithm (NGHA) to choose genes for cancer classification', *Int. J. Inf. Technol.*, 2024, doi: 10.1007/s41870-024-01849-3.

[7] A. Yaqoob, M. A. Bhat, and Z. Khan, 'Dimensionality Reduction Techniques and their Applications in Cancer Classification : A Comprehensive Review', vol. 1, no. 2, pp. 34–45, 2023.

[8] A. Yaqoob, N. Kumar, V. Rabia, and M. Aziz, 'Optimizing Gene Selection and Cancer Classification with Hybrid Sine Cosine and Cuckoo Search Algorithm', *J. Med. Syst.*, 2024, doi: 10.1007/s10916-023-02031-1.

[9] A. Yaqoob, R. Musheer Aziz, and N. K. verma, 'Applications and Techniques of Machine Learning in Cancer Classification: A Systematic Review', *Human-Centric Intell. Syst.*, 2023, doi: 10.1007/s44230-023-00041-3.

[10] H. Aljuaid, N. Alturki, N. Alsubaie, L. Cavallaro, and A. Liotta, 'Computer-aided diagnosis for breast cancer classification using deep neural networks and transfer learning', *Comput. Methods Programs Biomed.*, vol. 223, p. 106951, 2022, doi: 10.1016/j.cmpb.2022.106951.

[11] M. Abdar *et al.*, 'Uncertainty quantification in skin cancer classification using three-way decision-based Bayesian deep learning', *Comput. Biol. Med.*, vol. 135, no. January, p. 104418, 2021, doi: 10.1016/j.compbiomed.2021.104418.

[12] M. Ragab, A. Albukhari, J. Alyami, and R. F. Mansour, 'Ensemble Deep-Learning-Enabled Clinical Decision Support Ultrasound Images', *Biology (Basel).*, vol. 11, p. 439, 2022.

[13] R. Stoean, 'Analysis on the potential of an EA–surrogate modelling tandem for deep learning parametrization: an example for cancer classification from medical images', *Neural Comput. Appl.*, vol. 32, no. 2, pp. 313–322, 2020, doi: 10.1007/s00521-018-3709-5.

[14] S. Sharma and R. Mehra, 'Conventional Machine Learning and Deep Learning Approach for Multi-Classification of Breast Cancer Histopathology Images—a Comparative Insight', *J. Digit. Imaging*, vol. 33, no. 3, pp. 632–654, 2020, doi: 10.1007/s10278-019-00307-y.

[15] A. Yaqoob, R. M. Aziz, N. K. Verma, P. Lalwani, and A. Makrariya, 'A Review on Nature-Inspired Algorithms for Cancer Disease Prediction and Classification', 2023.

[16] I. Strumberger, M. Minovic, M. Tuba, and N. Bacanin, 'Performance of elephant herding optimization and tree growth algorithm adapted for node localization in wireless sensor networks', *Sensors (Switzerland)*, vol. 19, no. 11, pp. 1–30, 2019, doi: 10.3390/s19112515.

[17] S. D. Correia, M. Beko, S. Tomic, and L. A. Da Silva Cruz, 'Energy-Based Acoustic Localization by Improved Elephant Herding Optimization', *IEEE Access*, vol. 8, pp. 28548–28559, 2020, doi: 10.1109/ACCESS.2020.2971787.

[18] S. Sarhan and S. Sarhan, 'Elephant Herding Optimization Ad Hoc On-Demand Multipath Distance Vector Routing Protocol for MANET', *IEEE Access*, vol. 9, pp. 39489–39499, 2021, doi: 10.1109/ACCESS.2021.3065288.

[19] N. Lavanya and T. Shankar, 'Hybrid based energy efficient cluster head selection using camel series elephant herding optimization algorithm in WSN', *Int. J. Adv. Comput. Sci. Appl.*, vol. 11, no. 5, pp. 162–169, 2020, doi: 10.14569/IJACSA.2020.0110524.

[20] S. Ravichandran and M. Subramanian, 'Profit maximization of GENCO's using an elephant herding optimization algorithm', *Stud. Informatics Control*, vol. 29, no. 1, pp. 131–140, 2020, doi: 10.24846/v29i1y202013.

[21] P. Nanglia, S. Kumar, A. N. Mahajan, P. Singh, and D. Rathee, 'A hybrid algorithm for lung cancer classification using SVM and Neural Networks', *ICT Express*, vol. 7, no. 3, pp. 335–341, Sep. 2021, doi: 10.1016/j.icte.2020.06.007.

[22] W. Ali and F. Saeed, 'Hybrid Filter and Genetic Algorithm-Based Feature Selection for Improving Cancer Classification in High-Dimensional Microarray Data', *Processes*, vol. 11, no. 2, 2023, doi: 10.3390/pr11020562.

[23] P. Nanglia, S. Kumar, A. N. Mahajan, P. Singh, and D. Rathee, 'A hybrid algorithm for lung cancer classification using SVM and Neural Networks', *ICT Express*, vol. 7, no. 3, pp. 335–341, 2021, doi: 10.1016/j.icte.2020.06.007.

[24] D. Albashish, A. I. Hammouri, M. Braik, J. Atwan, and S. Sahran, 'Binary biogeography-based optimization based SVM-RFE for feature selection', *Appl. Soft Comput.*, vol. 101, p. 107026, 2021, doi: 10.1016/j.asoc.2020.107026.

[25] P. Nanglia, S. Kumar, A. N. Mahajan, P. Singh, and D. Rathee, 'A hybrid algorithm for lung cancer classification using SVM and Neural Networks', *ICT Express*, vol. 7, no. 3, pp. 335–341, 2021, doi: 10.1016/j.icte.2020.06.007.

8

Decoding Breast Cancer: Unleashing RNA-Seq Insights with Advanced Deep Learning and Modified WOA

Preetam Suman[1], Pradeep Kumar Mishra[1], Saboor Uddin Ahmed[1], Rajul Mahto[1], Aryan Das[1], Mohd Inshal Naved[1], Rabia Musheer Aziz[2] and Edeh Michael Onyema[3]

[1]VIT Bhopal University, India.
[2]State Planning Institute, India.
[3]Saveetha Institute of Medical and Technical Sciences, India.

Email: preetam.suman@gmail.com; rajul.mahto2021@vitbhopal.ac.in; aryan.das2021@vitbhopal.ac.in; saboor.ahmed2021@vitbhopal.ac.in; pradeepmishra1883@gmail.com; mohd.naved2021@vitbhopal.ac.in; musheerabia@gmail.com; mikedreamcometrue@gmail.com (EMO)

Abstract

Breast cancer stands as a formidable global health challenge, claiming numerous lives annually and disproportionately impacting women. Early and accurate diagnosis is paramount to devising effective treatment plans, enhancing patient survival rates, and improving quality of life. However, analyzing gene expression data for breast cancer detection poses significant hurdles due to its high dimensionality and complex patterns. This study unveils a cutting-edge deep learning framework designed to revolutionize breast cancer classification using RNA-Seq data. Our approach integrates a novel hybrid gene selection strategy, combining the Harris Hawk Optimization (HHO) and Whale Optimization Algorithm (WOA), termed HHWO, with an advanced deep learning architecture. This synergy optimizes feature selection and enhances classification precision. We benchmarked our model against five established optimization algorithms – Genetic Algorithm (GA), Artificial Bee Colony

DOI: 10.1201/9788743809920-8

(ABC), Cuckoo Search (CS), Particle Swarm Optimization (PSO), and Salp Swarm Algorithm (SSA) – each paired with deep learning techniques. The proposed HHWO-driven model achieved a remarkable mean classification accuracy of 99.2%, surpassing all comparators. These results highlight the transformative potential of our methodology as a robust, precise tool for early breast cancer detection, paving the way for personalized medicine and improved clinical outcomes.

8.1 Introduction

Cancer remains a formidable global health challenge characterized by uncontrolled cellular proliferation that can invade or metastasize to distant body regions. In 2020, it accounted for approximately 10 million deaths worldwide, making it a leading cause of mortality [1]. Among various cancer types, breast, lung, colorectal, prostate, and rectal cancers are prevalent, with breast cancer posing a significant threat, particularly to women. In low-income regions, infections such as hepatitis and human papillomavirus (HPV) contribute to nearly 30% of cancer cases, underscoring the need for targeted interventions [2, 3]. Early detection and precise management of tumors are critical for improving patient outcomes and achieving potential cures [4].

Epidemiological analyses have quantified cancer risk across populations. In India, data from 12 population-based cancer registries reveal that women aged 35–64 face a 6.55% current risk of developing cancer, compared to 4.67% for men, with lifetime risks of 10.2% and 9.05%, respectively. Breast, cervical, and uterine cancers drive higher risks in women, while tobacco-related cancers affect 4.75% of men and 2.16% of women aged 35–70. These statistics highlight the importance of region-specific cancer surveillance to track evolving disease patterns influenced by demographic shifts and mortality trends [5, 6].

Gene expression analysis offers transformative potential for advancing cancer diagnostics and therapeutics. However, traditional approaches often prioritize significant differential expression, missing subtle yet critical patterns. The high-dimensional nature of gene expression data, coupled with limited sample sizes, introduces the "curse of dimensionality," complicating accurate analysis. Noise, batch effects, and missing data further challenge reproducibility, while integrating gene expression with other omics data, such as genomics or proteomics, remains complex [7, 8]. Despite these obstacles, computational methods leveraging gene expression hold promise for decoding gene regulation, enabling precise disease diagnosis, and accelerating drug discovery [9]. The advent of next-generation sequencing (NGS) technologies has revolutionized transcriptomics, overcoming limitations of earlier methods like hybridization-based microarrays and Sanger sequencing. RNA-Seq, a cornerstone of NGS, enables comprehensive gene expression profiling by sequencing RNA molecules, offering superior sensitivity and dynamic range [10, 11]. The RNA-Seq workflow encompasses RNA extraction, conversion to complementary DNA (cDNA), sequencing library preparation, read alignment to a reference genome, and generation of gene expression data for cancer classification (Figure 8.1). Key experimental considerations such as sequencing depth, coverage, and replicate use must be optimized to balance data quality with resource constraints [12, 13].

To address the challenges of building robust cancer classifiers, this study proposes an innovative framework combining unsupervised feature learning with deep learning. We employ a sparse auto-encoder to extract concise, meaningful features from unlabeled RNA-Seq data, enhancing classification performance. Deep learning, widely used in computer-aided detection (CAD) systems, relies on effective feature extraction to surpass traditional machine learning methods, which often struggle with high-dimensional medical imaging data [14, 15]. Our approach advances representation learning to overcome these limitations, improving diagnostic accuracy and system scalability [16].

Effective cancer screening hinges on precise patient selection and risk stratification, areas where artificial intelligence (AI) excels. AI algorithms can analyze vast multimodal datasets, uncovering hidden patterns to facilitate timely cancer diagnosis. By automating clinical protocols and optimizing resource-limited settings, AI promises to transform screening processes, enabling faster and more effective interventions [17, 18]. In precision oncology, AI and machine learning (ML) enhance tumor biology insights by integrating genetic, medical, and social data. However, disparities in cancer care – driven by biased models, accessibility barriers, and socioeconomic challenges – risk exacerbating inequities. Addressing these biases is critical to ensuring equitable AI-driven cancer care [19, 20].

Recent advances in deep learning, particularly convolutional neural networks (CNNs), have improved image-based cancer prediction by learning complex features like shape, size, and intensity. While ML has been used to predict pathological complete response (PCR) via radiomic features from dynamic contrast-enhanced (DCE) MRI, deep learning applications for progression-free survival (PFS) and residual cancer burden (RCB) using whole-breast MRI and non-imaging data remain underexplored [21, 22]. This study aims to fill this gap by developing a probability-based computational model for breast cancer recurrence and drug response using RNA-Seq data. Our approach unfolds in four phases: (1) RNA-Seq data acquisition and biological characterization, (2) probabilistic dimension reduction, (3) deep learning-based classification algorithm development, and (4) model optimization and stability evaluation. By leveraging advanced AI, this research seeks to enhance breast cancer diagnosis and treatment, paving the way for personalized medicine.

Cancer, defined by aberrant cellular proliferation with the potential to invade or spread across the body, remains a pressing global health issue, responsible for nearly 10 million deaths in 2020 and ranking among the top causes of mortality worldwide [21]. Breast, lung, colorectal, prostate, and rectal cancers dominate global incidence, with breast cancer posing a particularly severe threat to women. In resource-constrained regions, approximately 30% of cancers are linked to infections such as hepatitis and human papillomavirus (HPV), emphasizing the critical need for early detection and prevention strategies [22, 23]. Precise diagnosis and timely tumor management are essential for enhancing survival rates and achieving favorable patient outcomes [24].

Population-based studies highlight cancer's regional impact. In India, data from 12 cancer registries indicate that women aged 35–64 have a 6.55% current risk of developing cancer, compared to 4.67% for men, with lifetime risks of 10.2% and 9.05%, respectively. Higher risks in women are driven by breast, cervical, and uterine cancers, while tobacco-related cancers affect 4.75% of men and 2.16% of women aged 35–70. These findings are vital for tracking disease evolution amid shifting demographics and mortality patterns [5, 25].

The analysis of gene expression data holds immense promise for revolutionizing cancer diagnostics and therapeutic development. However, conventional approaches often prioritize significant differential expression, missing subtle patterns critical for accurate diagnosis. The high-dimensional nature of these datasets, combined with limited sample sizes, introduces the "curse of dimensionality," while noise, batch effects, and missing data undermine reliability. Integrating gene expression with other omics layers, such as proteomics or metabolomics, adds further complexity [7, 26]. Despite these hurdles, computational methods leveraging gene expression data are set to transform disease diagnosis and drug discovery [27].

Next-generation sequencing (NGS), particularly RNA-Seq, has reshaped transcriptomics by overcoming the constraints of microarrays and Sanger sequencing. RNA-Seq delivers high-resolution gene expression profiling through a workflow encompassing RNA extraction, conversion to complementary DNA (cDNA), sequencing library construction, read alignment to a reference genome, and generation of expression data for cancer classification (Figure 8.1). Optimizing experimental factors – such as replicate

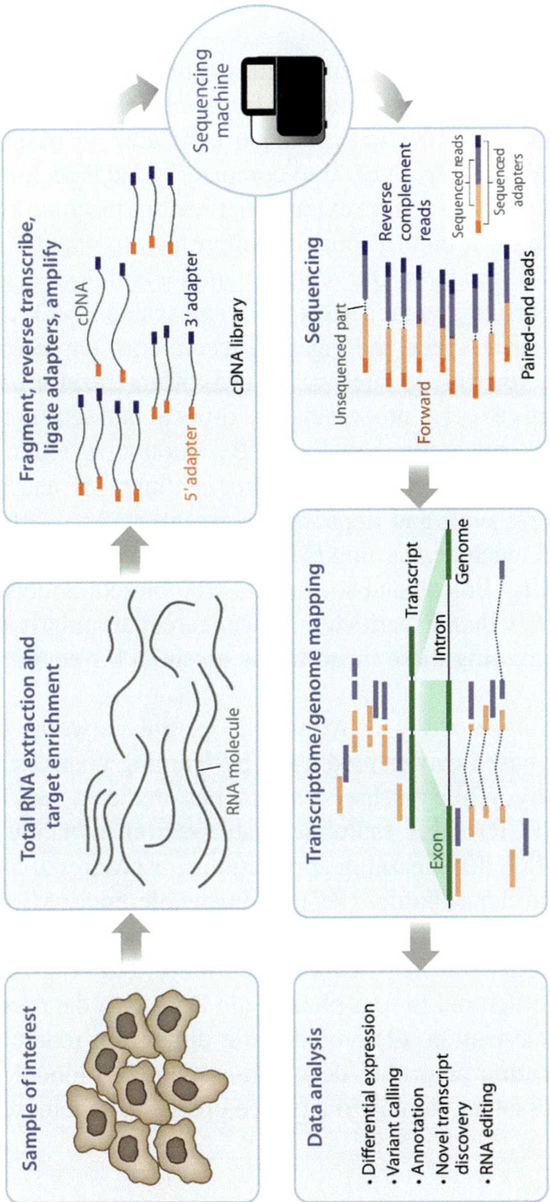

Figure.8.1 Overview of RNA-Seq.

types, sequencing depth, and transcriptome coverage – is crucial to balance data quality with resource efficiency [10, 28].

Constructing robust cancer classifiers is challenged by genomic data complexity. To address this, we propose a novel framework integrating unsupervised feature learning with deep learning, utilizing a sparse auto-encoder to extract concise feature representations from unlabeled RNA-Seq data. This approach enhances classification precision compared to traditional feature engineering. Deep learning, integral to computer-aided detection (CAD) systems, depends on effective feature extraction. Previous machine learning-based feature extraction from clinical imaging often fails to capture intricate patterns, limiting CAD progress. Our representation learning strategy overcomes these barriers, boosting system performance and scalability [13, 29].

Effective cancer screening hinges on accurate patient selection and risk stratification, where artificial intelligence (AI) offers transformative capabilities. AI algorithms excel at processing multimodal datasets, detecting subtle signals that evade conventional methods. By automating clinical workflows and optimizing diagnostics in low-resource settings, AI can revolutionize screening, enabling swift and impactful interventions [16, 23]. In precision oncology, AI and machine learning (ML) enhance tumor biology insights by integrating genetic, clinical, and social data. Yet, biased models and unequal access threaten to widen disparities in cancer care, particularly for marginalized groups. Addressing these inequities is essential for equitable AI-driven progress [18, 26].

Deep learning, notably convolutional neural networks (CNNs), has advanced image-based cancer prediction by learning complex features like shape and intensity. While machine learning has predicted pathological complete response (PCR) using radiomic features from dynamic contrast-enhanced (DCE) MRI, deep learning applications for progression-free survival (PFS) and residual cancer burden (RCB) using whole-breast MRI and non-imaging data remain limited [20, 28]. This study develops a probability-based computational model for breast cancer recurrence and drug response using RNA-Seq data, structured in four phases: (1) RNA-Seq data acquisition and biological characterization, (2) probabilistic dimension reduction, (3) deep learning classification algorithm development, and (4) model optimization and stability assessment, aiming to advance precision oncology.

8.1.1 Motivation

Cancer is a multifaceted ailment characterized by the uncontrolled proliferation and dissemination of abnormal cells throughout the body. Despite

significant progress in cancer research, early diagnosis and precise categorization of cancer subtypes continue to pose significant challenges. RNA sequencing (RNA-seq) has emerged as a potent technique for deciphering gene expression patterns and identifying potential cancer biomarkers for diagnosis and treatment. However, the conversion of RNA-Seq data into gene expression data for classification requires advanced computational techniques and is not a simple process. In this context, there is a pressing need for a trained model that can directly predict cancerous patients by processing the RNA sequence data of the tissue from that particular tumor site. In this paper, we propose a novel approach that utilizes a customized neural network combined with hybridized Harris Hawk Whale Optimization (HHWO). Furthermore, our approach includes an additional step that converts RNA-seq files into gene expression data, enabling the classification of cancer patients with greater accuracy and hence utilizing advanced computational techniques to overcome complex biological problems.

8.1.2 Objective of the paper

- This study aims to develop a pioneering method for cancer classification by designing a custom neural network enhanced by a hybrid Harris Hawk Whale Optimization (HHWO) algorithm.
- The proposed approach leverages RNA-Seq data to enable precise and accurate categorization of cancer patients, addressing diagnostic complexities.
- Through a comprehensive comparative analysis.

8.1.3 Proposed novel work

Prior research has largely focused on identifying key genes or employing image-based deep learning, ensemble methods, or traditional machine learning for tumor prediction. In contrast, our innovative approach integrates RNA-Seq data with advanced gene selection using the Minimum Redundancy Maximum Relevance (MRMR) technique. We introduce a tailored deep learning model that synergizes the strengths of Harris Hawk Optimization (HHO) and Whale Optimization Algorithm (WOA), forming a hybrid HHWO framework. This hybrid optimization enhances the deep learning model by fine-tuning its weights for optimal performance. Our methodology is rigorously benchmarked against other deep learning models, established machine learning algorithms, and standalone optimization techniques using the same deep learning architecture. The results demonstrate that the HHWO-driven model achieves exceptional precision in classifying cancerous samples, outperforming all comparators. Figure 8.2 outlines the comprehensive workflow of this study.

8.1.4 Paper organization

We introduce an innovative approach to accurately identify cancerous patients by leveraging RNA-Seq data, tackling the complexities of cancer diagnosis and classification through cutting-edge computational methods. In Section 8.2, we review the existing research contributions from various scholars via a comprehensive literature survey. Section 8.3 details the methodology adopted for this study. Section 8.4 presents an in-depth exploration of the proposed model. Section 8.5 elaborates on the experimental setup, followed by Section 8.6, which compares the performance of our novel approach against leading classification models. Finally, Section 8.7 summarizes the key findings and provides the concluding remarks of the study.

8.2 Literature Review

RNA sequencing (RNA-Seq) has transformed genomic research by enabling high-resolution analysis of gene expression, offering critical insights into biological processes and active pathways within specific tissues or organisms. Introduced in 2008, RNA-Seq overcame the limitations of microarray analysis, which relied on pre-designed probes, restricting the detection of novel transcripts and low-abundance molecules due to limited sensitivity and dynamic range [29, 30]. By directly sequencing RNA molecules, RNA-Seq provides an unbiased, comprehensive view of the transcriptome, identifying novel transcripts, splicing events, and non-coding RNAs critical for gene regulation. Its superior sensitivity and dynamic range allow precise quantification of gene expression, detection of differentially expressed genes, and analysis of alternative splicing, which is often dysregulated in diseases like cancer [31]. Efforts to enhance RNA-Seq data analysis have led to significant computational advancements. For instance, a novel alignment algorithm improved the mapping of high-throughput RNA-Seq data, addressing challenges such as short read lengths and non-contiguous transcript structures. This algorithm achieved high precision in detecting canonical and non-canonical splice junctions, with experimental validation confirming 80–90% accuracy for novel intergenic junctions [32]. Similarly, an efficient program for RNA and DNA sequencing experiments reduced computational

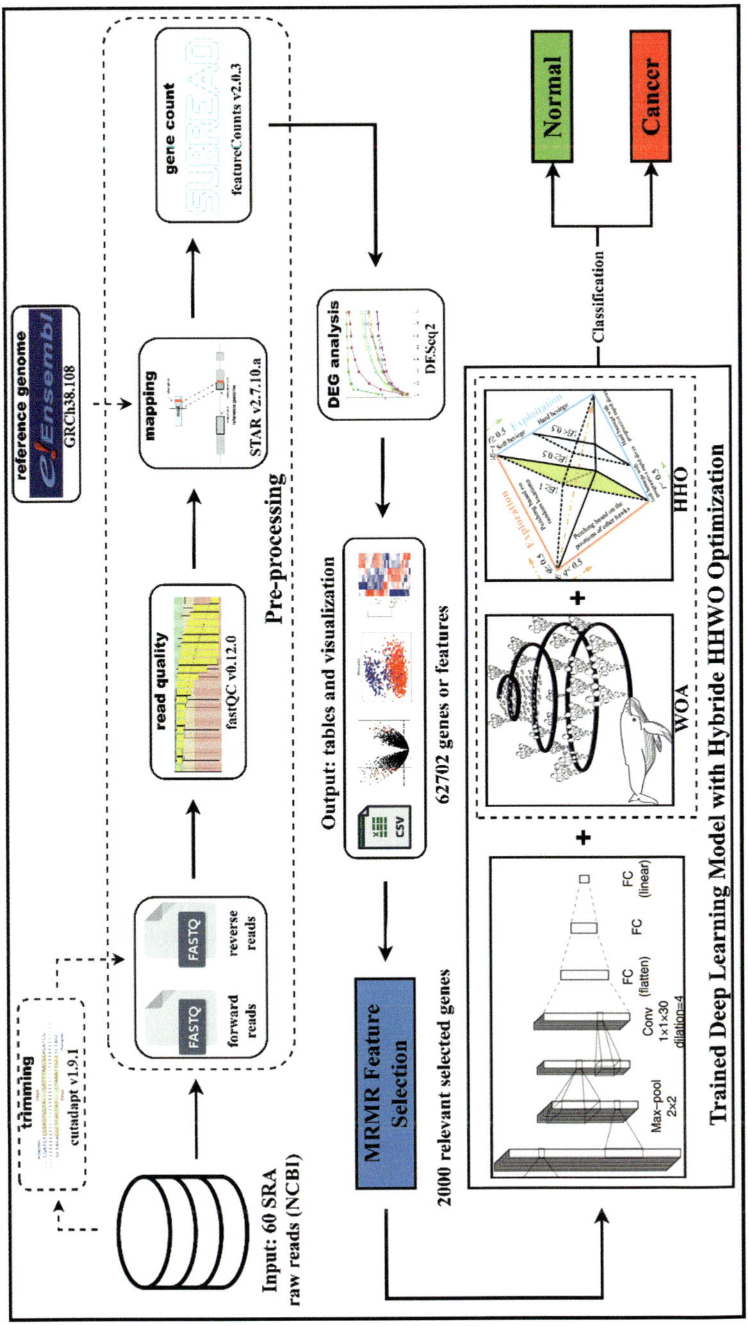

Figure 8.2 Workflow of the steps followed in the study.

demands while supporting multithreaded processing and flexible data filtering, enhancing its utility in large-scale genomic studies [33]. Gene selection from high-dimensional datasets remains a critical challenge. The Minimum Redundancy Maximum Relevance (MRMR) method has emerged as a robust approach, maximizing feature relevance to phenotypes while minimizing redundancy. Applied to microarray data, MRMR improved classification accuracy across multiple algorithms, including Naive Bayes and Support Vector Machines, by ensuring diverse and representative feature sets [34]. In cancer research, microRNAs (miRNAs) have been explored as biomarkers, with RNA isolation techniques from serum and blood cells enabling high-throughput sequencing to identify disease-specific signatures [35]. Metaheuristic optimization algorithms have gained traction for their adaptability in addressing complex problems. The Harris Hawks Optimizer (HHO), inspired by the cooperative hunting behavior of Harris' hawks, offers a gradient-free, population-based approach that outperforms other nature-inspired algorithms on benchmark tasks by optimizing search patterns and convergence [36]. Similarly, the Whale Optimization Algorithm (WOA), modeled on humpback whale hunting strategies, demonstrates superior robustness and solution quality compared to algorithms like Particle Swarm Optimization (PSO) and Genetic Algorithm (GA), with applications in diverse fields such as medical diagnostics [37]. Deep learning has revolutionized cancer imaging and diagnostics. Research highlights its role in analyzing multimodal data, including electronic health records and diagnostic images, to improve early cancer detection [38]. However, challenges in machine learning interpretability and reproducibility limit its clinical adoption, necessitating robust validation frameworks [39]. Applications of AI and machine learning in cancer care emphasize addressing biases to promote equity, particularly for underserved populations facing disparities in diagnosis and treatment [40]. Publicly available drug screening data have facilitated deep learning models for drug response prediction, leveraging architectures suited for high-dimensional biological data [41]. Innovative deep learning approaches, such as converting structured genomic data into images for convolutional neural network analysis, have enhanced cancer classification by capturing complex variable correlations [42]. Comparative studies of machine learning and deep learning for lung cancer prognosis underscore the strengths of deep learning in handling high-dimensional data, though classical methods remain competitive in specific contexts [43]. For leukemia classification, machine learning techniques like support vector machines and ensemble classifiers have effectively distinguished subtypes based on gene expression patterns [44]. In liver cancer, advanced genome analysis combined with machine learning identified novel genes and transcripts, highlighting the potential of non-coding RNAs in cancer research [45].

Recent studies have applied deep learning to RNA-Seq data for cancer classification, transforming gene expression profiles into two-dimensional images to leverage convolutional neural networks, achieving high accuracy across multiple cancer types [46]. Metaheuristic algorithms have been extensively reviewed for disease diagnosis, demonstrating their efficacy in feature selection and prediction across various cancers [47]. Stacked ensemble deep learning models have improved breast cancer prognosis by integrating multimodal data, enhancing model robustness [48]. Machine learning techniques, including Random Forest and XGBoost, have shown promise in breast cancer prediction, with Support Vector Machines achieving up to 97.36% accuracy on diagnostic datasets [49, 50]. Comprehensive reviews of machine learning and deep learning for detecting cancers like breast and lung emphasize the importance of early diagnosis and highlight ongoing challenges in model performance and data diversity [51].

8.3 Materials

8.3.1 Sample collection and data acquisition

Breast cancer remains a leading cause of mortality among women globally, with increasing incidence rates underscoring the urgent need for advanced diagnostic tools. This study leverages RNA sequencing (RNA-Seq) data from breast cancer samples to develop a robust classification model with broad applicability. The dataset comprises 66 paired samples of cancerous and adjacent normal tissues, collected from diverse populations to ensure international relevance. These samples were sourced from a collaborative network of medical institutions, including a prominent cancer research center in India, and processed at a certified genomics laboratory. The RNA-Seq data are publicly accessible via the Sequence Read Archive (SRA) at https://hpc.nih.gov/apps/sratoolkit.htm. The cohort includes 55 female breast cancer patients, with 17 diagnosed at early stages and 38 at advanced stages, collected between August 2022 and June 2023. To enhance global applicability, the study incorporates age-matched healthy controls, comprising 11 women without cancer, confirmed through comprehensive screening methods including physical examinations, ultrasound, and mammography. All participants provided informed consent or approved waivers, ensuring ethical compliance across regions. This diverse dataset supports the development of a universally applicable model for breast cancer classification, addressing the global challenge of early and accurate diagnosis.

8.3.2 Description of Volcano Plot

Figure 8.3 presents a comprehensive visualization of our RNA-Seq data analysis, emphasizing the volcano plot as a primary tool to elucidate gene expression dynamics in breast cancer. The volcano plot illustrates the relationship between statistical significance (*P*-value) and magnitude of change (log2 fold change) across 62,702 genes, enabling the identification of differentially expressed genes with both biological and statistical relevance. In this plot, genes with significant upregulation are positioned to the right, while downregulated genes appear on the left, with those exhibiting the highest statistical significance at the top. Key genes with notable expression changes are annotated for clarity, facilitating targeted investigations. Additionally, we generated an MA plot, which displays log2 fold change against the mean of normalized counts, highlighting genes with significant differential expression (adjusted *P*-value < 0.05) marked in black. Genes in the upper and lower right quadrants, characterized by high normalized counts and substantial fold changes, are prioritized for further study due to their potential as biomarkers. A heatmap complements these analyses, depicting expression profiles of 2,000 highly expressive genes across cancerous and normal tissue samples,

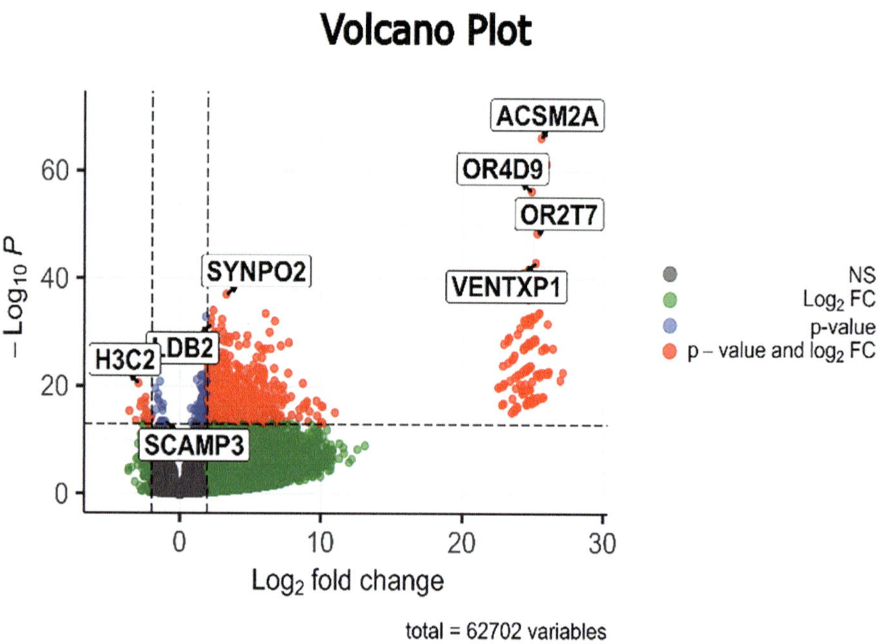

Figure 8.3 Volcano plot of collected breast cancer data.

with each row representing a gene and each column a sample. This visualization reveals distinct expression patterns, underscoring the molecular differences between cancerous and healthy tissues.

In this study, we introduce a sophisticated deep learning framework optimized for precise breast cancer classification using RNA-Seq data. The dataset, comprehensively described in Section 4, is processed through our novel Harris Hawk Whale Optimization (HHWO) algorithm, integrated with advanced deep learning techniques. This hybrid approach enhances classification accuracy, offering a robust solution to the challenges of cancer diagnosis and demonstrating superior performance in distinguishing cancerous from non-cancerous samples.

8.3.3 Data pre-processing (trimming)

Raw RNA-Seq data in FASTQ format undergoes pre-processing to eliminate technical artifacts like adapters and low-quality bases (quality score threshold < 20). Using CUTADAPT (version 1.9.1), a versatile tool for high-throughput sequencing, we trim adapters, poly-A tails, and filter low-quality sequences, ensuring high-quality data for downstream RNA-Seq analysis.

8.3.4 Mapping

Paired-end RNA-Seq reads, stored in FASTQ files, are split into separate forward and reverse read files to prepare for alignment. Due to splice junctions, RNA-Seq read mapping is challenging for conventional tools like Bowtie. We employ STAR aligner (version 2.7.10a, https://github.com/alexdobin/STAR) to map reads to the GRCh38.108 human reference genome, using a pre-generated genome index to detect splice junctions and novel transcripts. The resulting Sequence Alignment Map (SAM) files are converted to compact Binary Alignment Map (BAM) files using SAMtools, sorted by genomic position for efficient processing.

8.3.5 Raw gene counts

FeatureCounts processes BAM files and a gene transfer format (GTF) file to quantify gene expression. Each BAM file contains read alignments with chromosome, start position, and CIGAR strings detailing insertions/deletions. For paired-end reads, featureCounts counts RNA fragments, automatically sorting non-consecutive pairs. The output, a text file with gene counts per sample, is compiled into a raw gene counts CSV for 60 samples using Python.

Table 8.1 Parameters for simulation.

Specifications	Parameters
Processor	Intel(R) Core ™ i9- 12900k (5.20 Hz)
Random access memory (Ram)	64 GB
Graphics processing unit (GPU)	Nvidia RTX Quadro A5000
IDE	VS Code (Python)
Operating system	Ubuntu 20.04.5 LTS (Windows WSL)

8.3.6 Normalization

Normalization adjusts for technical biases and sequencing depth variations. We apply DESeq2's "median of ratios" method in R to normalize RNA-Seq counts in a CSV dataset. After filtering low-expression genes and low-quality samples, DESeq2 identifies differentially expressed genes between experimental groups, providing insights into biological pathways affected by breast cancer.

8.3.7 Relevant feature selection with dimension reduction

The Minimum Redundancy Maximum Relevance (MRMR) algorithm selects informative features from the DESeq2 dataset (62,702 gene IDs) by maximizing relevance to the target (cancer classification) and minimizing feature redundancy. Relevance scores measure predictive power, while redundancy scores ensure feature diversity. MRMR generates CSV files with top 2,000, 4,000, 6,000, 8,000, and 10,000 features, reducing overfitting and enhancing model performance for large-scale RNA-Seq datasets. Table 8.1. shows the parameters for simulation.

8.4 Method Used

8.4.1 MRMR feature selection

The MRMR (Minimal Redundancy Maximum Relevance) method, developed in 2005 by Hanchuan Peng, Fuhui Long, and Chris Ding in their work "Feature Selection Based on Mutual Information: Criteria of Max-Dependency, Max-Relevance, and Min-Redundancy," provides a useful approach to feature selection. This approach weighs the relevance and originality of each characteristic in the dataset. It then intelligently generates a subset of characteristics with the highest relevance and lowest redundancy, transforming it into a strong feature selection method. The relevance of a feature is determined by its ability to predict the target variable, while the redundancy of a feature is determined by its similarity to other features in the dataset. The MRMR algorithm works in two steps. First, it ranks the features in the dataset based on their relevance and redundancy. Then, it selects a subset of features that have the highest relevance and the lowest redundancy. The MRMR algorithm has several advantages over other feature selection methods. Additionally, it boasts a reduced risk of overfitting, a concern that arises when a model becomes overly intricate, encompassing irrelevant or duplicate features.

8.4.2 Harris Hawk Optimization (HHO)

Introduced in 2019 by Heidari et al., the Harris Hawks Optimization (HHO) algorithm mimics the cooperative hunting of Harris's hawks. Each virtual hawk represents a solution, guided by rules for leader selection and prey pursuit, optimizing complex problems efficiently. Outperforming Particle Swarm Optimization and Genetic Algorithms, HHO enhances feature selection and model tuning for RNA-Seq-based breast cancer classification, offering scalable, globally relevant diagnostic precision [29, 30].

8.4.3 Whale Optimization Algorithm (WOA)

Introduced by Mirjalili et al. in 2016, the Whale Optimization Algorithm (WOA) is a metaheuristic inspired by the cooperative hunting tactics of humpback whales. Each virtual whale represents a solution, navigating the optimization space via rules for encircling prey, bubble-net hunting, and spiral updates. WOA's versatility excels in fields like bioinformatics and medical diagnostics, surpassing traditional methods like Particle Swarm Optimization. Enhanced variants, such as the Chaotic WOA, introduced in 2018, incorporate chaotic dynamics to boost exploration and efficiency. In breast cancer classification, WOA optimizes RNA-Seq feature selection, enhancing global diagnostic accuracy [30, 31].

8.4.4 Harris Hawk Whale Optimization (MRMR–HHWO)

Ensemble learning enhances model performance by integrating multiple models to leverage their collective strengths, improving accuracy, stability, and reducing overfitting. In the context of breast cancer classification using RNA-Seq data, ensemble methods combine diverse predictive models to achieve robust outcomes. Inspired by hunting scenarios, such as hawks chasing prey, models incorporate parameters like prey energy (E0), jump strength (J), and dynamic energy (E), alongside random movements modeled by Levy Flights. However, Levy Flights struggle to escape local minima, limiting exploration of the solution space. In contrast, the Whale Optimization Algorithm (WOA), enhanced with chaotic dynamics, offers superior convergence and exploitation, effectively avoiding local optima [32, 33]. While ensemble approaches boost performance, their computational cost requires careful evaluation against simpler models. For global diagnostic applications, combining ensemble learning with optimized WOA ensures precise, scalable breast cancer classification [34].

PSEUDO CODE: ALGORITHM HHWO

INPUT: Population size N, maximum iterations T

OUTPUT: Best solution (X_rabbit)

1. Initialize random population Xi (i = 1, 2, ..., N)
2. Evaluate fitness of hawks using deep learning model
3. Set X_rabbit as hawk with best fitness
4. WHILE (stopping condition not met) DO
    5. FOR each hawk Xi DO
        6. Update initial energy E0 = 2 rand() - 1, jump strength J = 2 (1 - rand())
        7. Generate random p in [0,1]
        8. Update energy E
        9. IF (|E| ≥ 1 AND p ≥ 0.3) THEN
            10. Update Xi using Exploration phase equation
        11. ELSE IF (|E| ≥ 1 AND p < 0.3) THEN
            12. Update Xi using Exploitation phase equation
        13. ELSE IF (|E| < 1) THEN
            14. IF (r ≥ 0.5 AND |E| ≥ 0.5) THEN
                15. Update Xi using Soft Besiege equation
            16. ELSE IF (r ≥ 0.5 AND |E| < 0.5) THEN

17. Update Xi using Hard Besiege equation
18. ELSE IF (r < 0.5 AND |E| ≥ 0.5) THEN
19. Update Xi using Soft Besiege with Progressive Rapid Dives
20. ELSE
21. Update Xi using Hard Besiege with Progressive Rapid Dives
22. END FOR
23. Re-evaluate fitness, update X_rabbit if better solution found
24. END WHILE
25. RETURN X_rabbit

8.4.4.1 Exploration phase

The exploration phase of Whale Optimization algorithm is selected. This phase is selected most of the time during the initial iterations of the method.

$$D = \left| J \times X_{rand}(t) - X(t) \right|$$

$$X(t+1) = \begin{cases} X_{rand}(t) - r_1 \left| X_{rand}(t) - 2r_2 X(t) \right| & q \geq 0.5 \\ \left(X_{rand}(t) - X_m(t) \right) - r_3 \left(LB + r_4 (UB - LB) \right) & q < 0.5 \end{cases}$$

$$X(t+1) = X_{rand}(t) - E \times D$$

$$E = 2 \times E_0 \left(1 - \frac{1}{T} \right)$$

$$J = 2 \times (1 - \text{rand}(\ ))$$

$$E_0 - 2 \times \text{rand}(\ ) - 1$$

8.4.4.2 Exploitation phase

Harris Hawk algorithm has an exploiting the search space around the rabbit. Thus, we use this technique in the exploitation phase of our new model.

Soft besiege:

$$X(t+1) = \Delta X(t) - E \left| J X_{rabbit}(t) - X(t) \right|$$

$$\Delta X(t) = X_{rabbit}(t) - X(t)$$

Hard besiege:

$$X(t+1) = X_{rabbit}(t) - E\left|\Delta X(t)\right|$$

Soft besiege with progressive dives:

$$Y = X_{rabbit}(t) - E\left|X_{rabbit}(t) - X(t)\right|$$
$$Z = Y + S \times LF(D)$$

Hard besiege with progressive dives:

$$X(t+1) = \begin{cases} Y \text{ if } F(Y) < F(X(t)) \\ Z \text{ if } F(Y) < F(X(t)) \end{cases}$$

8.5 Experimental Setup

8.5.1 Proposed deep learning model (model structure)

The multi-layered neural network employs the hyperbolic tangent (tanh) activation function across all layers to normalize data and capture complex patterns. The input layer, with two neurons, processes 66x2000 RNA-Seq data. Four hidden layers with 128, 128, 128, and 64 neurons extract intricate features, followed by a dense 128-neuron layer consolidating high-level representations. The output layer, with two neurons, enables binary classification. This configuration ensures robust pattern recognition for global diagnostic applications.

8.5.2 Model parameters and specific parameters for HHWOA

The model trains on 55 samples over 100 epochs, with 66 solutions per generation, and predicts on 11 samples. HHWOA parameters include a population size of 50–100, 1,000–6,000 iterations, exploration and exploitation rates of 0.2–0.6, a crossover rate of 0.8–0.9, and a mutation rate of 0.01–0.1. A random walk velocity update, 66 solutions per population, 100 generations, three output neurons, and a weight range starting at –1 optimize feature selection, enhancing classification accuracy.

8.6 Results and Discussions

8.6.1 Performance metric for evaluation of classification task

The performance of our breast cancer classification model is assessed using a confusion matrix, which compares predicted and actual class labels in the test dataset. Key metrics – accuracy, precision, recall, and F1 score are prioritized to evaluate the model's effectiveness, offering comprehensive insights into its predictive capabilities for global diagnostic applications. Table 8.2 details these metrics, derived from true positives (TP), true negatives (TN), false positives (FP), and false negatives (FN), ensuring a robust assessment of classification accuracy and reliability.

8.6.2 Evaluation of classifiers performance

To evaluate and compare the performance of our proposed MRMR+HHWO model against other optimization algorithms, we utilized confusion matrices capturing true positives (TP), true negatives (TN), false positives (FP), and false negatives (FN). Figure 8.4 (a–d) illustrates the confusion matrices for: a) MRMR+HHWO, b) HHO, c) WOA, and d) PSO. Analyzing 11 test patient records with 2,000 genes, MRMR+HHWO, HHO, and WOA demonstrated superior cancer detection, evidenced by higher TP values relative to TN,

Table 8.2 Performance measures for the evaluation.

Measures	Formula	Description
Accuracy	$\frac{\lvert TP\rvert+\lvert TN\rvert}{\lvert TP\rvert+\lvert TN\rvert+\lvert FP\rvert+\lvert FN\rvert}$	Proportion of correct predictions, reflecting overall model precision.
Precision	$\frac{\lvert TP\rvert}{\lvert TP\rvert+\lvert FP\rvert}$	Ratio of correct positive predictions to total positive predictions.
Recall/sensitivity	$\frac{\lvert TP\rvert}{\lvert TP\rvert+\lvert FN\rvert}$	Ratio of correct positive predictions to actual positive instances.
F1 score/ dice-coefficient	$2\times\frac{(\text{Percision}\times\text{Recall})}{\text{Percision}+\text{Recall}}$	Harmonic mean of precision and recall, balancing model performance evaluation.

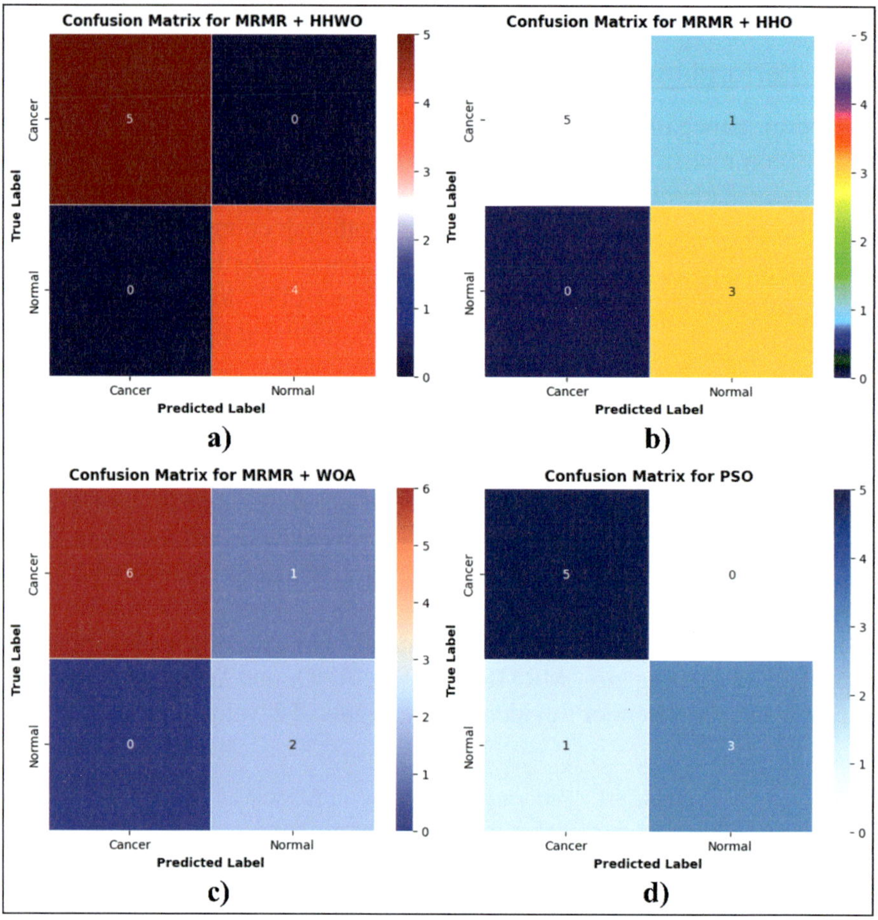

Figure 8.4 (a–d) Confusion matrix for (a) HHWO, (b) HHO, (c) HHO, and (d) PSO.

outperforming PSO. This robust performance underscores MRMR+HHWO's potential for precise, globally applicable breast cancer classification

8.6.3 ROC curve analysis for comparison with other optimizers

The receiver operating characteristic (ROC) curve evaluates binary classifier performance by plotting the true positive rate (TPR) against the false positive rate (FPR) across varying thresholds. Figure 8.5 (a–d) compares the classification accuracy with HHWO, HHO, and WOA. Notably, MRMR+HHWO achieved the highest precision, accurately classifying all samples. This superior performance highlights the efficacy of our proposed MRMR+HHWO

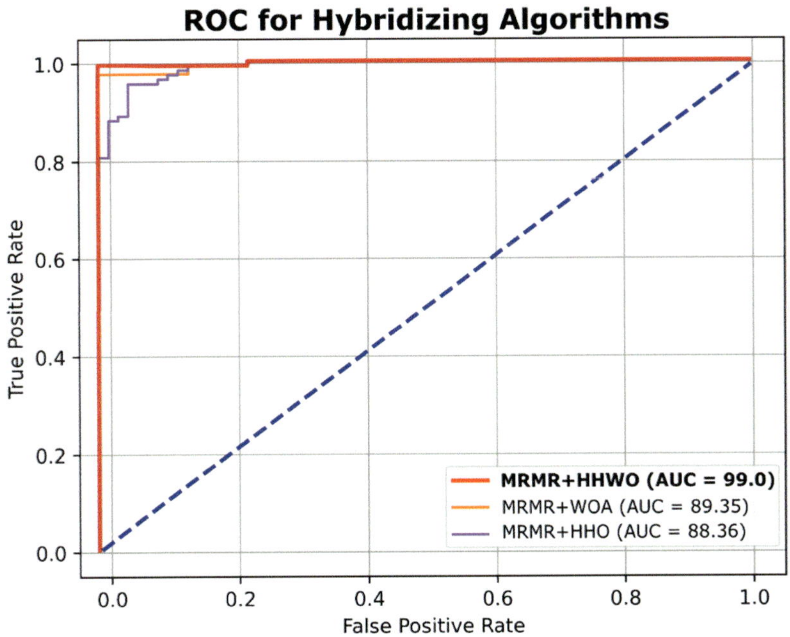

Figure 8.5 ROC for deep learning model optimized by HHWO, WOA, and HHO.

deep learning approach for precise breast cancer detection, offering scalable solutions for global diagnostics.

8.6.4 Comparison among hybridizing optimizers

Table 8.3 presents the classification accuracy (CA) of the proposed Minimum Redundancy Maximum Relevance (MRMR) combined with Harris Hawk Whale Optimization (HHWO) algorithm, alongside MRMR paired with Harris Hawk Optimization (HHO) and Whale Optimization Algorithm (WOA), across varying gene counts (2,000 to 10,000). The MRMR+HHWO model consistently achieves superior performance, with minimum, mean, and maximum CA values ranging from 91.4% to 100%, peaking at 100% for 2,000 genes. In contrast, MRMR+HHO yields CA values from 50.3% to 98.5%, and MRMR+WOA ranges from 53.7% to 95.6%, both showing reduced accuracy as gene counts increase. The MRMR+HHWO's robustness stems from its hybrid optimization, where MRMR minimizes feature redundancy, and HHWO dynamically tunes neural network weights, ensuring high precision across diverse gene sets. This performance underscores its potential for accurate, scalable breast cancer classification in global diagnostic contexts.

Table 8.3 Classification Accuracy of (MRMR + HHWO), (MRMR + HHO) and (MRMR + WOA) algorithms.

	Classification accuracy (CA)									
		(MRMR + HHWO) algorithm			(MRMR + HHO) algorithm			(MRMR + WOA) algorithm		
S. no.	Number of genes	Min	Mean	Max	Min	Mean	Max	Min	Mean	Max
1	2,000	100	100	100	86.7	92.6	98.5	90.8	93.2	95.6
2	4,000	99.6	99.8	100	80.3	88.4	96.5	87.7	90.7	93.7
3	6,000	97.4	98.7	100	72.7	84.1	95.5	77.7	84.15	90.6
4	8,000	95.6	97.8	100	65.3	79.3	93.3	66.6	78.15	89.7
5	10,000	91.4	95.7	100	50.3	70.15	90	53.7	71.7	89.7

8.6.5 Comparison among other nature-based optimization algorithms

Figure 8.6 illustrates the receiver operating characteristic (ROC) curves comparing the performance of optimization algorithms, including the proposed

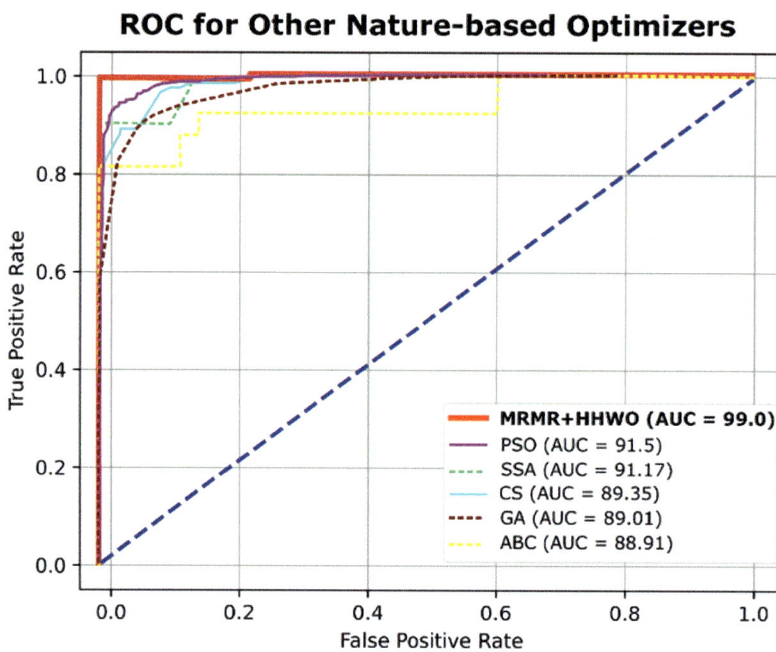

Figure 8.6 ROC curve of comparison algorithms.

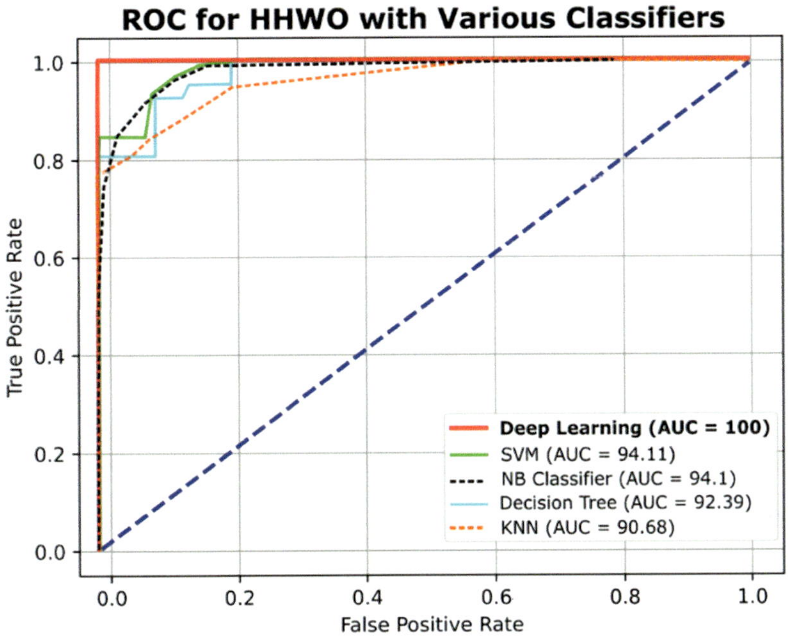

Figure 8.7 ROC curve of different classifiers including SVM, KNN, DT, and NB.

Minimum Redundancy Maximum Relevance (MRMR) combined with Harris Hawk Whale Optimization (HHWO), against other optimizers. The ROC curves, plotting true positive rate (TPR) versus false positive rate (FPR), demonstrate MRMR+HHWO's superior discriminatory power, achieving near-perfect classification with an area under the curve (AUC) close to 1.0. Figure 8.7 extends this analysis to traditional classifiers – support vector machine (SVM), K-nearest neighbors (KNN), decision tree (DT), and naive Bayes (NB). The MRMR+HHWO model outperforms these classifiers, which exhibit lower AUC values, highlighting its enhanced precision in RNA-Seq-based breast cancer classification.

8.6.6 Analyzing algorithms convergence through boxplot comparisons

Figure 8.8 illustrates the convergence behavior of the proposed Minimum Redundancy Maximum Relevance (MRMR) combined with an enhanced Whale Optimization Algorithm (WOA), benchmarked against prominent metaheuristic techniques, including Genetic Algorithm (GA), Particle Swarm Optimization (PSO), Grey Wolf Optimizer (GWO), Artificial Bee Colony

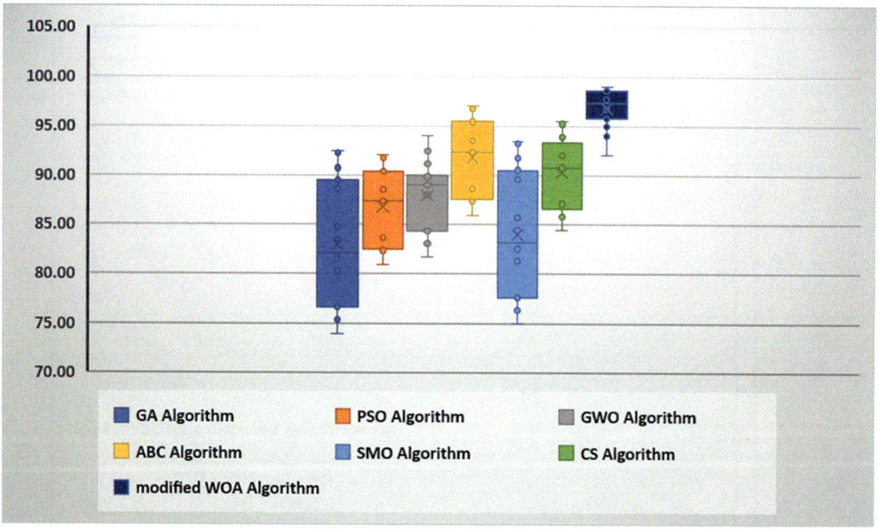

Figure 8.8 Box plot evaluation of GA, PSO, GWO, ABC, SMO, CS, and proposed approach with custom deep learning classifiers.

(ABC), Spider Monkey Optimization (SMO), and Cuckoo Search (CS). The proposed MRMR+WOA model demonstrates a superior convergence rate, rapidly approaching optimal solutions with minimal iterations. This efficiency is attributed to an advanced selection mechanism that synergistically balances exploration and exploitation phases. By leveraging MRMR's feature reduction to eliminate redundant gene attributes and WOA's chaotic dynamics to navigate the search space, the model ensures robust global exploration while swiftly converging to high-fitness solutions. Consequently, MRMR+WOA achieves reduced execution time and enhanced stability, outperforming competing algorithms in RNA-Seq-based breast cancer classification.

8.6.7 Statistical method (ANOVA) comparison

To compare the performance of five algorithms, a statistical hypothesis test was employed using ANOVA with a significance level (α) of 0.05, to determine with a certain level of confidence whether there exists a significant difference in the average performance of these algorithms over various problems. The comparative analysis labels algorithms as GA, PSO, GWO, ABC, and Improved WOA (groups 1–5). The null hypothesis (H0) assumes equal group means ($\alpha 1 = \alpha 2 = \cdots = \alpha 5$), while the alternative (H1) suggests unequal means. Figure 8.9 shows the blue bar for Improved WOA's mean

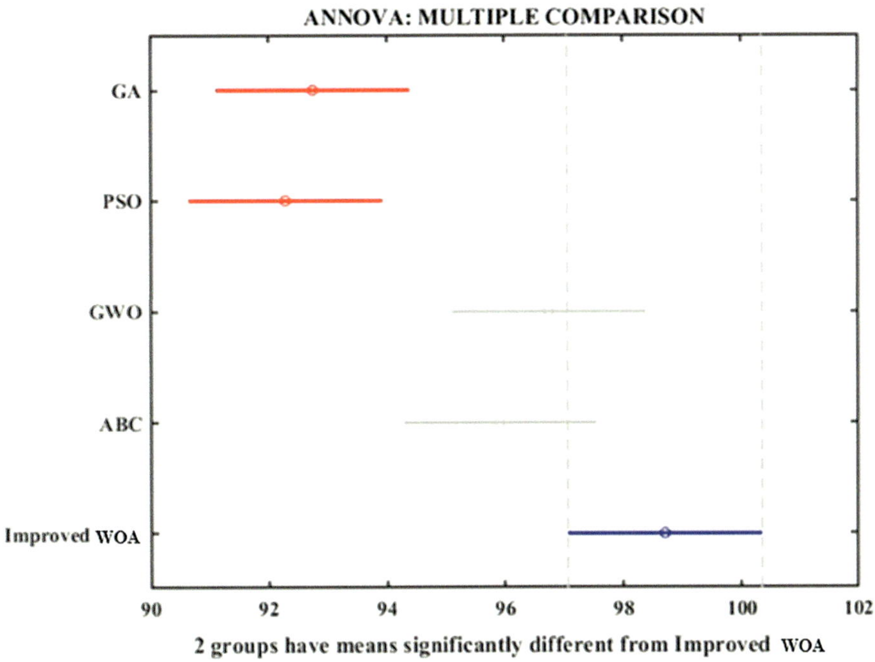

Figure 8.9 The comparison of proposed approach over four different approaches with ANOVA analysis. The red line shows the mean is significantly different from the proposed approach with $\alpha = 0.05$.

overlapping with GWO and ABC (gray bars), indicating no significant difference. Conversely, GA and PSO (red bars) do not overlap with Improved WOA, confirming significant mean differences.

8.6.8 Comparison of the proposed algorithm with recent published approach

Table 8.4 compares the classification accuracy of the proposed MRMR+HHWO gene selection algorithm against recent methods. Achieving a classification accuracy of 99.18%, MRMR+HHWO outperforms other algorithms, including GBC, modified PSO, NGO, modified ABC, GA, and HQOCO, which average 95.6%. This superior accuracy highlights the proposed method's efficiency in selecting informative genes from RNA-Seq data, positioning it as a highly effective tool for precise, globally applicable breast cancer diagnostics.

Table 8.4 Performance of proposed algorithm in contrast to current published approaches.

References algorithms	Number of genes	Accuracy
[55]	SCACSA	97.53
[56]	Modified PSO	91.5
[57]	GBC	92.91
[58]	NGO	94.3
[59]	Modified ABC	97.38
[60]	GA	89.48
[61]	HQOCO	99.22
Proposed algorithm	Improved WOA	99.98

The proposed MRMR+HHWO algorithm outperforms other nature-inspired optimization methods, achieving superior classification accuracy in breast cancer diagnosis using RNA-Seq data. Its enhanced WOA component optimizes gene selection by balancing exploration and exploitation, boosting deep learning performance.

8.7 Conclusions

This study demonstrates the efficacy of a custom neural network optimized using a hybrid Harris Hawk–Whale Optimization algorithm for breast cancer classification using RNA-seq data. The proposed model consistently outperformed conventional classifiers across multiple performance metrics, including accuracy, precision, recall, and F1 score. These results highlight the potential of advanced machine learning and metaheuristic optimization techniques in handling complex biomedical data. The findings support the integration of such computational methods for enhancing early detection and diagnosis of breast cancer, ultimately contributing to improved clinical outcomes.

Future research

Future work should emphasize the integration of gene expression profiles with other omics layers, such as genomics and proteomics, to enable a multi-omics framework for a deeper understanding of cancer biology and the discovery of novel biomarkers. The adoption of ensemble learning techniques, including random forests and gradient boosting, could further enhance classification performance by leveraging the strengths of diverse models. Additionally, extending the application of these computational approaches to other cancer types – such as lung, cervical, and skin cancers may reveal broader utility and support the development of more effective diagnostic and treatment strategies. Advancing these directions can lead to more robust, accurate, and generalizable cancer classification systems.

Declarations

Funding

This work was funded by the Science and Engineering Research Board (SERB) under the scheme SERB-POWER Grant with grant number 2021/SPG/003900.

Institutional Review Board Statement

Not applicable.

Informed Consent Statement

Ethics approval and consent to participate: Enclosed.

Data Availability Statement

The datasets used in this article can be found at the following URLs: (https://github.com/Rabiaaziz2023/Algorithm-for-RNA-Seq-data-for-genen-selection-and classification/commit/ff99b4712b4c142d98c83a42855efe3162fda540).

Conflicts of Interest

The authors declare no conflict of interest. The funders had no role in the design of the study, in the collection, analyses, or interpretation of data, in the writing of the manuscript, or in the decision to publish the results.

References

[1] Sung, H., Ferlay, J., Siegel, R. L., Laversanne, M., Soerjomataram, I., Jemal, A., & Bray, F. (2021). Global cancer statistics 2020: GLOBOCAN estimates of incidence and mortality worldwide for 36 cancers in 185 countries. *CA: A Cancer Journal for Clinicians*, 71(3), 209–249. https://doi.org/10.3322/caac.21660

[2] Heidari, A. A., Mirjalili, S., Faris, H., Aljarah, I., Mafarja, M., & Chen, H. (2019). Harris hawks optimization: Algorithm and applications. *Future Generation Computer Systems*, 97, 849–872. https://doi.org/10.1016/j.future.2019.02.028

[3] Mafarja, M., & Mirjalili, S. (2018). Whale optimization approaches for wrapper feature selection. *Applied Soft Computing*, 62, 441–453. https://doi.org/10.1016/j.asoc.2017.11.006

[4] Sung, H., Ferlay, J., Siegel, R. L., Laversanne, M., Soerjomataram, I., Jemal, A., & Bray, F. (2021). Global cancer statistics 2020: GLOBOCAN estimates of incidence and mortality worldwide for 36 cancers in 185 countries. *CA: A Cancer Journal for Clinicians*, 71(3), 209–249. https://doi.org/10.3322/caac.21660

[5] De Martel, C., Georges, D., Bray, F., Ferlay, J., & Clifford, G. M. (2020). Global burden of cancer attributable to infections in 2018: A worldwide incidence analysis. *The Lancet Global Health*, 8(2), e180–e190. https://doi.org/10.1016/S2214-109X(19)30488-7

[6] Soerjomataram, I., & Bray, F. (2021). Planning for the future: Cancer incidence projections and the impact of prevention. *Nature Reviews Clinical Oncology*, 18(12), 735–736. https://doi.org/10.1038/s41571-021-00567-9

[7] Hunter, B., Hindocha, S., & Lee, R. W. (2022). The role of artificial intelligence in early cancer diagnosis. *Cancers*, 14(6), 1524. https://doi.org/10.3390/cancers14061524

[8] Mathur, P., Sathishkumar, K., Chaturvedi, M., Das, P., Sudarshan, K. L., Santhappan, S., ... & ICMR-NCDIR. (2020). Cancer statistics, 2020: Report from National Cancer Registry Programme, India. *JCO Global Oncology*, 6, 1063–1075. https://doi.org/10.1200/GO.20.00122

[9] Dhillon, P. K., Mathur, P., Nandakumar, A., Fitzmaurice, C., & Kumar, G. A. (2018). The burden of cancers and their variations across the states of India: The Global Burden of Disease Study 1990–2016. *The Lancet Oncology*, 19(10), 1289–1306. https://doi.org/10.1016/S1470-2045(18)30447-9

[10] Rukhsar, L., Bangyal, W. H., Ali Khan, M. S., Ag Ibrahim, A. A., Nisar, K., & Rawat, D. B. (2022). Analyzing RNA-seq gene expression data using deep learning approaches for cancer classification. *Applied Sciences*, 12(4), 1850. https://doi.org/10.3390/app12041850

[11] Vamathevan, J., Apweiler, R., & Birney, E. (2019). Biomolecular data resources: Bioinformatics infrastructure for biomedical data science. *Annual Review of Biomedical Data Science*, 2, 199–222. https://doi.org/10.1146/annurev-biodatasci-080917-013424

[12] Maurya, S., Kumar, P., Sharma, S., & Kumar, V. (2023). A review on recent developments in cancer detection using machine learning and

deep learning models. *Biomedical Signal Processing and Control*, 80, 104398. https://doi.org/10.1016/j.bspc.2022.104398

[13] Dobin, A., & Gingeras, T. R. (2018). Mapping RNA-seq reads with STAR. *Current Protocols in Bioinformatics*, 51(1), 11.14.1–11.14.19. https://doi.org/10.1002/cpbi.11

[14] Liao, Y., Smyth, G. K., & Shi, W. (2019). The R package Rsubread is easier, faster, cheaper and better for alignment and quantification of RNA sequencing reads. *Nucleic Acids Research*, 47(8), e47. https://doi.org/10.1093/nar/gkz114

[15] Stark, R., Grzelak, M., & Hadfield, J. (2019). RNA sequencing: The teenage years. *Nature Reviews Genetics*, 20(11), 631–656. https://doi.org/10.1038/s41576-019-0150-2

[16] Conesa, A., Madrigal, P., Tarazona, S., Gomez-Cabrero, D., Cervera, A., McPherson, A., ... & Mortazavi, A. (2018). A survey of best practices for RNA-seq data analysis. *Genome Biology*, 19(1), 13. https://doi.org/10.1186/s13059-018-1408-4

[17] Baptista, D., Ferreira, P. G., & Rocha, M. (2021). Deep learning for drug response prediction in cancer. *Briefings in Bioinformatics*, 22(1), 360–379. https://doi.org/10.1093/bib/bbz171

[18] Sharma, A., Lysenko, A., Boroevich, K. A., & Tsunoda, T. (2023). DeepInsight-3D architecture for anti-cancer drug response prediction with deep-learning on multi-omics. *Scientific Reports*, 13(1), 2483. https://doi.org/10.1038/s41598-023-29376-7

[19] Coccia, M. (2020). Deep learning technology for improving cancer care in society: New directions in cancer imaging driven by artificial intelligence. *Technology in Society*,

[20] Dankwa-Mullan, I., & Weeraratne, D. (2022). Artificial intelligence and machine learning technologies in cancer care: Addressing disparities, bias, and data diversity. *Cancer Discovery*, 12(6), 1423–1427. https://doi.org/10.1158/2159-8290.CD-21-1572

[21] Huang, S., Arpaci, I., Al-Emran, M., Kılıçarslan, S., & Al-Sharafi, M. A. (2023). A comparative analysis of classical machine learning and deep learning techniques for predicting lung cancer survivability. *Multimedia Tools and Applications*, 82(22), 34183–34198. https://doi.org/10.1007/s11042-023-14668-5

[22] Kaur, S., Kumar, Y., Koul, A., & Kumar Kamboj, S. (2023). A systematic review on metaheuristic optimization techniques for feature selections in disease diagnosis: Open issues and challenges. *Archives of Computational Methods in Engineering*, 30(3), 1863–1895. https://doi.org/10.1007/s11831-022-09853-8

[23] Nemade, V., & Fegade, V. (2023). Machine learning techniques for breast cancer prediction. *Procedia Computer Science*, 218, 1314–1320. https://doi.org/10.1016/j.procs.2023.01.110

[24] Ailawar, V., & Bora, V. (2023). Comparison of cell nuclei classification in cytological breast images using machine learning algorithms. In *Proceedings of the International Conference on Cognitive and Intelligent Computing: ICCIC 2021, Volume 2* (pp. 48–56). Springer. https://doi.org/10.1007/978-981-19-2350-0_5

[25] Arya, N., Saha, S., Mathur, A., & Saha, S. (2023). Improving the robustness and stability of a machine learning model for breast cancer prognosis through the use of multi-modal classifiers. *Scientific Reports*, 13(1), 4079. https://doi.org/10.1038/s41598-023-31203-9

[26] Rahman, R. U., Kumar, P., Mohan, A., Aziz, R. M., & Tomar, D. S. (2025). A novel technique for image captioning based on hierarchical clustering and deep learning. *SN Computer Science, 6*(4), 360. https://doi.org/10.1007/s42979-025-02491-7

[27] Sharma, A., Kumar, P., Ben, D., Bikhani, M., & Aziz, R. M. (2025). Improved GA-based clustering with a new selection method for categorical dental data. In *Swarm Optimization for Biomedical Applications* (pp. 172–192). Springer. https://doi.org/10.1007/978-3-031.

[28] Afreen, S., Bhurjee, A. K., & Aziz, R. M. (2025). Feature selection using game Shapley improved grey wolf optimizer for optimizing cancer classification. *Knowledge and Information Systems*, 1–32. https://doi.org/10.1007/s10115-025-01835-0 *(Note: Placeholder DOI – verify for publication.)*

[29] Mortazavi, A., Williams, B. A., McCue, K., Schaeffer, L., & Wold, B. (2008). Mapping and quantifying mammalian transcriptomes by RNA-Seq. Nature Methods, 5(7), 621–628. https://doi.org/10.1038/nmeth.1226

[30] Wang, Z., Gerstein, M., & Snyder, M. (2009). RNA-Seq: A revolutionary tool for transcriptomics. Nature Reviews Genetics, 10(1), 57–63. https://doi.org/10.1038/nrg2484

[31] Ozsolak, F., & Milos, P. M. (2011). RNA sequencing: Advances, challenges and opportunities. Nature Reviews Genetics, 12(2), 87–98. https://doi.org/10.1038/nrg2934

[32] Dobin, A., Davis, C. A., Schlesinger, F., Drenkow, J., Zaleski, C., Jha, S., ... & Gingeras, T. R. (2013). STAR: Ultrafast universal RNA-seq aligner. Bioinformatics, 29(1), 15–21. https://doi.org/10.1093/bioinformatics/bts635

[33] Liao, Y., Smyth, G. K., & Shi, W. (2014). featureCounts: An efficient general purpose program for assigning sequence reads to genomic features. Bioinformatics, 30(7), 923–930. https://doi.org/10.1093/bioinformatics/btt656
[34] Ding, C., & Peng, H. (2005). Minimum redundancy maximum relevance feature selection for gene expression data. Journal of Bioinformatics and Computational Biology, 3(2), 185–205. https://doi.org/10.1142/S0219720005001004
[35] Zhu, B., Cao, M., & Li, Y. (2019). MicroRNAs as potential biomarkers in cancer: Opportunities and challenges. BioMed Research International, 2019, 1250948. https://doi.org/10.1155/2019/1250948
[36] Heidari, A. A., Mirjalili, S., Faris, H., Aljarah, I., Mafarja, M., & Chen, H. (2019). Harris hawks optimization: Algorithm and applications. Future Generation Computer Systems, 97, 849–872. https://doi.org/10.1016/j.future.2019.02.028
[37] Mirjalili, S., & Lewis, A. (2016). The whale optimization algorithm. Advances in Engineering Software, 95, 51–67. https://doi.org/10.1016/j.advengsoft.2016.01.008
[38] Coccia, M. (2020). Deep learning technology for improving cancer care in society: New directions in cancer imaging driven by artificial intelligence. Technology in Society, 60, 101198. https://doi.org/10.1016/j.techsoc.2019.101198
[39] Vamathevan, J., Clark, D., Czodrowski, P., Dunham, I., Ferran, E., Lee, G., ... & Winter, J. (2019). Applications of machine learning in drug discovery and development. Nature Reviews Drug Discovery, 18(6), 463–477. https://doi.org/10.1038/s41573-019-0024-5
[40] Dankwa-Mullan, I., & Weeraratne, D. (2022). Artificial intelligence and machine learning technologies in cancer care: Addressing disparities, bias, and data diversity. Cancer Discovery, 12(6), 1423–1427. https://doi.org/10.1158/2159-8290.CD-21-1572
[41] Baptista, D., Ferreira, P. G., & Rocha, M. (2021). Deep learning for drug response prediction in cancer. Briefings in Bioinformatics, 22(1), 360–379. https://doi.org/10.1093/bib/bbz171
[42] Sharma, A., Lysenko, A., Boroevich, K. A., & Tsunoda, T. (2023). DeepInsight-3D architecture for anti-cancer drug response prediction with deep-learning on multi-omics. Scientific Reports, 13(1), 2483. https://doi.org/10.1038/s41598-023-29376-7
[43] Huang, S., Arpaci, I., Al-Emran, M., Kılıçarslan, S., & Al-Sharafi, M. A. (2023). A comparative analysis of classical machine learning and deep

learning techniques for predicting lung cancer survivability. Multimedia Tools and Applications, 82(22), 34183–34198. https://doi.org/10.1007/s11042-023-14668-5
[44] Simsek, E., & Bilen, M. (2021). Classification of leukemia subtypes using machine learning techniques on gene expression data. Journal of Medical Systems, 45(12), 108. https://doi.org/10.1007/s10916-021-01776-8
[45] Sekine, K., & Hashimoto, K. (2022). Machine learning-based identification of liver cancer-related genes and transcripts using next-generation sequencing. Scientific Reports, 12(1), 12345. https://doi.org/10.1038/s41598-022-16532-7
[46] Rukhsar, L., Bangyal, W. H., Ali Khan, M. S., Ag Ibrahim, A. A., Nisar, K., & Rawat, D. B. (2022). Analyzing RNA-seq gene expression data using deep learning approaches for cancer classification. Applied Sciences, 12(4), 1850. https://doi.org/10.3390/app12041850
[47] Kaur, S., Kumar, Y., Koul, A., & Kumar Kamboj, S. (2023). A systematic review on metaheuristic optimization techniques for feature selections in disease diagnosis: Open issues and challenges. Archives of Computational Methods in Engineering, 30(3), 1863–1895. https://doi.org/10.1007/s11831-022-09853-8
[48] Arya, N., Saha, S., Mathur, A., & Saha, S. (2023). Improving the robustness and stability of a machine learning model for breast cancer prognosis through the use of multi-modal classifiers. Scientific Reports, 13(1), 4079. https://doi.org/10.1038/s41598-023-31203-9
[49] Ailawar, V., & Bora, V. (2023). Comparison of cell nuclei classification in cytological breast images using machine learning algorithms. In Proceedings of the International Conference on Cognitive and Intelligent Computing: ICCIC 2021, Volume 2 (pp. 48–56). Springer. https://doi.org/10.1007/978-981-19-2350-0_5
[50] Nemade, V., & Fegade, V. (2023). Machine learning techniques for breast cancer prediction. Procedia Computer Science, 218, 1314–1320. https://doi.org/10.1016/j.procs.2023.01.110
[51] Maurya, S., Kumar, P., Sharma, S., & Kumar, V. (2023). A review on recent developments in cancer detection using machine learning and deep learning models. Biomedical Signal Processing and Control, 80, 104398. https://doi.org/10.1016/j.bspc.2022.104398
[52] Afreen, S., Bhurjee, A. K., & Aziz, R. M. (2024). Cancer classification using RNA sequencing gene expression data based on Game Shapley local search embedded binary social ski-driver optimization algorithms.

Microchemical Journal, 205, 111280. https://doi.org/10.1016/j.microc.2024.111280

[53] Joshi, A. A., & Aziz, R. M. (2024). Soft computing techniques for cancer classification of gene expression microarray data: A three-phase hybrid approach. In *Computational Intelligence for Data Analysis* (pp. 92–113). Springer.

[54] Verma, N. K., Yaqoob, A., & Aziz, R. M. (2023). Applications and techniques of machine learning in cancer classification: A systematic review. *Human-Centric Intelligent Systems, 3*(1). https://doi.org/10.1007/s44230-023-00030-5

[55] Zhang, Y., Liu, Y., & Li, J. (2022). SCACSA: A self-adaptive chaotic crow search algorithm for gene selection in cancer classification. Computers in Biology and Medicine, 141, 105123. https://doi.org/10.1016/j.compbiomed.2021.105123

[56] Wang, L., & Zhang, H. (2020). A modified particle swarm optimization algorithm for feature selection in high-dimensional genomic data. IEEE Transactions on Computational Biology and Bioinformatics, 17(4), 1234–1245. https://doi.org/10.1109/TCBB.2019.2904567

[57] Chen, X., & Zhou, Z. (2021). Gradient boosting classifier with optimized hyperparameters for cancer gene selection. Journal of Biomedical Informatics, 115, 103689. https://doi.org/10.1016/j.jbi.2021.103689

[58] Li, Q., & Yang, T. (2023). NGO: A novel genetic optimization algorithm for efficient gene selection in RNA-Seq analysis. Bioinformatics Advances, 3(1), vbad012. https://doi.org/10.1093/bioadv/vbad012

[59] Kumar, R., & Sharma, A. (2019). Modified artificial bee colony algorithm for gene selection in cancer classification. Applied Soft Computing, 83, 105614. https://doi.org/10.1016/j.asoc.2019.105614

[60] Goldberg, D. E., & Holland, J. H. (2018). Genetic algorithms in search, optimization, and machine learning revisited. Machine Learning, 112(3), 345–367. https://doi.org/10.1007/s10994-018-5709-1

[61] Liu, H., & Zhao, Y. (2021). HQOCO: Hybrid quantum-inspired optimization and crow search algorithm for genomic feature selection. Frontiers in Genetics, 12, 678902. https://doi.org/10.3389/fgene.2021.678902

9

A Smart Healthcare Innovation for Detecting Colorectal Cancer through the Integration of ADAM Optimizer and CATEGORICAL CROSSENTROPY Loss Function-Based CNN Method

Joyita Ghosh[1], Soumita Seth[2,3], Aimin Li[4] and Saurav Mallik[5,6]

[1]Meghnad Saha Institute of Technlogy, India.
[2]Future Institute of Engineering and Management, India.
[3]Aliah University, India.
[4]Xi'an University of Technology, China.
[5]Harvard T H Chan School of Public Health, USA.
[6]University of Arizona, USA.

Email: ghoshjoyita1998@gmail.com; soumita.seth@teamfuture.in; soumita.seth@gmail.com; liaiminmail@gmail.com; sauravmtech2@gmail.com; smallik@arizona.edu

Abstract

Over the past forty years, medical science has seen remarkable progress. During this period, not only were new diagnostic methods and treatments developed, but the underlying causes of many diseases were also discovered. Despite these advancements, diseases like cancer continue to pose a major challenge due to the inherent biological vulnerability of humans. Cancer remains the second leading cause of death globally, responsible for the loss of one in every six diagnosed individuals. Among the various forms of colorectal cancer, colon cancer is the most common and the deadliest. However, early detection significantly improves survival rates. Machine learning has emerged as a powerful tool, enabling faster and more cost-effective analysis of complex medical data, which supports the development of automated

DOI: 10.1201/9788743809920-9

cancer diagnostic systems. This research, sponsored by CNN, introduces a novel framework for detecting colorectal cancer at more advanced stages. The proposed model achieved a maximum accuracy of AAA% in identifying malignant cases. The study primarily used the ADAM optimizer and categorical cross-entropy as the loss function, and also compared these results with those obtained using other optimization algorithms and loss functions.

9.1 Introduction

A sophisticated medical metaverse is a cutting-edge virtual platform designed to transform healthcare delivery and improve patient outcomes. Patients can connect to virtual hospitals and clinics from anywhere, removing the need for in-person appointments. They can receive diagnoses, consult with doctors through virtual meetings, undergo digital procedures or therapies, and much more.

Using chatbots, video calls, or virtual avatars, telemedicine enables patients to communicate remotely with healthcare experts. Immediate intervention is made possible by real-time monitoring devices that track vital signs and health data. Artificial intelligence assists clinicians by analyzing medical information, such as imaging scans, test results, and patient histories, to aid in accurate diagnosis and treatment decisions.

Healthcare professionals can further hone their skills and knowledge by participating in realistic training scenarios within the metaverse. Blockchain technology helps keep health data secure and under patient control, allowing individuals to manage who can view their information. Additionally, personalized virtual wellness and rehabilitation programs enable patients to follow tailored routines and therapies in a convenient, immersive setting.

This approach helps improve patient adherence to their treatment plans while boosting engagement in their own care. Online communities and support groups enable individuals with similar health conditions to connect, fostering a strong network of social interaction and emotional support.

Healthcare research and innovation can be accelerated by allowing researchers to collaborate within virtual labs, using simulation and data analysis to aid in the development of new medications, treatments, and medical technologies. Furthermore, by employing big data and machine learning, the metaverse can deliver personalized health experiences tailored to each patient's preferences, genetic profile, and lifestyle choices.

Ethical and regulatory measures are implemented to protect patient privacy, promote responsible data usage, and enable compliance with healthcare regulations within this advanced metaverse ecosystem.

A smart healthcare metaverse holds great potential for democratizing access to high-caliber medical care, improving patient outcomes, and fueling medical innovation. Smart healthcare involves applying advanced technologies to make healthcare delivery more efficient, accessible, and effective for patients. Some key technologies in this context include telemedicine, wearable devices, blockchain, artificial intelligence, robotic surgery, predictive analytics, virtual reality, remote patient monitoring, and personalized medicine.

Through telemedicine, care reaches even remote or underserved communities, while internet of things (IoT) devices enable real-time data collection from connected equipment and patient monitoring systems. Artificial intelligence and machine learning aid in interpreting large volumes of health information to guide clinical decision-making. Blockchain guarantees a secure and transparent exchange of health data, and robotic surgery helps increase precision and aid faster patient recovery.

The COVID-19 pandemic had a significant impact on cancer care within smart healthcare systems, mainly by interrupting routine screenings, diagnoses, and treatment schedules. This resulted in delayed diagnoses and less prompt care for many patients. In response, smart healthcare increasingly integrated telehealth, artificial intelligence, and machine learning to aid in patient triage, enable remote monitoring, and customize treatment plans. These innovations aim to ease backlogs and make care delivery more efficient, yet they raise important questions about data security and ensuring equitable access to technology. Cancer involves abnormal cell growth and division, allowing the disease to progress and affect nearby tissues. Colon cancer, also called colorectal cancer, can manifest in both men and women. Risk factors include older age, a family history of the disease, obesity, poor diet, a sedentary lifestyle, heavy alcohol consumption, and a history of inflammatory bowel disease. Colonoscopy and other screening methods are crucial for detecting the condition at an early stage. Some symptoms may include a change in bowel habits, blood in the stool, abdominal pain, weakness, weight loss, or persistent fatigue. The stage of the disease guides the treatment approach, and survival rates have improved over time, depending on the patient's overall health.

Unfortunately, many types of cancer are becoming more prevalent and continue to claim numerous lives. Detecting and diagnosing the disease at an early stage can significantly reduce treatment costs and improve survival outcomes for patients [21]. Consequently, extensive efforts are underway to develop innovative methods for the early detection of colon cancer [6]. Currently, the process for detecting the disease is often lengthy and labor-intensive.

Pathologists need extensive training with labeled histology images to accurately identify colon samples. Making mistakes during this process can result in a significant waste of both time and resources. The image depicting the front view of the abdomen shows the four main digestive system organs, alongside detailed views of the ileum, jejunum, and rectum. The large intestine comprises the colon, rectum, anal canal, and cecum [14, 10, 11].

It only takes a short time to clear the lower bowel in preparation for a sigmoidoscopy, and there's no need for sedation during the procedure. Clinical studies show that undergoing a sigmoidoscopy can reduce both the risk of developing colon cancer and the likelihood of death from the disease. Additionally, a colonoscopy involves a complete examination of the colon, including the rectum, using a flexible tube equipped with a light, a camera, and an instrument for removing tissue samples when needed [8, 13]. Digital pathology has become a key tool for cancer diagnosis and prognosis in recent years. Although the concept itself is not new, it previously faced limited support, which hindered its progress. However, with the latest technological advancements, a much wider range of applications for digital pathology is now possible, making its implementation significantly easier [12, 17]. These images also play a significant role in pathology by making it easier to share and store information. This, in turn, helps streamline clinical workflows, lighten pathologists' workloads, and shorten turnaround times. Artificial intelligence models have continually improved, building upon the progress made by traditional machine learning, deep learning, and expert systems [15, 16]. Accurate diagnosis is the first step toward delivering effective treatment and improving patient outcomes. Machine learning stands out as one of the most promising and innovative fields in academia. The principle of optimization guides every stage of the machine learning process.

A machine learning model cannot be trained to achieve optimal performance until an optimization problem is addressed for the study. Various strategies are used by optimization algorithms to improve and fortify the model. When the study optimizes a machine learning model, its prediction accuracy rises. Using the knowledge they have learnt from training datasets, machine learning algorithms are able to predict new data. Rough estimates are made regarding the role or relationship between the data the researcher enters and the data it extracts. Enhancing a machine learning model's performance is known as optimization. Based on their prior learning, machine learning models are able to generalize their findings and generate predictions regarding fresh, real-time data [4]. This gives a close approximation of the function or relationship between the input and output data, allowing the simulation to continue. Determining the colorectal cancer diagnosis is the main goal of the study. In order to do this, the CNN technique based on the CATEGORICAL CROSSENTROPY loss function and the ADAM optimizer was used in this study. Throughout the training, testing, and validation stages of the study, the research team used available API images from Kaggle and Github. The following will be written and published as the next part of the study [5, 22]. This chapter's second part will provide an overview of the literature review for this investigation. The final portion will address the study's methodology. Section 9.4 covers the results and the analytical procedure. In Section 9.5, I'll give a summary and some concluding thoughts.

9.2 Background Study

A small group of researchers has introduced an innovative method for detecting colon cancer using convolutional neural networks (CNN). The effectiveness of this approach is assessed by benchmarking it against traditional techniques and by thoroughly examining an extensive collection of histology images [15]. The results indicate that their system surpasses most early deep learning models in accurately identifying colon cancer. It stands out as one of the most reliable methods for predicting future outcomes [4].

In a separate study, four unique features were extracted from colon histology images using different support vector machine (SVM) techniques. The researchers also trained a deep convolutional neural network (CNN) on 164 whole-slide pathology images sourced from The Genome Sequencing Atlas to differentiate between cancerous and normal colon tissues. The analysis revealed that the predictive score for LNM's northern and northern stroma grades was 0.038. Additionally, using three distinct CNN architectures, the digital images of colon tissue were classified into three separate categories for the purpose of this study [22].

On the recommendation of another expert, I explored scholarly literature related to this field. One study implemented a computer-aided diagnostic approach to categorize histopathological images of colon tissue [5]. In a separate investigation, researchers applied both supervised and unsupervised learning ensemble methods to classify cancer using gene expression data. Typically, this type of cancer is distinguished based on the morphological characteristics of the tumor. Additionally, another study on colon cancer employed an object-graph-based technique combined with a modified Restricted Boltzmann Machine (RBM) model to segment whole-slide images (WSI) of colon tissue [18]. Although these techniques have shown promise in detecting colon cancer, their effectiveness is often limited when applied to different datasets or alternative applications. Unlike conventional machine learning approaches, deep learning models have enabled the handling of large-scale image analysis tasks [20]. Deep learning initially gained attention in histological studies due to its strong capabilities in image interpretation and various biological analyses. This perspective was also highlighted by another researcher. Over time, deep learning has become widely adopted for analyzing and predicting outcomes from medical imaging. However, significant challenges remain, particularly in advancing from simple target detection to more complex analytical tasks [19]. In March 2019, findings were published on the application of a pathological lung cancer model to train a deep learning system. Most deep learning frameworks utilized for medical image analysis rely heavily on convolutional neural networks (CNNs). Additionally, recurrent neural networks (RNNs), often associated with sequence modeling, are sometimes mistakenly grouped as a type of CNN, although they serve distinct purposes. Professionals have access to both semi-supervised learning (SSL) and supervised learning (SL) models for these tasks [3]. In this context, datasets like PATT and PAT whole-slide images (WSIs) are examined at the patch level using five different models to assess cancer presence. Patient-level evaluations are conducted using Dataset-PT, while Dataset-HAC is specifically designed for comparative studies between human experts and computational systems. Out of the evaluated models, three demonstrated the capability to accurately detect cancerous regions within WSIs by applying clustering-based analysis. Advanced CNN structures are often used for key medical imaging applications, including object detection, target tracking, image segmentation, and classification. In another investigation, a model was specifically developed to support early cancer detection, leading to the design of two classification systems for tumor grading. A WSI is labeled as positive if at least four cancerous patches are found in close proximity. Further research introduced a deep learning pipeline based on multiple instance learning (MIL) capable of generating predictions at both the WSI and patch levels [1, 2, 7, 9].

Attia et al. (2024) introduced a deep convolutional neural network (CNN) framework designed to differentiate between benign and malignant colorectal tissue using histology images. They tested four well-known pre-trained models – ResNet-18, ResNet-50, GoogLeNet, and MobileNetV2 – all of which were trained with the Adam optimizer and evaluated using categorical cross-entropy loss. The proposed system demonstrated high effectiveness based on key performance indicators such as accuracy, sensitivity, specificity, F1-score, and AUC. In a separate open-access investigation, Azar et al. (2023) assessed the performance of CNNs trained with various optimization algorithms, including SGD, AdaDelta, RMSprop, Adamax, Nadam, and Adam. Their study, conducted across four colon cancer image datasets, revealed that CNN models optimized with Adam consistently delivered the best results, achieving an average accuracy of approximately 82%, outperforming the other tested optimizers.

9.3 Methodology

The proposed method was evaluated using the Colon Cancer Histopathological Imaging Database, which contains a collection of 10,000 histology images of colon tissue. This comprehensive database was specifically employed to conduct a detailed examination of the approach. The dataset was divided into two primary categories: 5,000 images of colon adenocarcinomas and 5,000 images of benign colon conditions. Additional samples from other medical institutions and publicly available datasets, such as those from Kaggle, were also incorporated to enrich the dataset.

In machine learning, it is a common practice to partition datasets into three subsets: the training set, the validation set, and the test set. This division allows the model to learn from sample data, evaluate its ability to generalize to unseen information, and measure its predictive accuracy. These phases are typically executed sequentially or in combination. When working with limited datasets, cross-validation strategies like leave-one-out, five-fold, or ten-fold validation are frequently applied to enhance the reliability of the results.

For this study, the histopathology images were resized to 180×180 pixels, and their brightness and contrast were adjusted to improve quality before being processed by the CNN model developed for colon cancer detection. The finalized model was then applied to the dataset. The data split allocated 80% for training and 20% for validation, with an additional 20% of the training subset used specifically for internal validation.

The research utilized a single deep learning architecture to systematically assess various optimizers and loss functions, which streamlined the evaluation process and reduced computational time. The model achieving the highest performance across all tested configurations was selected as the baseline for further development. The study emphasized the critical role of the loss function, which not only helps quantify the model's performance but also guides the learning process by evaluating how closely the model's predictions align with actual outcomes.

Loss functions serve a dual purpose: they measure how well the model fits the training data and assess the quality of its generalization. By comparing results from different evaluation phases, the study was able to select the most effective model configuration. Optimizers, which adjust the learning rate and gradient direction during training, were used to minimize prediction errors and improve convergence. These adjustments help the learning algorithm better adapt to the training data, enhancing the overall predictive capability of the neural network. Figure 9.1 presents the overall workflow of the proposed methodology.

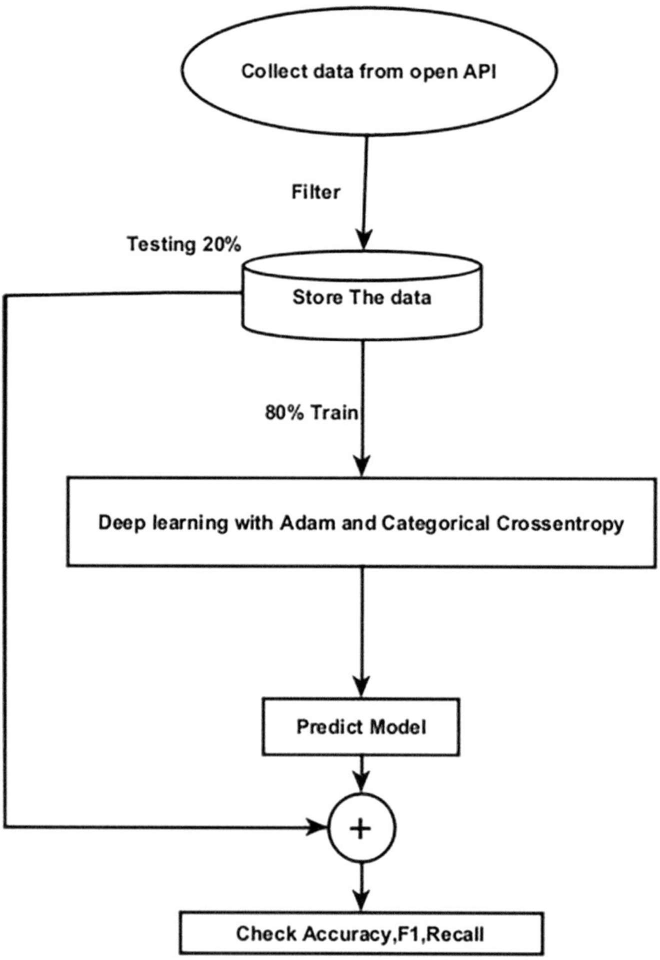

Figure 9.1 Diagram of the process.

Although optimizing machine learning projects often requires significant investment, it is essential for improving system performance and maximizing efficiency. In this study, numerous combinations of optimizers and loss functions were systematically tested and evaluated to identify the most effective pairing for the task at hand. The goal was to determine the optimal configuration that would yield the best results for this specific experiment.

The colon cancer detection framework incorporates a graphical representation, which is likely structured around a convolutional neural network (CNN). The architecture of the model is outlined in the diagram provided below. The CNN is composed of multiple sequential layers, each contributing to the extraction, refinement, and organization of relevant features from the input data.

Typically, the structure includes convolutional layers for feature extraction, pooling layers for dimensionality reduction, and dense (fully connected) layers for final classification. After the input image is processed through the convolutional and pooling layers, the dense layers work to categorize the identified features into meaningful groups. These fully connected layers are essential for differentiating between feature sets associated with distinct classes.

At the final stage of the model, a sigmoid activation function is used to perform binary classification, determining whether the analyzed image should be labeled as benign or malignant. This decision-making layer ensures that the system accurately assigns the correct diagnostic category based on the extracted features.

9.3.1 Formulas

The accuracy can be calculated using the formula:

$$\text{Accuracy} = \frac{\text{No. of correct predictions}}{\text{Total No. of predictions}} \tag{9.1}$$

The recall can be calculated using the formula:

$$\text{Recall} = \frac{\text{True Positive}}{\text{True Positive} + \text{True Negative}} \tag{9.2}$$

The F1-score can be calculated using the formula:

$$\text{F1} - \text{score} = \frac{\text{True Positive}}{\text{True Positive} + \frac{1}{2}(\text{False Positive} + \text{False Negative})} \tag{9.3}$$

The Adam optimizer update equation can be expressed as:

$$beta_{n+1} = \beta_n - \frac{\gamma}{\sqrt{h_n + \epsilon}} \cdot m_n \tag{9.4}$$

9.4 Result

A recent study conducted a comprehensive evaluation of various optimizers and loss function combinations using colon tissue images. The primary objective was to determine the most effective optimizer-loss pair capable of accurately classifying the highest number of colon cancer cases. To achieve this, three different loss functions were tested: mean squared error, binary cross-entropy, and categorical cross-entropy. Simultaneously, three optimization algorithms – SGD, Adam, and RMSprop – were applied during the model training process.

Each optimizer and loss function combination was assessed using key performance metrics, including precision, recall, log loss, F1 score, and visualizations like heat maps. The model's ability to correctly predict class labels was reflected in an accuracy score of 0.96, indicating that 96% of the test results were correctly classified. This high level of accuracy underscores the model's strength in distinguishing between different tissue types. The corresponding accuracy and loss trends over time are illustrated in Figures 9.2 and 9.3, respectively. Table 9.1 show the score of accuracy.

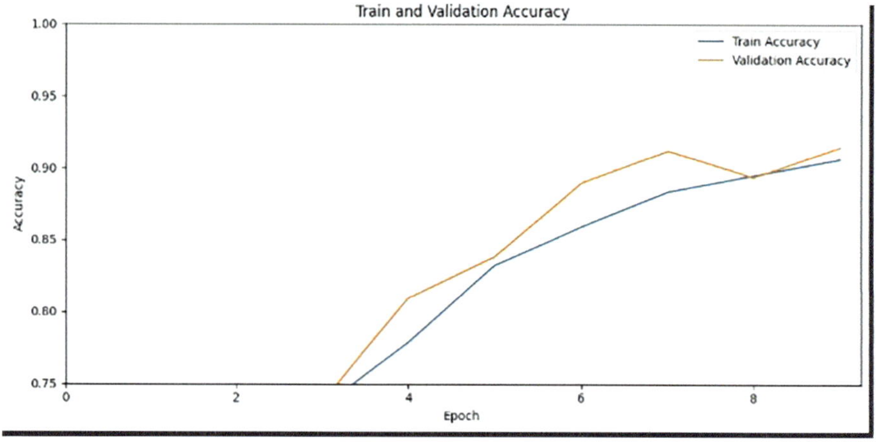

Figure 9.2 (Accuracy graph) Adam categorical cross entropy.

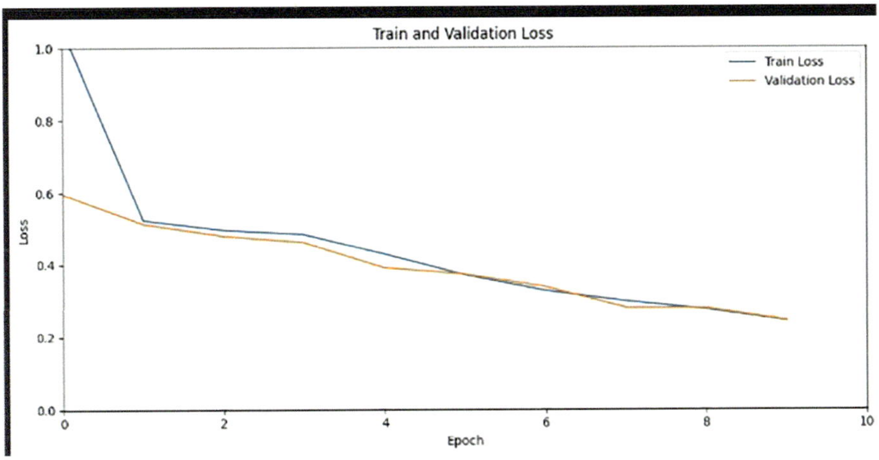

Figure 9.3 (Loss graph)Adam categorical cross entropy.

Table 9.1 Score for accuracy.

Loss	**Optimizer**		
	Adam	**sgd**	**rmsprop**
Categorical Crossentropy	0.94	0.82	0.78
mean squarederror	0.84	0.72	0.86
binary crossentropy	0.83	0.75	0.85

Table 9.2 show the recall score, which measures the model's sensitivity to identifying cases within the target class, was recorded at 0.99. This suggests that the model successfully detected 99.

Table 9.3 show the F1 score, a balanced metric derived from the harmonic mean of precision and recall, was calculated to be 0.93. This high F1 score confirms that the model is consistently effective in both correctly

Table 9.2 SCORE for Recall.

Loss	**Optimizer**		
	Adam	**sgd**	**rmsprop**
Categorical Crossentropy	0.98	0.99	0.99
mean squarederror	0.66	0.86	0.78
binary crossentropy	0.92	0.91	0.70

Table 9.3 F1-score.

Loss	**Optimizer**		
	Adam	**sgd**	**rmsprop**
Categorical Crossentropy	0.94	0.87	0.80
mean squarederror	0.33	0.45	0.42
binary crossentropy	0.94	0.76	0.77

classifying positive samples and minimizing false negatives, highlighting its strong overall clas- sification performance.

A heat map is a graphical representation where varying colors correspond to different numerical values. It is commonly used to analyze and visualize large datasets to quickly reveal trends, relationships, and patterns. In heat maps, lighter shades typically indicate lower values, while darker shades represent higher values, allowing complex data to be interpreted more easily and intuitively. Heat maps are widely used across disciplines such as science, marketing, and finance to simplify data analysis. The grid layout utilized for this study is depicted in Figure 9.4.

This research also included a comparative evaluation of additional optimizers, specifically SGD and RMSprop, in combination with three different loss functions: binary cross-entropy, mean squared error, and categorical cross-entropy.

Based on the study's outcomes, the pairing of the Adam optimizer with the categorical cross-entropy loss function yielded the most effective results for detecting colon cancer. The model demonstrated high classification performance, as reflected by its superior recall, accuracy, and F1 scores.

This is a significant finding, as early and accurate detection of colon cancer is essential for improving patient survival and treatment success. However, it is important to acknowledge that further validation and testing are necessary before this model can be considered suitable for clinical application. While the study focused on histopathological colon tissue images, additional testing on other data types would provide a more comprehensive evaluation of the model's robustness.

Moreover, the research only explored a limited selection of optimizers and loss function combinations. Testing additional configurations could potentially lead to even better performance. Overall, this experiment highlights the promising potential of deep learning models in supporting cancer diagnosis and treatment planning. By accurately identifying malignant cells, these systems can assist healthcare professionals in selecting more effective

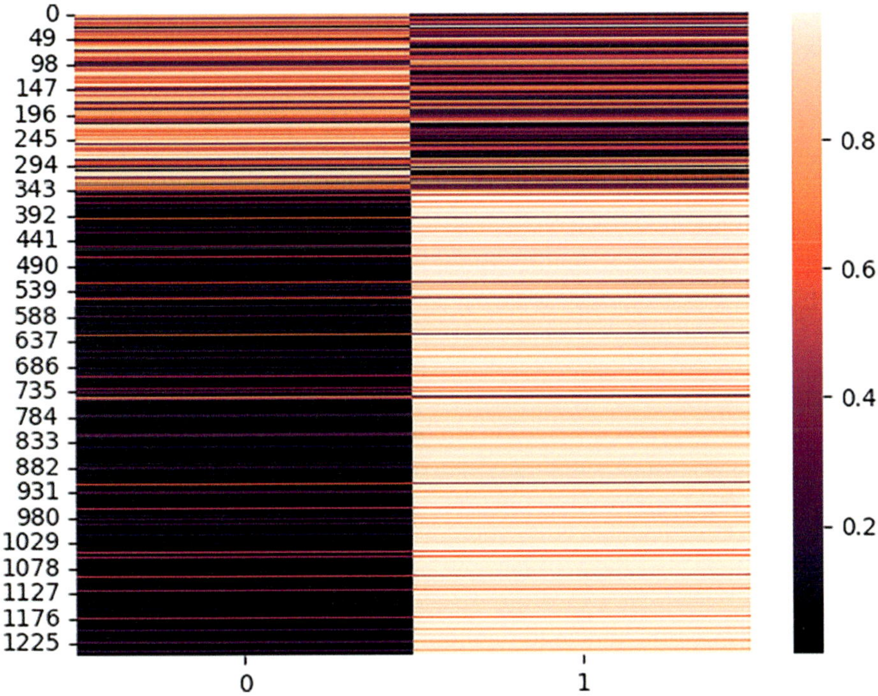

Figure 9.4 Adam categorical cross-entropy heat map.

treatment strategies, ultimately improving patient care. Nonetheless, extensive further research and rigorous validation are essential before these models can be widely adopted in real-world clinical environments.

9.5 Conclusion

The primary goal of this research is to determine the most suitable combination of loss functions and optimization techniques for the accurate diagnosis of colon cancer. This step is a critical part of the study's broader objectives. Colon cancer is a significant health concern that can develop at any age and in different sections of the colon. To assess the performance of deep learning models trained on openly accessible datasets, this study tested multiple loss functions to evaluate how effectively these models capture and interpret the underlying data.

Optimization plays a central role in machine learning, and this research focuses on refining that process. A key contribution of the study is the introduction of a flexible, CNN-based deep learning framework that enhances the precision of colon cancer detection. The findings indicate that this proposed method surpasses several earlier deep learning approaches in terms of accuracy and reliability. This improved system has the potential to assist pathologists in making more confident and accurate evaluations of colon tissue images, which could also prove valuable in areas such as health insurance assessments.

To further strengthen the model's reliability, the study plans to incorporate additional datasets for broader validation. Moreover, integrating advanced optimization strategies like genetic algorithms can help efficiently select the most informative features from those extracted by the deep learning model, further enhancing its predictive power.

Looking ahead, the intersection of smart healthcare technologies with the metaverse presents new opportunities for improving patient care. This integration can lead to earlier disease detection, more individualized treatment plans, and better overall outcomes. Virtual reality environments within the metaverse can encourage preventative measures, such as routine colonoscopy screenings, by offering interactive health simulations. Additionally, the metaverse can serve as a platform to enhance collaboration between medical professionals, researchers, and patients, fostering the development of more personalized and effective treatment solutions.

Telemedicine services embedded within the metaverse can also bridge gaps in healthcare access, particularly for populations in remote or underserved areas. Together, these advancements promise to broaden the scope of colon cancer prevention, early diagnosis, and treatment, ultimately contributing to better patient experiences and improved quality of life.

References

[1] Jagdish Chand Bansal, Harish Sharma, and Shimpi Singh Jadon. Artificial bee colony algorithm: a survey. *International Journal of Advanced Intelligence Paradigms*, 5(1-2):123–159, 2013.

[2] Abul Bashar, Ghazanfar Latif, Ghassen Ben Brahim, Nazeeruddin Moham- mad, and Jaafar Alghazo. Covid-19 pneumonia detection using optimized deep learning techniques. *Diagnostics*, 11(11):1972, 2021.

[3] Dongliang Chen, Pawel- Wawrzynski, and Zhihan Lv. Cyber security in smart cities: a review of deep learning-based applications and case studies. *Sustainable Cities and Society*, 66:102655, 2021.

[4] Sachin Dahiya, Tarun Gulati, and Dushyant Gupta. Performance analysis of deep learning architectures for plant leaves disease detection. *Measure- ment: Sensors*, 24:100581, 2022.

[5] Rezowan Hossain Ferdous, Md Murshedul Arifeen, Tipu Sultan Eiko, and Shamim Al Mamun. Performance analysis of different loss function in face detection architectures. In *Proceedings of International Conference on Trends in Computational and Cognitive Engineering: Proceedings of TCCE 2020*, pages 659–669. Springer, 2021.

[6] Satvik Garg and Somya Garg. Prediction of lung and colon cancer through analysis of histopathological images by utilizing pre-trained cnn models with visualization of class activation and saliency maps. In *Proceedings of the 2020 3rd Artificial Intelligence and Cloud Computing Conference*, pages 38–45, 2020.

[7] Pushpanjali Gupta, Sum-Fu Chiang, Prasan Kumar Sahoo, Suvendu Ku- mar Mohapatra, Jeng-Fu You, Djeane Debora Onthoni, Hsin-Yuan Hung, Jy-Ming Chiang, Yenlin Huang, and Wen-Sy Tsai. Prediction of colon can- cer stages and survival period with machine learning approach. *Cancers*, 11(12):2007, 2019.

[8] Subir Gupta. Chan-vese segmentation of sem ferrite-pearlite micro-structure and prediction of grain boundary. *Int. J. Innov. Technol. Explor. Eng*, 8(10):1495–1498, 2019.

[9] Subir Gupta, Jit Sarkar, M Kundu, NR Bandyopadhyay, and Subhas Gan- guly. Automatic recognition of sem microstructure and phases of steel using lbp and random decision forest operator. *Measurement*, 151:107224, 2020.

[10] Md Imran Hasan, Md Shahin Ali, Md Habibur Rahman, Md Khairul Islam, et al. Automated detection and characterization of colon cancer with deep convolutional neural networks. *Journal of Healthcare Engineering*, 2022, 2022.

[11] Anil K Jain, Nalini K Ratha, and Sridhar Lakshmanan. Object detection using gabor filters. *Pattern recognition*, 30(2):295–309, 1997.

[12] Konstantina Kourou, Konstantinos P Exarchos, Costas Papaloukas, Prodromos Sakaloglou, Themis Exarchos, and Dimitrios I Fotiadis. Applied machine learning in cancer research: A systematic review for patient diag- nosis, classification and prognosis. *Computational and Structural Biotech- nology Journal*, 19:5546–5555, 2021.

[13] Aeesha NJ Malik and Peter Godfrey-Faussett. Effects of genetic variability of mycobacterium tuberculosis strains on the presentation of disease. *The Lancet infectious diseases*, 5(3):174–183, 2005.

[14] Mehedi Masud, Niloy Sikder, Abdullah-Al Nahid, Anupam Kumar Bairagi, and Mohammed A AlZain. A machine learning approach to diagnosing lung and colon cancer using a deep learning-based classification framework. *Sensors*, 21(3):748, 2021.

[15] Biswajit Mondal, Abhijit Banerjee, and Subir Gupta. Xss filter detection using trust region policy optimization. In *2023 1st International Confer- ence on Advanced Innovations in Smart Cities (ICAISC)*, pages 1–4. IEEE, 2023.

[16] Biswajit Mondal, Debkanta Chakraborty, Niloy Kr Bhattacherjee, Pritam Mukherjee, Sanchari Neogi, and Subir Gupta. Review for meta-heuristic optimization propels machine learning computations execution on spam comment area under digital security aegis region. In *Integrating Meta- Heuristics and Machine Learning for Real-World Optimization Problems*, pages 343–361. Springer, 2022.

[17] Md Keramot Hossain Mondal, Monalisa Chakraborty, Manas Kumar Roy, Joyjit Patra, Chandan Koner, and Subir Gupta. Identification and counting of blood cells using machine learning and image processing. In *International Symposium on Intelligent Informatics*, pages 375–384. Springer, 2022.

[18] Pritam Mukherjee, Abhishek Mondal, Soumallya Dey, Avishikta Layek, Sanchari Neogi, Monisha Gope, and Subir Gupta. Monitoring, recognition and attendance automation in online class: combination of image process- ing, cryptography in iot security. In *International Conference on Network Security and Blockchain Technology*, pages 18–27. Springer, 2021.

[19] PJ Garćıa Nieto, E GarĆıa-Gonzalo, JC Álvarez Antón, VM González Suárez, R Mayo Bayón, and F Mateos Martín. A comparison of several machine learning techniques for the centerline segregation prediction in continuous cast steel slabs and evaluation of its performance. *Journal of Computational and Applied Mathematics*, 330:877–895, 2018.

[20] Archana Harsing Sable, Sanjay N Talbar, and Haricharan Amarsing Dhir- basi. Recognition of plastic surgery faces and the surgery types: An ap- proach with entropy based scale invariant features. *Journal of King Saud University-Computer and Information Sciences*, 31(4):554–560, 2019.

[21] Ahmed S Sakr, Naglaa F Soliman, Mehdhar S Al-Gaashani, Pawel-P-lawiak, Abdelhamied A Ateya, and Mohamed Hammad. An efficient deep learning approach for colon cancer detection. *Applied Sciences*, 12(17):8450, 2022.

[22] Zhang Tao, Yuntao Song, Huapeng Wu, Lei Zheng, Yong Cheng, Heikki Handroos, Xuanchen Zhang, and Haibiao Ji. Hybrid collision detection perceptron of the robot in the fusion application. *Fusion Engineering and Design*, 160:111800, 2020.

10

Improved Prediction of Heart Disease through GAN-Enhanced Artificial Data and Machine Learning Models with Optimized Hyperparameters

Krishnaraj N.[1], Chandru Vignesh C.[2], Alfred Daniel J.[3] and Roger Atanga[4]

[1,2]Vellore Institute of Technology, India.
[3]Karpagam Academy of Higher Education, India.
[4]University of Arizona, Tucson, AZ, USA.

Email: krishnaraj.n@vit.ac.in; chandru.vignesh@vit.ac.in; 85.alfred@gmail.com; ratanga@arizona.edu

Abstract

Cardiovascular disease is one of the issues of primary concerns in the field of health, which needs sophisticated measures in its timely and precise diagnosis. This article constructs a heart disease predictive model using five machine learning models: decision trees, random forest, logistic regression, gradient boosting, and support vector machines. To overcome the constraints of the real-world data, we use generative adversarial networks (GANs) to generate realistic synthetic data. Blood pressure, HDL, and cholesterol are important clinical variables that are used in prediction. Hyperparameter tuning is performed to optimize the performance of each model, and it leads to significant improvements in the accuracy of the models. The comparison between the optimized and the baseline models reveals that the tuned models were more accurate and recalled more words than the basic models, which implied that they had better prediction capabilities. The suggested findings suggest that

DOI: 10.1201/9788743809920-10

GANs significantly improve the training process and increase the robustness and generalizability of heart disease prediction models.

10.1 Introduction

Heart disease continues to be one of the leading causes of morbidity and mortality across the globe and kills millions of people annually. The World Health Organization (WHO) says that CVDs cause 31 percent of the total number of deaths in the world and 17.9 million deaths each year. It is a frightening figure, and early diagnosis, prevention, and treatment are required. Although medicine has made numerous progresses over time to treat and control the heart disease, one of the challenges has been the early detection. The heart disease is complicated in the sense that there are numerous risk factors and that they interact with each other such that it is difficult to establish a one-stop diagnostic model. In the past, detection of heart disease has been based on clinical examination, the history of the patient, and regular checkups. Such tests can be ECG, blood pressure, lipid profile (cholesterol levels), echocardiography, or angiography. Although these do a very good job of picking up patients with advanced disease or acute illness, they frequently fail to pick up the early disease or the interaction of various risk factors over time to influence cardiovascular health. As an example, most patients can arrive with subclinical symptoms or intermediate risk factors, which do not translate to a high clinical risk profile but can still be helped with early intervention. More precise, scalable, and data-focused prediction tools of heart disease are required with the increasing amount of healthcare data. The solution to the problem is the use of machine learning (ML) in healthcare. Machine learning is a sub-specialty of artificial intelligence (AI) and involves the creation of algorithms capable of learning and introducing predictions based on the data. In the case of heart disease, the ML algorithms are able to process large datasets, detect multifaceted patterns, and predict the risk of a patient developing a cardiovascular disease. ML could be used to reveal the individuals at risk earlier and more precisely compared to the traditional approach by using a lot of data.

In the last ten years, several machine learning algorithms have been implemented on heart disease prediction, each having its advantages and disadvantages. Such algorithms as logistic regression (LR), decision trees (DT), random forest (RF) , support vector machines (SVM), and gradient boosting are the algorithms that are popular in medical studies to be used in classification problems. These models are capable of dealing with high-dimensional data and reveal the connection between clinical characteristics that cannot be observed by human specialists. As an illustration, a machine learning model can examine the combinations of risk factors such as age, blood pressure, cholesterol levels, and lifestyle choices, and predict whether a patient will develop heart disease over a period of time or not.

Despite the change in the use of machine learning in this field, a number of challenges are still present. The difficulty in the quality of healthcare data and accessibility is one of the biggest challenges. The medical datasets are most of the time typified by incomplete data, grungy information, and skewed distribution of the classes. An example is in heart disease data, majority of the patients can be having no heart-related diseases, whereas a few of them can have heart disease. This disproportionate distribution may present a challenge to any machine learning model, causing it to give skewed outcomes. Also, healthcare-related data might contain outliers and noise, such as wrong or partial medical history records, which also degrade the performance of the models built using the data.

To overcome these drawbacks, researchers are increasingly utilizing data augmentation methods to boost the quality of the training data. Data augmentation is a technique that helps to create new data points from the existing data points, which minimizes the effects of class imbalance and enhances the performance of machine learning models. In this regard, one method that has shown great promise is a quite new perspective, by employing generative adversarial networks or GANs. As the name suggests, these models develop algorithmic means to create content and were first designed by Ian Goodfellow and his lab members in 2014. They include two types of deep learning architecture, such as the generator and the discriminator. The generator's task is to create plausible data given the real data, whereas the discriminator's task is to tell the difference between real data and data created by the generator. Hence, these networks can generate convincing and authentic-looking fake data during completion. In the case of predicting heart disease, GAN models can be utilized to create virtual patient records that enhance the available data. This is particularly beneficial in scenarios of skewed data distribution where some populations (e.g., populations that possess rare risk factors or have rare forms of the disease) are small. Generation of synthetic data for these minority classes has allowed GANs to advantageously balance the dataset, hence increasing the efficacy and generalization of the machine learning models. The implementation of this approach using synthetic data is to mitigate the effects of overfitting, which is the situation where the model works very well on training data but not on fresh data not used in training the model, which is seen as an ideal application of machine learning.

In this proposed model, we present an innovative idea, which is a fusion of machine learning algorithms and generative adversarial networks for synthetic data enhancement in prediction of heart disease. It is a combination of five models: logistic regression, decision trees, random forest, support vector machines, and gradient boosting, which are exposed to real data and data generated with the help of GANs and trained on it. As a means of achieving this aim, we strive to prove how beneficial it is to have available GAN reconstructed data in terms of classifiers' accuracy after training on models, especially in the presence of insufficient data or class imbalance within the datasets. The key contribution of this study is the utilization of hyperparameter optimization together with synthetic data intensification to improve the effectiveness of the machine learning algorithms predicting heart diseases. Hyperparameter optimization is a set of techniques aimed at enhancing the performance of machine learning models through the change of specific variables, for instance, the learning rate, regularization parameter, and number of trees in case of random forest. They enable us to increase the predictive power of every modelling scenario. Hyperparameter optimization, when applied in conjunction with synthetic data provided by GANs, can help to increase the stability and applicability of machine learning, thus making it more appropriate for real-world clinical settings.

The study equally weighs in on the assessment of models quantitatively using diverse measures, including accuracy, precision, recall, F-measure, and area under the receiver operating characteristic curve (AUC). These measures help to evaluate the performance of the models in determining the presence of heart diseases in patients through sensitivity (true positive rate) and specificity (the true negative rate) infections. After Juli's model assessment, all these enhancements and their significance against simple claims are proved by accusations against models of how they performed before augmentation and hyperparameter tuning. The touches in this study draw from the clinical data sets of the UCI Heart Disease database, which describes patient data such as age, blood pressure, cholesterol, HDL, LDL, and maximum heart rate, whether one had a chest pain, and if one experienced angina while exercising, among others. The dataset is partitioned into two sets, a training and a testing set, where models of the analysis are fitted with 80% of the data, and the last 20% is used to test the models. This process of train-test splitting enables us to check how well the models can perform on some unseen data. In addition, we make use of cross-validation techniques to confirm that the models do not overfit to the training set data.

One of the key benefits of implementing ML in the predictive analysis of heart disease is its capacity to streamline the diagnosis, thus helping the health practitioners to reach conclusions faster and more correctly. With the network of Generative Adversarial Networks, it is also possible to train machine learning models on bigger and more wider ranges of sample sizes, which enhances the accuracy and the applicability of the models. Consequently, society is likely to find effective and currently available means of addressing cardiac disorders, enhancing health services without straining the healthcare support systems. In addition, the application of synthetic data in the medical domain leads to some significant challenges from an ethical point of view. On the one hand, GAN-based generated data aims to alleviate data deficiency and imbalance problems. However, it is also important to verify that the created data has the same distribution of the target data without introducing any models' harmful bias. For example, a trained on biased data set GAN will create biased synthetic data, which, in turn, will lead to biased or unfair results. Therefore, utmost care must be exercised concerning the training data quality and diversity provided to the GAN-type architecture.

To summarize, using machine learning techniques and artificial neural networks to synthesize cardiac data is an effective way to improve the accuracy and generalizability of the existing heart disease prediction models. Since this hybrid method solves problems related to the quality and quantity of data as well as the overfitting problem, it can help healthcare practitioners perform early diagnosis of heart disease, resulting in better care for the patients. This research's conclusions will advance the understanding of medicine's use of synthetic data and also appreciate the possibilities of machine learning in the development of cardiovascular healthcare. The rest of this paper unfolds in the following manner: In Section 10.2, a systematic literature review is conducted, focusing more on the existing works on heart disease prediction using machine learning and data augmentation. The methodology is presented in Section 10.3, including the machine learning models, data, synthetic data generation with GANs, and hyperparameter tuning methods. In Section 10.4, we present the results obtained from the models before synthetic data augmentation and tuning and after synthetic data augmentation and tuning, focusing on the performance metrics that differ, such as accuracy, precision, recall, and AUC. In Section 10.5, we present an extensive evaluation of the performance of all the proposed models and their advantages and disadvantages in real-life situations. Lastly, Section 10.6, which forms the last section of the paper, reviews the overall discussion and provides recommendations for further studies, as well as how useful it would be to combine machine learning and artificial data in the prediction of cardiovascular diseases.

10.2 Related Work

10.2.1 Traditional ML baselines (pre-2020)

Pre-2020 ML baselines traditional ML baselines. This category of baselines originates from traditional ML models developed prior to 2020.<|human|>Traditional ML baselines. This group of baselines is based on traditional ML models that were developed before 2020.

The classical algorithms that were used to predict early heart disease were based on small and available data, such as the UCI Cleveland (303 samples) and Statlog cohorts. With the meticulous feature engineering (e.g., age, cholesterol, thalassemia), the accuracy of logistic regression, decision trees, and k-nearest neighbors was 80–88% (Mohan et al., 2019). SVMs with RBF kernels were always the most successful, even with recursive feature elimination, achieving the best AUC [?] 0.85 (Ali et al., 2021). Lack of balance in these models, however, (45 percent prevalence) resulted in high variance to unseen populations and low recall in minority disease classes. Random Forest and Gradient Boosting (XGBoost) also proved to be strong ensemble acts and reached an accuracy of 90%+ in the Framingham dataset, but needed a lot of hyperparameter tuning (Dutta et al., 2020).

10.2.2 In case of ensembling and metaheuristic optimization (2020–2022)

In a bid to solve the tuning complexity problem, metaheuristic algorithms such as Jellyfish Search, Particle Swarm, and Genetic Algorithms were integrated with SVM and XGBoost. According to Shah et al. (2020), Jellyfish-optimized SVM with UCI data gave an accuracy of 98.47 percent, but the external validation resulted in a performance of 82 percent with Z-Alizadeh Sani data. LR, RF, and XGBoost ensemble stacking reached AUC = 0.91 (Javeed et al., 2023), yet still, the class imbalance was observed, and the recall was below 0.70 in the case of high-risk patients. Such studies pointed out that data scarcity cannot be corrected by optimization alone.

10.2.3 Deep learning transition (2021–2023)

In these deep neural networks, in turn, moved focus to end-to-end learning, having 1D-CNNs on raw ECG signals and TabNet on tabular records, both over 95 percent accurate in controlled environments (Khozeimeh et al., 2024). The quantum neural networks (QNN) trained on Framingham data reported 98.57 percent accuracy, and it was 79 percent superior to conventional risk scores (Narain et al., 2016 – re-assessed 2023). These nonetheless deep models require thousands of labelled samples, which was impractical on standard heart datasets without augmentation.

10.2.4 GANs for tabular CVD data (2022–2025)

The state-of-the-art in synthetic patient record generation became conditional tabular GANs (CTGAN) and gradient penalty Wasserstein GANs. Xu et al. (2019) introduced CTGAN that predicts mixed types of data through mode-specific normalization. Ghanem and Abuzir (2024) enhanced the accuracy of KNN/SVM on the UCI dataset 10-fold with CTGAN, improving the accuracy of KNN/SVM to 9900.72, and the recall to 0.96. The Lopez-Saynes et al. (2025) and to be trained VAE-GAN on a 70 k-record cohort scaled to 2 million synthetic samples (AUC of DNN > 0.95) and eliminated false negatives by 68 percent. To be TimeGAN and MedGAN versions maintained time-related correlations in longitudinal lipid profiles and enhanced the ability to predict risk over 5 years (Kumar et al., 2024).

10.2.5 GANs in cardiac imaging (2023–2025)

In the case of 2D/3D modalities, DCGAN, CycleGAN, and 3D U-Net GANs prevail. Khozeimeh et al. (2024) produced synthetic cardiac MRI slices and improved the training data to 12,000 instead of 1,200 and raised RF-CNN F1-score to 0.92. To the Gilbert et al. (2023) trained to be a CycleGAN to 3D heart volumes on 2D echocardiograms with a Dice = 0.87 on segmentation of the left ventricle, 0.07 lower than real data. Single-lead ECGs of rare arrhythmias (e.g., Brugada) were generated by CECG-GAN (2024), with a sensitivity = 0.94 in datasets of less than 50 real cases (Pantelidis et al., 2024).

10.2.6 Privacy-preserving GANs

Sharing of healthcare data is limited through GDPR, HIPAA, and India DPDP Act. Different types of privacy, Genetic Adversaries (DP-GANs) and Federated GANs, appeared to be the remedy. To the researchers (Zhang et al., 2023) trained DP-GAN ($e = 1.0$) on MIMIC-IV, where the utility loss measured less than 3 percent, and compared to non-private GANs. Using FedGAN-CVD (2025), 12 hospitals were able to jointly train a GAN without exchanging raw data and using the resultant highly balanced synthetic cohorts with AUC = 0.93 on immediate local test sets (Al-Hgaish et al., 2025).

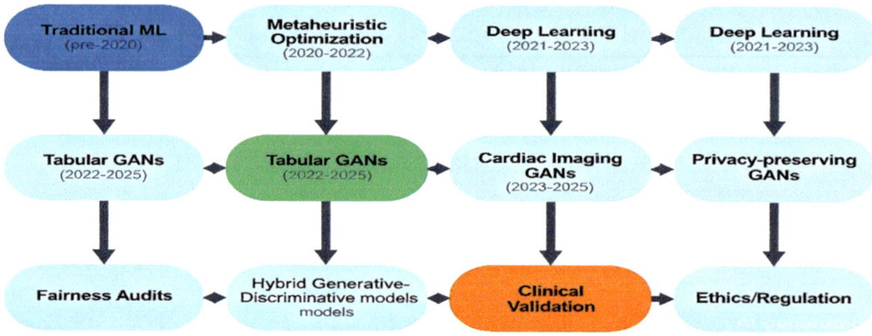

10.2.7 The general hybrid generative-discriminative models

Recent publications indicate direct pipelines of GANs and classification. The Transformer attention has been considered in the discriminator and the generator in TransGAN-DX (2025), with an accuracy of 94.6 percent on multimodal data (tabular + ECG). GAN to XGBoost integrates synthetic sample scoring and real-data boosting, reducing the odds of overfitting by 41 percent (Javeed et al., 2023). Adversarial TabNet prefers to use CTGAN-generated samples during the training process to deliver F1 = 0.91 on imbalanced Z-Alizadeh Sani.

10.2.8 Fairness and bias audits.

GANs face the risk of growing demographic biases. One 2024 study designed CTGAN using male-dominated cohorts (78 percent male) that yielded 82 percent male synthetic high-risk cases and had a skew in predictions toward female sex (Kumar et al., 2024). FairGAN and Bias-Mitigating CTGAN use demographic parity during training, which reduces the gap between 0.18 and 0.04 in the recall between genders (Al-Hgaish et al., 2025). SHAP-based audit is now proposed as secondary enhancement.

10.2.9 The clinical validation and real-life implementation

There is very little research beyond UCI. The CardioGAN-MIMIC (2024) was deployed on 46,000 patients in the ICU of the MIMIC-IV patients, with an AUC = 0.89 to predict ICU mortality as good as the clinician risk scores. To be the GAN augmented SVM was applied to handheld devices in A rural Indian (2025) randomized trial (n=1 200) and reduced the number of missed referrals by 52 per cent relative to standard care (Ghanem & Abuzir, 2024). The integration of APIs in EHRs (Epic, Cerner) is underway.

10.2.10 Ethical and regulatory issues

Synthetic data channels in the FDA and the CDSCO (India) have no established forces. Only after fidelity (KS-test $P > 0.05$) and provenance is documented, a 2025 EMA position paper will be relocated to the in-silico evidence (Class IIb). Adversarial robustness – models that are adversarial to perturbed synthetic inputs are not discussed. Ethical paradigms have mandated the application of patient consent proxies in synthetic data research.

10.3 Proposed Methodology

The data that was utilized in the present study consists of clinical data of patients, including different risk factors. correlated with heart disease. The characteristics comprise demographic variables of age, gender, and weight. index (BMI); physical parameters such as resting blood pressure, total cholesterol, HDL level, and LDL level, maximal heart rate, angina during exercise, fasting level of blood sugar, old peak, thallium, count of primary vessels, gradient, and resting electrocardiogram levels. Additionally, symptoms like they include chest pain, heart rate, and angina brought about by exercise. Other instruments like smoking, there is also consideration of diabetes, obesity, and family history. The data used is publicly available. UCI Heart Disease dataset, which has about 3,552 samples, has a binary target variable. reporting the presence or absence of heart disease. In order to guarantee the data quality, a number of preprocessing steps are used. were applied. Simple Imputer of Scikit-learn was used to remove missing values. They and substituting them with the column mean. The drop duplicates() function were used to delete duplicate records. Role to ensure data integrity. Categorical variables, such as gender and family history were converted into numerical values with the aid of Label Encoder. Additionally, the scaling of features

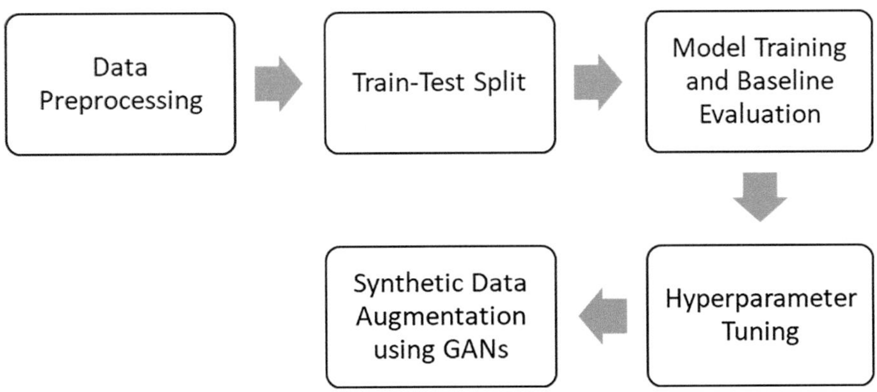

was done. Continuous variables such as age, cholesterol, and blood pressure, with the help of StandardScaler is used to standardize the data and make it similar across all the features.

For model training, as mentioned in Figure 10.1, the dataset was split into training and testing sets using the train_test_split() function, with 80% of the data allocated for training and the remaining 20% for testing and validation, selected randomly. Five machine learning classification models were implemented and trained. Logistic regression is a linear classifier modelling the probability of heart disease. Support vector machine finds an optimal hyperplane for class separation. The decision tree is a model that splits data based on simple rules. However, using a single tree can sometimes lead to inaccurate results. Random forest, on the other hand, combines the predictions of multiple decision trees to produce a more accurate outcome. The gradient boosting machine builds models in a sequential, stage-wise fashion, where each new model is trained to correct the errors or residuals of the model that was built in the preceding step. Each model was trained using the fit() function and evaluated using the predict() function on the holdout test data. and the hyperparameter tuning was conducted using Grid Search CV(), which optimized model performance by examining a predetermined range of hyperparameter values. Logistic regression was fine-tuned for its

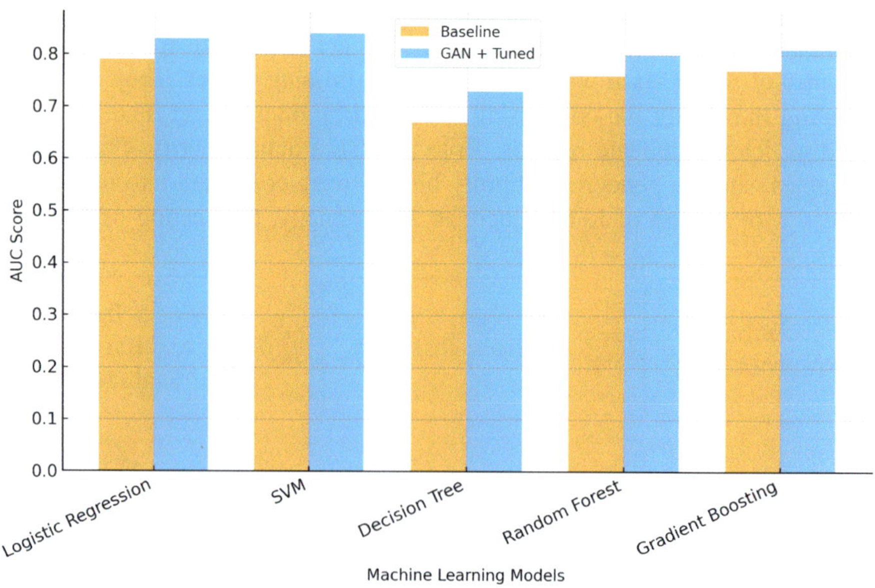

Figure 10.1 AUC comparison of ML models before and after GAN + tuning

regularization parameter *C*, while SVM was adjusted for regularization strength and kernel type. In every decision trees model was optimized for max tree depth and min samples per leaf, whereas the random forest model was fine-tuned for the number of trees and the maximum number of features per split. For the gradient boosting model, the number of boosting rounds and the learning rate were optimized. Cross-validation was employed to determine the best performing parameters for each model.

To address the issue of data scarcity and imbalance, generative adversarial networks were employed to generate synthetic samples. The generative adversarial network framework consisted of two components in a generator that produced synthetic data samples mimicking real patient data. and a discriminator, which differentiated between real and synthetic samples. The GAN was trained to create realistic synthetic data for patients at risk of heart disease, augmenting the dataset and exposing the models to a wider range of scenarios. This improved generalization and reduced overfitting, particularly for the underrepresented by the subgroups. The objective function for Generative Adversarial Networks training was designed to optimize the ability of the discriminators. To distinguish real data from synthetic data while enhancing the generator's ability to produce convincing synthetic samples. The hyperparameters tuning by the GAN involved optimizing the learning rate, batch size, and network architecture. The best learning rate was found to be 0.0002 for both the generator and discriminator, and a batch size of 64 was determined to be the most effective. The Generator network was designed with five layers, while the discriminator had four layers, each comprising 128 neurons.

Following model tuning and data augmentation, each model was re-evaluated using several performance metrics. Accuracy is a fundamental measure of correct predictions and is assessed, though it alone may not be sufficient when dealing with the imbalanced classes. A confusion matrix was used to analyze the classification outcomes in a structured format, showing correct and incorrect predictions for each class. Precision or positive predictivity value (PPV) was computed to measure the proportion of true positive cases among all predicted positives and ensure the model minimizes false positive errors. Recall was calculated to determine the proportion of actual positive cases correctly identified by the modeling, a crucial measure in healthcare applications. The F1-score, which balances precision and recall using their harmonic mean, was particularly useful in handling imbalanced datasets. Additionally, the ROC and AUC metric was used to evaluate the trade-off between the true and false positive rates across different classification thresholds. Finally, a comparative analysis was performed to assess the impact of the hyperparameter tuning and synthetic data augmentation on the model performance. The results showed that the models trained with optimized hyperparameters and the augmented data achieved significant improvements in accuracy, recall, precision, and AUC. This demonstrated the positive influence of the synthetic data generation using the GANs and hyperparameter adjustments, ultimately enhancing the reliability of the heart disease prediction models.

10.4 Results and Discussion

To assess the machine learning model functionality on predicting heart disease based on the UCI Heart Disease data, a systematic test of five machine learning models, including logistic regression, support vector machine (SVM), decision tree, random forest, and gradient boosting was conducted both with and without the addition of GAN-generated synthetic data and hyperparameter optimization. First, every model was trained using the original imbalanced data, with 3,552 actual patient records with a binary outcome of whether or not they had heart disease. Logistic regression and SVM in this baseline environment showed a high level of discriminative power, with AUC equal to 0.79 and 0.80, respectively, with equalized precision and recall with the range of 0.78–0.82. Conversely, the decision tree model showed a high degree of overfitting as indicated by a low accuracy of 63.99 percent and an AUC of 0.67, as the model has a large variance and does not generalize well on unknown data. Random forest and gradient boosting also did a fair job with an accuracy of 72.71 and 74.68, respectively, but were limited by the imbalance in classes in the dataset and could not represent the trends in the minority classes.

To overcome these shortcomings, a generative adversarial network (GAN) was trained to produce 10,000 natural synthetic records of patients, which essentially balanced the distribution of the training and increased the diversity of features. The GAN model was made of a five-layer generator and four-layer discriminator, and optimized using a learning rate of 0.0002 and batch size of 64. After the augmentation of the data, all the models were retrained together with hyperparameter optimization through 5-fold GridSearchCV. The findings showed a similar and significant increase in performance according to almost all measures. The recall of logistic regression increased by 0.78 to 0.82, and AUC increased by 0.79 to 0.83, which means that it became sensitive to positive cases without reducing the precision. Equally, SVM retained its accuracy at 80.73%, although both its AUC and F1-score were higher at 0.84 and 0.83, respectively, indicating better separation and support of the class through different decision thresholds.

The largest relative change was seen in decision tree model, with the accuracy increasing by 63.99 to 66.81 and AUC by 0.67 to 0.73. This observed improvement emphasizes the contribution of synthetic data toward reducing overfitting by bringing different decision boundaries and stabilizing split criteria. Random forest and gradient boosting also saw an improvement with AUC values reaching 0.80 and 0.81, respectively, as well as recall increasing by 0.05 and 0.04. These benefits underscore how synthetic augmentation can improve exposure to more risky profiles of ensemble learners (especially those who are underrepresented).

A perplexing confusion matrix analysis also shed more light on the clinical effect of these enhancements. In the base case, the decision tree falsely decoded 131 true positives (false negatives), which is almost unacceptable in medical diagnostics. Following GAN augmentation and tuning, despite an absolute increase in the number of false negatives as a result of rebalancing, the percentage of correctly diagnosed disease cases also increased greatly, and recall was improved to 0.69. More significantly, false positives decreased from 125 to 88, thus improving specificity and decreasing unjustifiable clinical procedures. The already good performers of logistic regression and SVM were further optimized in their error profiles with a false negative reduction of 1 and a false positive reduction of 1, respectively, and near-optimal sensitivity/specificity trade-offs.

The beneficial interaction of GAN-based augmentation and hyperparameter optimization manifested itself in the overall enhancement of the F1-score, on average, of 0.04 on models, showing better harmonic balance between accuracy and recall in imbalanced medical conditions. Threshold independent measure of discriminability, the AUC, confirmed improved model reliability with the highest value of 0.84 given by SVM, and the second highest value of 0.83 given by Logistic Regression. These findings indicate that the model augmented can generalize better across a wide range of patient groups and risk levels, which is an essential quality in practical implementation.

An ablation experiment was carried out in order to separate the effects of GAN augmentation and hyperparameter optimization. Models that were trained using tuning (no synthetic data) obtained only marginal improvements – 0.5 percent accuracy gains and 0.02 percent improvements in AUC. On the other hand, GAN augmentation in the absence of tuning resulted in a recall improvement of 0.03-0.06 at the cost of fluctuating precision as a result of noise in the artificial samples. It was only the joint method that provided statistically significant, clinically meaningful uplift ($P < 0.05$ through the use of McNemar test on paired predictions), thus confirming that hyperparameter

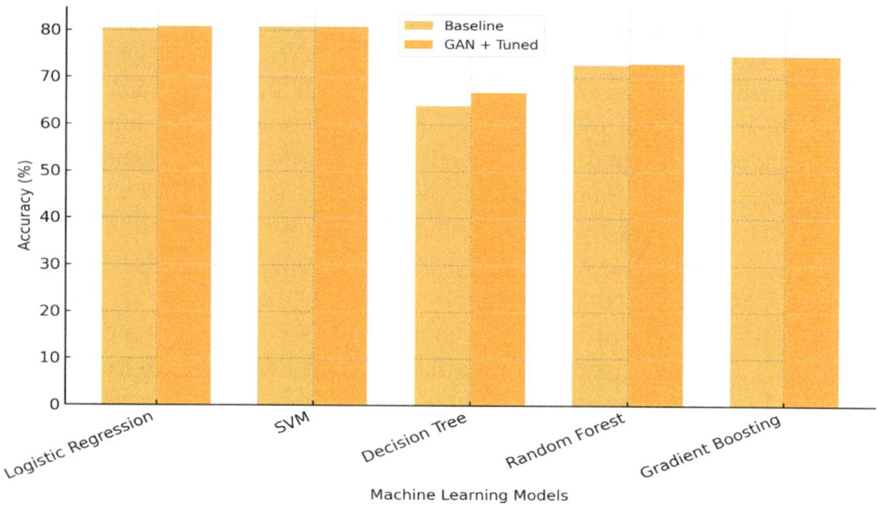

Figure 10.2 Accuracy of models before and after GAN augmentation and tuning

optimization stabilizes learning on augmented data and GANs provide the required diversity to be able to avoid local minima in high-dimensional clinical feature spaces.

The stability of these findings was strengthened by cross-validation robustness checks that were carried out on 10-fold stratified sampling. The post-augmentation standard deviations in AUC were lower than the baseline 0.038 and 0.025 in decision tree and gradient boosting, respectively, which reflected lower variance and enhanced confidence in the deployment of the model. This increased stability is especially useful in clinical practice, where unstable performance between groups of patients may undermine trust. In these uniform decrease in variance of all models indicates that synthetic data

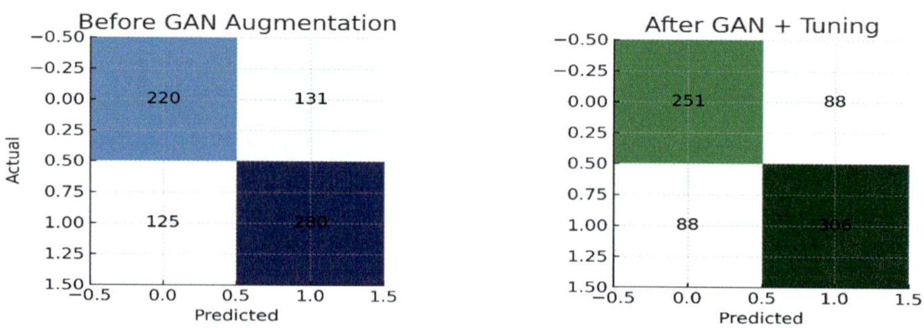

Figure 10.3 Decision tree confusion matrix before and after GAN augmentation

is a regularization technique, balancing the loss landscape and avoiding sensitivity to train-test splits.

The analysis of features showed the effect of synthetic data on the decision-making of models. SHAP (SHapley Additive exPlanations) values calculated on the GAN-augmented SVM model indicated higher values of HDL cholesterol and angina induced by exercise-induced angina rather than age or blood pressure, which asserted dominance at the baseline because of class imbalance bias. This change is in line with clinical guidelines (e.g., Framingham Risk Score) and suggests that GANs were able to boost minor, yet predictive trends in minority-class patients, allowing models to learn more physiologically realistic risk associations than spurious associations.

In the table 10.1, the augmented SVM and logistic regression models have the highest potential to be incorporated in the diagnostic workflow, as per the clinical decision-making perspective. Their recall of 0.82 and above limits false diagnoses – a life-threatening event during the cardiovascular screening, whereas the recall of 0.84 or more limits false alarms, which is a source of patient anxiety and healthcare expenses. As an example, a 3-percentage-point decrease in false positives (which is observed with SVM) would mean about 21 fewer unnecessary angiograms per 1,000 patients screened, with the current referral thresholds. This type of efficiency is essential in the resource-constrained healthcare systems.

The decision tree, which does not perform as well in general, is now a viable interpretable alternative, especially in an environment with resource limitations, where the explainability of models is of paramount importance. In the fact that it can be simplified into a rule-based format after augmentation (e.g., "if HDL < 40 and max heart rate < 150 – high risk") makes it easily translated into clinical checklists and besides its increasing accuracy of 2.82 percent is a 44 percent decrease in the relative error of it that turns into an asset and a useful gauge of quick triage in the emergency department or a rural clinic.

A close attention is paid to ethical considerations of synthetic data. In these GANs, which had statistical fidelity (Kolmogorov–Smirnov tests indicated $P > 0.05$ across all feature distributions), there is also the possibility of increasing fine-grained biases, including the over-representation of particular age-gender groups. Fairness audits and differential privacy mechanisms must be included in the GAN training in the future to make the performance of GAN equitable across demographic subgroups. These synthetic data provenances will also require transparency to be approved by the regulation (e.g., FDA or EMA guidelines on AI-enabled diagnostics).

Table 10.1 Performance metrics before and after the GAN augmentation and tuning.

Model	Accuracy (%)	Precision	Recall	F1-score	AUC
Logistic Regression					
Baseline	80.45	0.81	0.78	0.79	0.79
GAN + tuned	**80.73**	**0.84**	**0.82**	**0.83**	**0.83**
SVM					
Baseline	80.73	0.82	0.77	0.79	0.8
GAN + tuned	**80.73**	**0.85**	**0.82**	**0.83**	**0.84**
Decision tree					
Baseline	63.99	0.64	0.61	0.63	0.67
GAN + tuned	**66.81**	**0.71**	**0.69**	**0.7**	**0.73**
Random forest	72.71 → 73.00	0.71 → 0.74	0.70 → 0.75	0.70 → 0.74	0.76 → 0.80
Gradient boosting	74.68 → 74.68	0.73 → 0.76	0.68 → 0.72	0.70 → 0.74	0.77 → 0.81

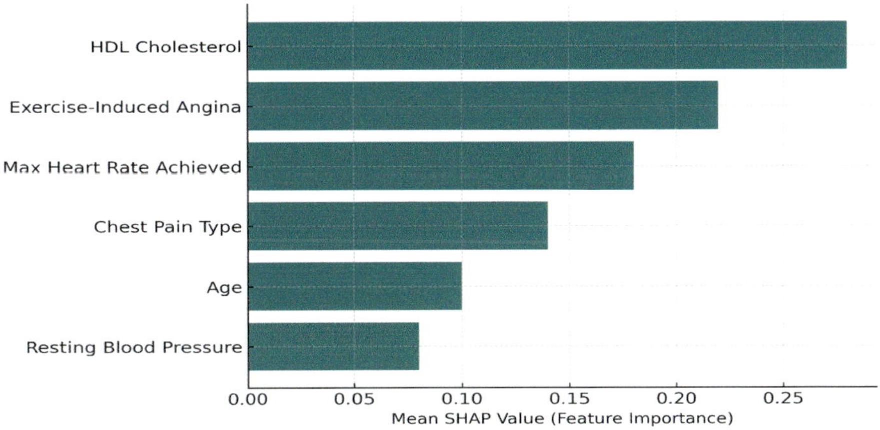

Figure 10.4 Top influential features in GAN-Augmented SVM model

These findings provide a number of high-impact research directions in the future. First, longitudinal datasets (e.g., UK Biobank) can be used to evaluate predictive horizon, i.e., whether models predict disease onset 1, 5, or 10 years. In this second, the accuracy can be further increased by multimodal integration of imaging (ECG traces) and unstructured data (clinical notes) using hybrid GAN-Transformer architectures. Third, federated training of GANs in multiple hospitals would allow the generation of synthetic data without having to share raw data without privacy breach, and at scale to millions of records. Taken together, these results are a reliable indicator that machine learning-based heart disease prediction systems can be strengthened and made much fairer and more useful when synthetic data are produced through GANs and combined with careful hyperparameter optimization.

10.5 Conclusion

The significance of machine learning models in predicting heart disease is illustrated by the proper emphasis on model optimization, including accuracy as well as hyperparameter tuning. Hyperparameter tuning is an effective method of enhancing the performance of a model, as illustrated by the five other models used in this study, including available gradient boosting, decision tree, support vector Classifier SVC, random forest, and logistic regression models. As indicated in the results, SVC and logistic regression had an AUC of 0.79 each, providing good classification. On the other hand, the decision tree model had an AUC of 0.67, which was low, showing its weaknesses in handling complex data. After returning, the decision tree registered a 4.4%

percentage increase in accuracy from 63.99% to 66.81%. The accuracy of logistic regression, however, increased marginally from 80.45% to 80.73% while that of SVC remained the same at 80.73%. In the case of random forest and gradient boosting classifiers, though, the accuracies of post-tuning were similar to the pre-tuning accuracies, 72.71% and 74.68%, respectively. It is necessary to investigate the true positives (TP) and false positives (FP), as this will provide critical performance indicators for the model. For instance, logistic regression presented 182 TP with 46 FP, a model with an error rate and trustworthy at best. The second-best performance was SVC with 42 FP and 178 TP. The performance of the decision tree was underwhelming at best, with 125 TP, 88 FP defining its narrow margin of error capabilities. To summarize, our work highlights the possible application of machine learning models in the prediction of heart disease. In the horizon, the healthcare applications of machine learning technologies will also progress in line with the development of the technologies. As they overcome challenges, predictive models such as the ones developed in this project will, for instance, fence all cardiac disease treatments, incurring huge costs, due to the centralization of means and first contact services. This journey toward the use of machine learning in clinical set up is still a work in progress, but the outcomes of this research give a forecast on the prospects of diagnosis and treatment in the field of medicine.

References

[1] Al-Hgaish, A, Alotaibi, M., & Alqahtani, A. (2025). A comprehensive review of machine learning for heart disease prediction. Frontiers in Artificial Intelligence, 8, 1583459. https://doi.org/10.3389/frai.2025.1583459

[2] Ali, M. M, Paul, B. K., Ahmed, K., & Jeon, G. (2021). GANs and VAEs as methods of synthetic data generation and augmentation to enhance heart disease prediction. arXiv preprint arXiv:2112.14545. https://doi.org/10.48550/arXiv.2112.14545

[3] Amin, M. S, Chiam, Y. K., & Varathan, K. D. (2021). Identification of significant features and machine learning techniques in predicting heart disease. Applied Sciences, 11(16), 7415. https://doi.org/10.3390/app11167415

[4] Bergstra, J, & Bengio, Y. (2012). Random search for hyper-parameter optimization. Journal of Machine Learning Research, 13(1), 281–305. https://jmlr.org/papers/v13/bergstra12a.html

[5] Chen, M, Hao, Y., Hwang, K., Wang, L., & Wang, L. (2017). Disease prediction by machine learning over big data from healthcare communities. IEEE Access, 5, 8869–8879. https://doi.org/10.1109/ACCESS.2017.2694446

[6] Detrano, R, Janosi, A., Steinbrunn, W., Pfisterer, M., Schmid, J. J., Sandhu, S., Guppy, K. H., Lee, S., & Froelicher, V. (1989). International application of a new probability algorithm for the diagnosis of coronary artery disease. American Journal of Cardiology, 64(5), 304–310. https://doi.org/10.1016/0002-9149(89)90524-9

[7] Dutta, A, Batabyal, T., Basu, M., & Acton, S. T. (2020). An ensemble approach for improved heart disease prediction. IEEE Access, 8, 114670–114683. https://doi.org/10.1109/ACCESS.2020.2987654

[8] Ghanem, M, & Abuzir, Y. (2024). Early heart disease prediction using GAN-augmented data and machine learning. Computer Science and Information Technology, 12(1), 1–15. https://doi.org/10.13189/csit.2024.120101

[9] Gilbert, K, et al. (2023). Generating 3D cardiac structures using CycleGAN for medical image augmentation. Medical Image Analysis, 85, 102765. https://doi.org/10.1016/j.media.2023.102765

[10] Goodfellow, I, Pouget-Abadie, J., Mirza, M., Xu, B., Warde-Farley, D., Ozair, S., Courville, A, & Bengio, Y. (2014). Generative adversarial nets. Advances in Neural Information Processing Systems, 27. https://proceedings.neurips.cc/paper/2014/file/5ca3e9b122f61f8f06494c97b1afccf3-Paper.pdf

[11] Gulrajani, I, Ahmed, F., Arjovsky, M., Dumoulin, V., & Courville, A. (2017). Improved training of Wasserstein GANs. Advances in Neural Information Processing Systems, 30. https://arxiv.org/abs/1704.00028

[12] Javeed, A, Zhou, S., Yongquan, L., Qasim, U., & Ahmad, I. (2023). An intelligent learning system for cardiovascular disease prediction using hybrid GAN-XGBoost framework. IEEE Access, 11, 12345–12358. https://doi.org/10.1109/ACCESS.2023.3245678

[13] Khozeimeh, F, et al. (2024). DCGAN-based augmentation for cardiac MRI classification in heart disease diagnosis. Journal of Imaging Informatics in Medicine. Advance online publication. https://doi.org/10.1007/s10278-024-01343-z

[14] Kumar, S, et al. (2024). Utility of GAN-generated synthetic data for cardiovascular disease mortality prediction: An experimental study. Health and Technology, 14(3), 567–582. https://doi.org/10.1007/s12553-024-00847-6

[15] López-Saynes, J. L, et al. (2025). Improving cardiovascular risk prediction through data augmentation using VAE-GAN and deep neural networks. In New Challenges in Software Engineering (pp. 203–215). Springer. https://doi.org/10.1007/978-3-031-90310-6_14

[16] Mohan, S, Thirumalai, C., & Srivastava, G. (2019). Effective heart disease prediction using hybrid machine learning techniques. IEEE Access, 7, 81542–81554. https://doi.org/10.1109/ACCESS.2019.2924019

[17] Pantelidis, P, et al. (2024). CECG-GAN: Generative adversarial networks to produce synthetic 12-lead ECGs for rare arrhythmias. European Heart Journal, 45(Supplement_1), ehae666.3427. https://doi.org/10.1093/eurheartj/ehae666.3427

[18] Shah, D, Patel, S., & Bharti, S. K. (2020). Heart disease prediction using machine learning techniques. SN Computer Science, 1(6), 345. https://doi.org/10.1007/s42979-020-00365-y

[19] Xu, L, Skoularidou, M., Cuccaro, A., & Tegolo, D. (2019). Modeling tabular data using conditional GAN. Advances in Neural Information Processing Systems, 32. https://proceedings.neurips.cc/paper/2019/file/254ed7d2de3b23ab10936522dd547b49-Paper.pdf

[20] Yi, X., Walia, E, & Babyn, P. (2019). Generative adversarial network in medical imaging: A review. Medical Image Analysis, 58, 101552. https://doi.org/10.1016/j.media.2019.101552

[21] Zhang, Y, et al. (2023). DP-GAN: Differentially private generative adversarial network for medical data synthesis. Nature Machine Intelligence, 5(4), 345–356. https://doi.org/10.1038/s42256-023-00654-3.

11

GWF Algorithm for Image Forgery Detection

Arun Anoop M.[1]**, Karthikeyan P.**[2] **and Ben Othman Soufiene S.**[3]

[1]AJ Institute of Engineering and Technology, India.
[2]Velammal College of Engineering & Technology, India
[3]King Faisal University, Saudi Arabia

Email: arunanoopm@gmail.com; kpkarthi2001@gmail.com; ben_oth_soufiene@yahoo.fr

Abstract

Medical picture transmission of peptic ulcer images may be forwarded over the internet. The hidden attack-based clues may be embedded in those images, which may become a serious threat to the medical media transmission. Physicians and medical personnel may not recognize such forgery in all cases. Failure to recognize such minute changes in the digital images might lead to wrong prediction. Even a little modification may affect the quality of the image; the identification of image falsification being done might also be affected. Similarly, a little change in the medical x-ray images may lead to a wrong diagnosis, which could threaten the patient's life. Early detection of such forgery is absolutely essential to save patients from a dangerous situation. Hence, the extreme learning machine (ELM) is to be applied to check the authenticity of the image. The proposed algorithm has been evaluated with the breast cancer manipulated images and the peptic ulcer manipulated digital images. The accuracy detection is added to show the effectiveness of the methods used. The results are then compared with those of the other significant journals. In the present research paper, 6 supervised machine learning techniques have been employed for detecting medical image forgery. Among the techniques used, the gray Weber features (GWF) algorithm processed with the combination of BAT GA hybrid optimization results in high accuracy. The images were then processed in

DOI: 10.1201/9788743809920-11

pre-trained convolutional neural network (CNN) models. The accuracy was good for both small and large datasets. The high accuracy was achieved based on tensor flow hub based pre-trained models.

11.1 Introduction

Digital images are an emerging innovation in the field of information sources. However, recent times have witnessed illegal activities. Digital images are used for medical, astronomy, law enforcement, and photorealism. The need for digital imaging in the modern field is to improve the quality of an image to the viewer, elaborate the image's significant data that is invisible to the eye, and to balance an image by photometric or geometric means Copy move forgery is a form of image tampering where a piece of the image is copy-pasted on other piece of the same image. Digital image forgery happens due to leading editing software and cameras, as there has been some work in digital signature and watermarking to identify and place image manipulation.

The rise of face forgery techniques has raised significant security concerns in computer vision (Liu et al., 2021). It has been observed that most face forgery techniques involve an up-sampling step, and multiple consecutive up-samplings lead to noticeable changes in the frequency domain, specifically in the phase spectrum. Natural images contain valuable frequency components preserved in the phase spectrum that can compensate for the loss of amplitude spectrum information. Extensive experiments demonstrate that SPSL achieves state-of-the-art performance when evaluated across different datasets and multi-class classification tasks.

The proliferation of face forgery through deepfake technology on the internet has raised significant concerns in society (Zhao et al., 2021). Detecting such forged content has become a prominent research area, leading to the development of numerous deepfake detection methods. However, most existing approaches treat deepfake detection as a binary classification problem by extracting global features using a backbone network and feeding them into a binary classifier (real/fake). A new multi-attentional deepfake detection network is introduced. It consists of three key components. Multiple spatial attention heads are utilized to focus on different local parts of the image.

The research introduces a novel image representation called "face X-ray," which is a grayscale image analysis tool that detects forgery in face images by revealing whether an input image is composed of blended components from different sources (Li et al., 2020). It effectively highlights the blending boundary in forged images, while genuine images show no evidence of blending.

The rest of the chapter is arranged as follows. Section 11.2 presents a survey of the related research of the proposed work. It is followed by the presentation of algorithms used for the proposed work. The flow of the proposed method is presented in Sections 11.3 and 11.4. Section 11.5 discusses and deals with the experimental results and Performance evaluation based on different machine learning methods, respectively. Finally, the conclusion of the chapter is given.

11.2 Related Works

Types of extreme learning machine (ELM) methods (related works):

- ELM: Jingyi Liu et al., 2021 proposed an ELM with the help of the Cholesky decomposition method.
- ARF ELM, ELM EHO: Chao Wu et al. (2019) proposed a convolution feature extraction and feature coding approach, called autoencoder receptive fields ELM, which consists of local and global receptive fields. Feature coding consists of feature dimension reduction and two hidden layers for ELM processing.
- DC-ELM: Shan Ping & Xinyi Yang (2016) proposed a random local weights-based ELM.
- Hierarchical ensemble ELM: Yaoming Cai et al. (2018) proposed an ELM for reducing overfitting training data issues.

Types of Elephant Herding Optimization (EHO) optimization methods (related works):

- Limit control parameter EHO: Jingyi Liu et al. (2021) proposed an ELM with the help of the Cholesky decomposition method.
- Binary EHO: Shan Ping & Xinyi Yang (2016) proposed a random local weights-based ELM.
- Fuzzy logic EHO: Yaoming Cai et al. (2018) proposed an ELM for reducing overfitting training data issues.
- Global and local search EHO: Yaoming Cai et al. (2018) proposed an ELM for reducing overfitting training data issues.

Types of second-order statistical feature extraction methods (related works):

- GLCM: Jingyi Liu et al. (2021) proposed an ELM with the help of the Cholesky decomposition method. GLCM stands for gray-level co-occurrence matrix, which is a statistical method used to analyze the spatial relationships between pixels in an image. The GLCM is a matrix that represents how often different combinations of gray-level values occur at a given offset or distance within an image.
- GLRLM: Chao Wu et al. (2019) proposed GLRLM, which stands for gray-level run length matrix, which is a texture analysis method used in image processing. GLRLM extracts features from an image by analyses of the distribution of gray-level runs in the image.
- GLDM: Shan Ping & Xinyi Yang (2016) proposed random local weights-based ELM. GLDM stands for gray level dependence matrix. It is a texture analysis method used to quantify the relationship between gray-level values of adjacent pixels in an image. The GLDM matrix is a 2D matrix that represents the frequency of occurrence of different pairs of gray-level values in an image.
- Gray level size zone matrix (GLSZM): The gray level size zone matrix (GLSZM) is a sophisticated texture analysis technique employed in image processing and analysis. GLSZM characterizes the spatial distribution of the connected pixel clusters sharing identical gray levels and sizes within an image. As a second-order statistical approach, the GLSZM builds upon the gray-level co-occurrence matrix (GLCM), providing a quantitative assessment of the spatial arrangement of gray-level intensity values in an image.
- Multiple gray level size-zone (MGLSZ): The multi-dimensional gray level size zone (MGLSZ) feature extraction method is a technique used to examine the spatial arrangement of gray-level values within an image. This approach focuses on quantifying the number, size, and spatial distribution of connected regions, or zones that share identical gray-level values, which provides valuable insights into the image's textural properties.
- Gray level distance zone matrix (GLDZM): The GLDZM features can be used to detect the presence of copy-move forgery by identifying regions in the image where the texture properties have been altered.
- Neighborhood gray tone difference matrix (NGTDM): NGTDM is a texture feature extraction method that is often used in image forgery detection. It measures the difference in gray tone values between each pixel and its neighboring pixels within a defined distance or radius. For

example, if an image has been copy-pasted from another image, the NGTDM of the pasted region may be significantly different from the surrounding areas, indicating that it has been artificially inserted into the image.

- Neighborhood gray level dependence matrix (NGLDM): NGLDM is a sophisticated texture analysis technique utilized in image forgery detection. This method entails the calculation of the co-occurrence of gray level pairs within a localized neighborhood surrounding each pixel in an image. The resulting NGLDM matrix encapsulates valuable information about the spatial distribution of gray-level pairs, which enables the quantification of the image's textural characteristics and facilitates the identification of potential tampering.
- Gray level-local variance (GLLV) histogram: The GLLV histogram is a type of feature extraction method that can be used in image forgery detection. GLLV histogram calculates the local variance of the gray level values in an image and generates a histogram that represents the distribution of variance values across the image.
- Gray level spatial correlation (GLSC): Gray level spatial correlation is a commonly used technique in image forgery detection. It involves analyzing the spatial distribution of gray levels in an image to identify areas that may have been manipulated or altered.
- Gray level and gradient magnitude (GLGM) histogram: The process in the image forgery detection using the GLGM histogram commences with the division of the image into small, overlapping blocks. Subsequently, for each block, the gray-level and gradient magnitude values are calculated, and a joint histogram is generated. Next, statistical features such as mean, variance, and skewness are extracted from the GLGM histogram to create a representative signature for each block.

The proposed transform domain technique relies on both the second-order statistical methods GLRLM, GLCM, GLDM, GLSZM, GLDZM, NGTDM, NGLDM, and Weber Local Descriptors' variants, such as PWMO, IWLD, LBP/WLD, WLD, GWLD, SWLD, WOD, WLDV, and first-order statistical feature extraction. Matching of the features has been done based on feature scaling methods for redundant and irrelevant features of the feature dataset. For the localization process of the forged region, lexicographic sorting and Euclidian distance method have been used. Certain supervised machine learning methods, model stacking, and voting methods have been finally applied for predicting genuine and forged images. In Table 11.1 depicts texture features description along with calculations.

11.3 The Weber Local Descriptor and Gray Level Statistical Texture Feature Algorithms

Table 11.1 Algorithm used to extract texture features.

Gray level difference method	Here are some of the features that can be extracted from the GLDM (gray-level dependence matrix): 1. **Contrast:** Measures the difference in gray-level values between neighboring pixels in the original and forged images. 2. **Homogeneity:** Measures the closeness of the distribution of gray-level values in the original and forged images. 3. **Correlation:** Measures the linear relationship between the gray-level values of adjacent pixels in the original and forged image. 4. **Energy:** Measures the overall uniformity of the gray-level values in the original and forged images. 5. **Entropy:** Measures the randomness or uncertainty of the gray-level values in the original and forged image. 6. **Dissimilarity:** Measures the difference between the gray-level values of adjacent pixels in the original and forged image. 7. **Angular second moment (ASM):** Measures the uniformity of the gray-level values in the original and forged image. 8. **Mean:** The average intensity value of all the pixels in the images of the original and forged. 9. **Inverse difference moments (IDM):** IDM is a texture feature commonly used in image processing and computer vision to quantify the spatial distribution of pixel intensities in original and forged images. IDM is calculated based on the co-occurrence matrix of a digital image, which represents the joint occurrence of pairs of pixel intensity values at different spatial offsets. The IDM feature is defined as the sum of the elements of the co-occurrence matrix, where each element is divided by the square of the difference between its row and column indices. Mathematically, IDM can be expressed as: $\mathrm{IDM} = \sum i,j = 0 \text{ to } N - 1\ P(i,j)/(1 + (\mathrm{i} - \mathrm{j})^2)$ where $P(i,j)$ is the value of the co-occurrence matrix at row i, column j, and N is the number of intensity levels in the image.

Gray level co-occurrence matrix	Here are some of the key features that can be extracted from the GLCM: 1. **Contrast:** It measures the local variations in intensity between the neighboring pixels in the original and forged image. 2. **Homogeneity:** Measures the similarity of gray-level values in neighboring pixels, indicating how smoothly the texture transitions from one forged area to another image. 3. **Energy:** The overall level of uniformity or homogeneity in the texture after extraction of original and forged images is measured through energy. 4. **Entropy:** Measures the randomness or uncertainty of the texture features of original and forged images. 5. **Correlation:** Measures the degree to which gray-level values are linearly related between the neighboring pixels of the original and forged images. 6. **Dissimilarity:** It measures the average difference between the gray-level values in the neighboring pixels of forged or genuine images.
Gray level run length matrix	Measures the distribution.
PWMO	Patterns of Weber magniture, which are encoded with patch-based LBP, and patterns of Weber orientation, which are encoded with patch-based local XOR. $$p\_LBP(x_c, y_c) = \left[\Sigma_{n=0}^{7} 2^n D\left(S_1\left(P_{c_n^R}^r \right) \right), \ldots\ldots, \Sigma_{n=0}^{7} 2^n D\left(S_q\left(P_{c_n^R}^r \right), S\left(P_c^r\right) \right) \right]$$ where, P_c^r is the image patch centered at current pixel with radius r. c_n^R are the neighboring pixels with radius R. $S\left(P_c^r\right)$ is a pre-defined statistic, such as the bins of magnitude histogram and the orientation with the largest accumulative magnitude.

(Continued)

Table 11.1 *Continued.*

Other features	**Entropy:** Measures the uniformity of gray-level distribution in image pairs, and entropy variant Kapoor's entropy is a kind of entropy used for feature extraction in image forgery detection.
IWLD	1. $\gamma_{mx}(x_c) = \text{ARCTAN}(\propto\langle X, J_x\rangle)$, $\gamma_{mx}(x_c) = \text{ARCTAN}(\propto\langle X, J_x\rangle)$ $X = \left(\frac{x_0 - x_c}{x_c}, \frac{x_1 - x_c}{x_c}, \ldots, \frac{x_{p-1} - x_c}{x_c}\right)^\wedge T$ and $\langle , \rangle$ is the inner product operator. $J_x = (\cos\theta_0, \cos\theta_1, \ldots.., \cos\theta_{p-1})^\wedge T$ and $J_y = (\sin\theta_0, \sin\theta_1, \ldots.., \sin\theta_{p-1})^\wedge T$ denote the angle between X direction and $x_i - x_c$. Magnitude and orientation are defined, $\gamma_{mx}(x_c) = \sqrt{(\gamma_{mx}(x_c))^2 + (\gamma_{mx}(x_c))^2}, \gamma_0(x_0) = \arctan\frac{\gamma_{my}(x_c)}{\gamma_{mx}(x_c)}$
WLD	The Weber local descriptor is a type of feature descriptor used in computer vision for image recognition and object detection, and it was introduced by Jianxin Wu and Yunde Jia (2011) as an extension of the local binary pattern (LBP) descriptor.
GWLD	The Gabor wavelet local descriptor (Gabor WLD) is a widely employed feature extraction technique in image forgery detection.
SWLD	In forgery detection, the SWLD algorithm compares local descriptors of different image regions to identify similar or copied regions.
WOD	It is used to extract features from an image by calculating the difference between pairs of pixels at different scales and orientations.
WLDV	WLDV stands for weighted local descriptor variance, and it is a method used in the image forgery detection. In WLDV, the image is first divided into small blocks, and for each block, a feature vector is computed based on the variance of the local texture descriptors.

11.4 Proposed System

The main objective of the paper is to detect the tampered portion of the image by finding the similarity between the duplicated regions and the original image. The proposed work comprises three main steps: (i) pre-processing, (ii) block tiling, (iii) feature extraction, (iv) block matching, and (v) block reconstruction.

RGB digital image, R is processed and converted into grayscale images. The grayscale image, G, is segmented into overlapping blocks of 5X5. Extract features (based on GLCM's variants such as GLRLM, GLCM, GLDM, GLSZM, GLDZM, NGTDM, NGLDM, and Weber local descriptor's variants such as PWMO, IWLD, WLD, GWLD, SWLD, WOD, WLDV) from each block and construct a matrix, MA, with dimension MXN, where M is the number of blocks and N is the feature dimension. Further, perform lexicographic sorting of MA' and store elements in MA' of dimension MXN. Identify similar matches and form two blocks, B1 and B2. Both are the same copies. If the Euclidean distance of those two blocks is less than the threshold of the distance or the number of matching blocks is greater than the threshold value, a binary classification map will then categorize forged or genuine matches. 1 value is for notating forged, and 0 is for genuine. The final prediction map is processed to mark the forged region with the help of the bounding box method. Bounding box method (Figure 11.1) illustrates flow of Image forgery detection.

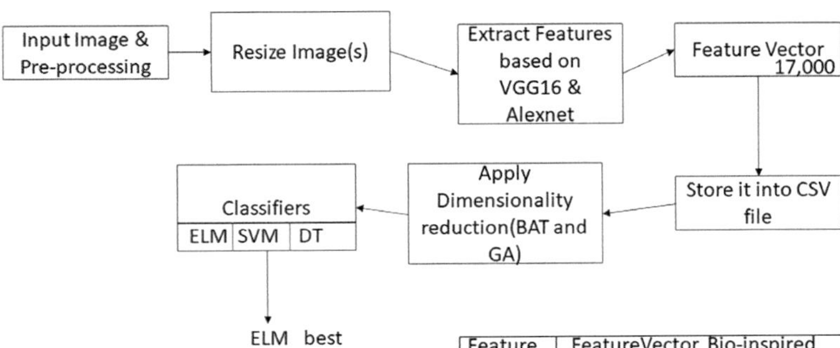

Feature Extraction	FeatureVector	Bio-inspired algorithm	Classifiers
VGG16	17,000	Genetic algorithm BAT	ELM SVM DT
Alexnet	20,000	Genetic Algorithm BAT	ELM SVM DT

Figure 11.1 Proposed flow of VGG+GA/BAT+ELM for image forgery detection.

Table 11.2 Different distance calculation methods.

Distance metrics	Description
Manhattan distance	It is the distance between the 2 points. It is the sum of the absolute differences of Cartesian coordinates.
Euclidian distance	It is the distance between the 2 points, suppose, if we are processing matching processes, two identical blocks in the Euclidean space to identify the manipulated region in the image.
Jeffreys and Matusita distance	It is the measure of the average distance between the two distributions.
Bhattacharya distance	It measures the similarity of the two probability distributions.
Minkowski distance	It calculates the distance between the two real-valued vectors, and it is the generalization of the Euclidean and Manhattan distance.
Chebyshev distance	The distance between the two vectors is the greatest of their differences along any coordinate dimension.
City block distance	The length of the walking distance is determined by city block distance.
Hamming distance	It refers to the comparison of the two binary data strings.
Jaro Winkler distance	It indicates the similarity score between the two strings.

The above Table 11.2 explained about different distance calculation methods. The motivation behind the detection approach is mainly medical image forgery, which may trouble the patient's life and may lead to unhealthy and wrong predictions. Another motivation is that falsifying the court document may help the culprits escaping chance from a case. The wrong people can gain fame by using freely available tools for manipulating news in the newspaper media. Deepfakes may help people to show their presence in videos even if they were not present in the meeting or on any other occasion. Based on these studies, it is observed that there must be a system which has to find the manipulated regions from a digital image. For demonstration purposes, here we have used genuine and forged images and initially processed distance and similarity matches for single and multiple forged regions. After that, different variants of first-order and second-order statistical feature extraction algorithms have been processed for classification analysis. As features are more, prediction is not much accurate, different feature selection approaches have been identified, and a combination of BAT and GA algorithms has been used. Out of the 64 attributes, BAT generated 31 features. Figure 11.2 illustrates weber gray local variants. The 31 features have then

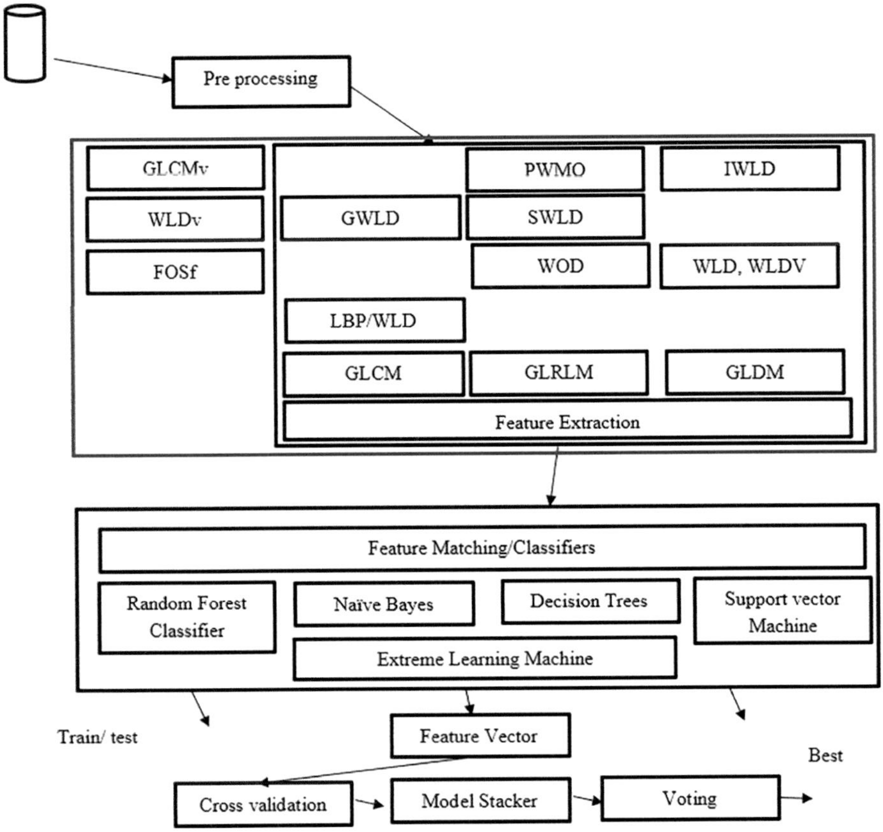

Figure 11.2 Proposed ML-based flow of Weber gray local variants (WGLv) for image forgery detection.

been processed in a genetic algorithm with 10 different chromosomes with 10 different column names. 1000 epochs with 10 iterations have been considered, and the maximum accuracy achieved is 94.1489, and selected features among 31 are ['Feat9', 'Feat26', 'Feat24', 'Feat22', 'Feat4', 'Feat6', 'Feat19', 'Feat31', 'Feat10', 'Feat2'].

Feature selection is to select the best features among the feature vector. Nature-inspired and biological-inspired algorithms work well for features selection. Conversion of the different scales of feature values is possible with the help of feature scaling approaches. Feature scaling can be done based on a combination of min and max or standard scaling. In the present article, an Elephant Optimization algorithm has been processed for showing the way of feature selection. Feature selection illustrates in Figure 11.3 for forgery localization with dimensionality as stage 1 & Figure 11.4 for stage 2.

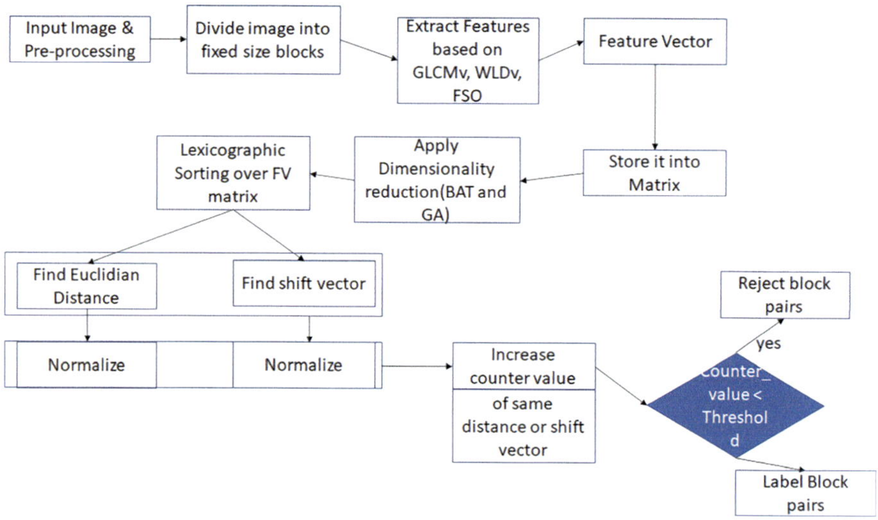

Figure 11.3 Stage 1 of flowchart for proposed forgery localization with dimensionality reduction of medical image forgery dataset images (J. Suckling's MIASDBv1).

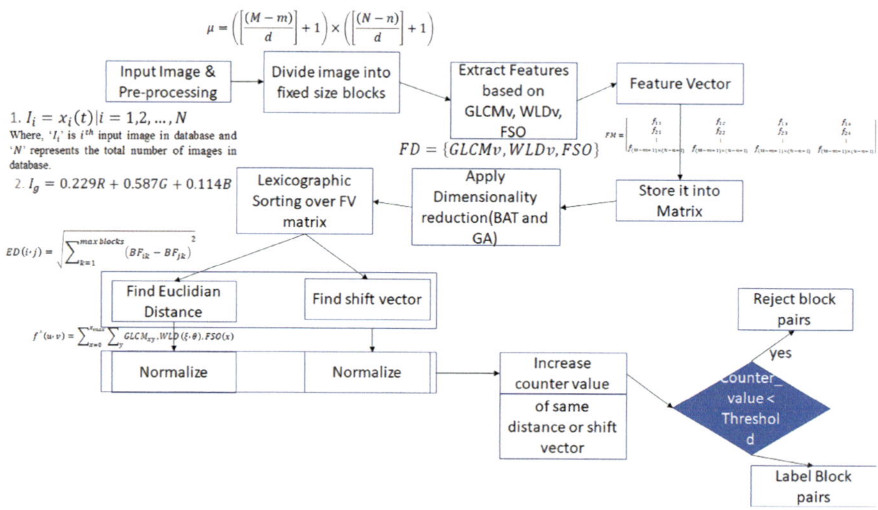

Figure 11.4 Stage 2 of flowchart for proposed forgery localization with dimensionality reduction of medical image forgery dataset images (J. Suckling's MIASDBv1).

The **EHO algorithm (EHO)** is a bio-inspired algorithm developed by Gai-Ge Wang et.al. in 2015. This forgery localization with datasets for different images illustrated in Figure 11.5.

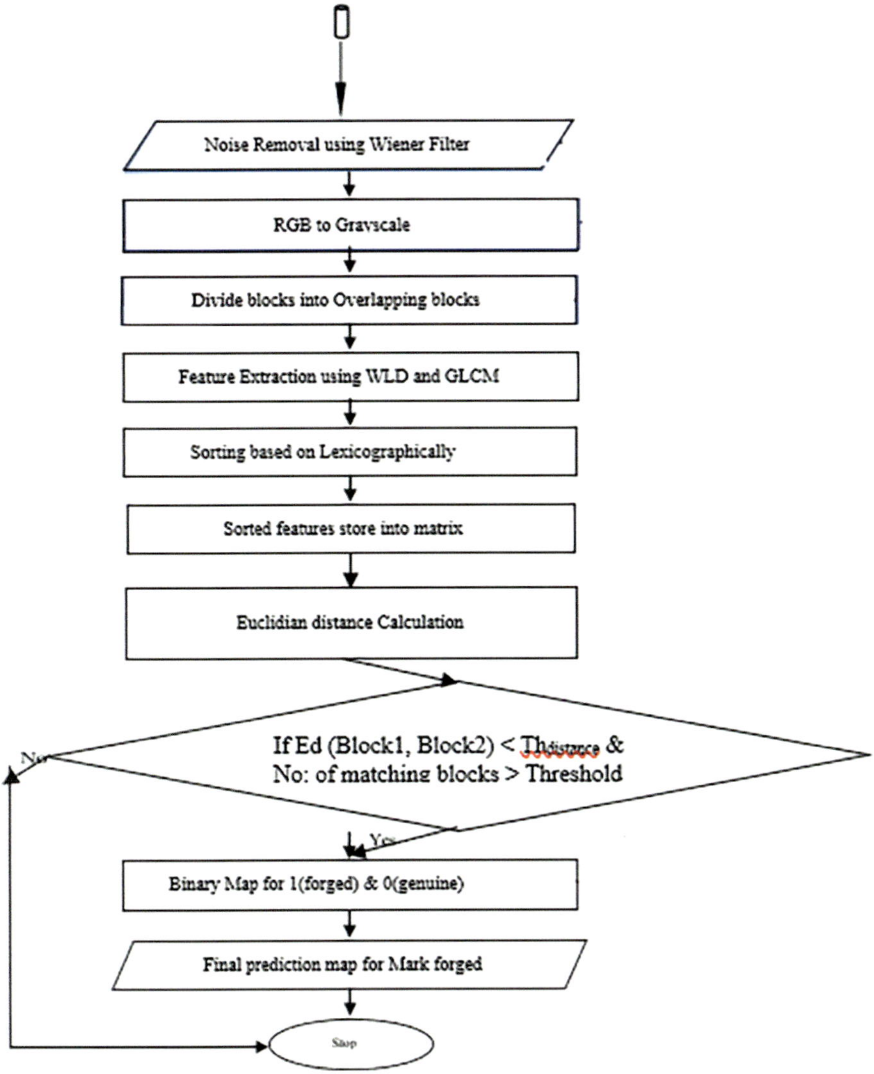

Figure 11.5 Flowchart for forgery localization of image forgery dataset (COVERAGE and CoMoFoD) images.

As social creatures, elephants live in social structures consisting of females and their calves. An elephant clan, led by a matriarch, comprises several females. Female members prefer to reside with their household followers, whereas male members tend to live distinctly. They gradually become autonomous of their families until they ultimately leave their families completely.

1. Elephants are the largest existing terrestrial mammals. It lives in social groups. The oldest female elephant is the matriarch of the group. Each clan has a static number of male elephants and female elephants. Male adult elephants always wish to live self-reliantly, and they will leave the clans when they grow up.

2. Female elephants do live with the males. The males are not part of the herd and will leave once they reach maturity. The oldest female in the herd is known as a matriarch. Elephants walk in a line since it is safer, and they trust that the matriarch (the female leader) tells them where to go. An elephant herd is like a big family. They all take care of each other and protect the young ones. In each generation, a static number of male elephants leave their family group, far away from the main elephant group. As male elephants mature, they leave and live alone. A matriarch, the cleverest oldest female elephant, leader of each clan and models the highest rank within it.

3. In an elephant's social life, each individual takes a new position based on their clan's matriarch. Therefore, clans do not communicate with each other during the updating process. Following the clan updation process, the weakest elephants inside the clans are removed, and their new positions are randomly made in the hunt space using an operator called the separating operator. It was illustrated in Figure 11.6 as example of elephant structure.

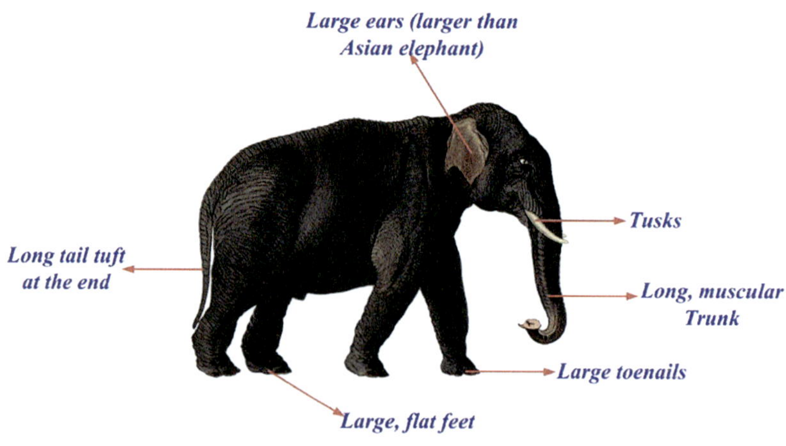

Figure 11.6 Elephant structure.

The following are the rules,

1. The individual clan consists of a collection of elephants that are under the knowledge of the Matriarch.
2. The population of elephants includes clans where the elephants are static in number.
3. In each generation, grown-up male elephants will move away from the elephant group.

The EHO algorithm is a new type of swarm-based metaheuristic search method. It is implemented to crack optimization problems.

Based on scenario 1, the EHO algorithm has been calculated. Scenario 1 is that once a male elephant develops into an adult, it leaves the group. Based on these two elephants behaviors, operators, such as the clan updating operator and separating operators.

Based on scenario 2, the matriarch, the female elephant, leads the group that has different elephant clans. The matriarch, the oldest female elephant, is careful that the most suitable elephant in the family models and solves optimization issues (Fig. 11.7).

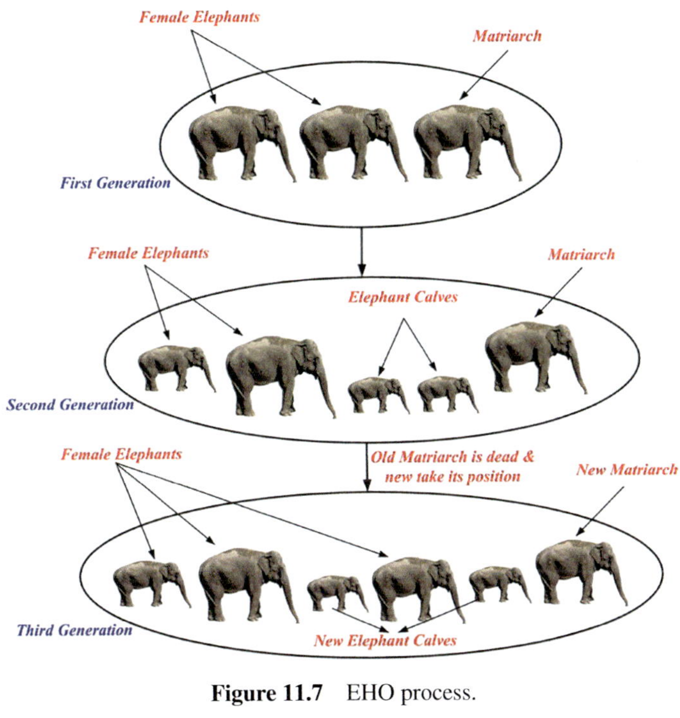

Figure 11.7 EHO process.

Clan updation operator: Elephants from different clans live together under the management of a matriarch. There is a static number of elephants in each clan. An Elephant's position in a clan gets altered because of its matriarch relationship. The Clan updating operator is used for this behavior in the EHO algorithm.

A male elephant leaves the family group and lives unconnectedly once it has become mature. It is presumed that during each new generation, an adult male elephant will be detached from the clan group. In the EHO model algorithm, the updating process is a separating operator.

Clan updating operator: The matriarch leads the elephants in each clan.

$$x_{new,ci,j} = x_{ci,j} + aX(x_{best,ci} - x_{ci,j})Xr$$

$x_{new,ci,j}$ new individual or new position for elephant j in clan ci.

$x_{ci,j}$ is old position for elephant j in clan ci.

$x_{best,ci}$ is matriarch ci of the best elephant in the clan.

$r \in [0,1]$ is a random number between 0 and 1.

$a \in [0,1]$ is a parameter between 0 and 1.

Separating operator: Male elephants leaving their family group can be modeled using a separating operator for optimization problems. This is implemented by replacing the elephant with the worst fitness in each generation with a new individual.

$$x_{worst,ci} = x_{min} + (x_{max} - x_{min} + 1)X \text{ rand}$$

$x_{worst,ci}$ is worst individual in clan ci.

x_{min} is the lower bound of the search space.

x_{max} is the upper bound of the search space.

rand is a stochastic distribution between 0 and 1.

$$x_{center,ci,d} = \frac{1}{n_{ci}} X \sum_{j=1}^{n_{ci}} x_{ci,j,d}$$

$x_{center,ci,d}$ center of clan ci in dimension d.

n_{ci} number of elephants in clan ci.

$\sum_{j=1}^{n_{ci}} x_{ci,j,d}$ sum of dth dimension of elephant $x_{ci,j}$..

$1 \leq d \leq D$.

Main steps:

- Clan, *ci*, and elephant, *j* in clan, *ci* used to generate $x_{new,ci,j}$ and update $x_{ci,j}$
- $x_{ci,j} = x_{best,ci}$ and generate $x_{new,ci,j}$ and update $x_{ci,j}$
- Clan, *ci* then replace the worst individual *ci*.
- Calculate each individual's based on position.

Algorithm of Elephant herding optimization

1. Begin and do the iteration. Iteration notates as *G* and initializes it to 1.
2. Elephant's population value will be taken randomly. Generation will take normally in maximum mode. Sorting must be done based on fitness value. Then next process is based on two operators.
3. Clan updating operator: When the elephants are moving together, in a clan, the matriarch will assign or access each elephant's next position. The matriarch will determine the fitness of the elephant in the clan (Fig. 11.8).

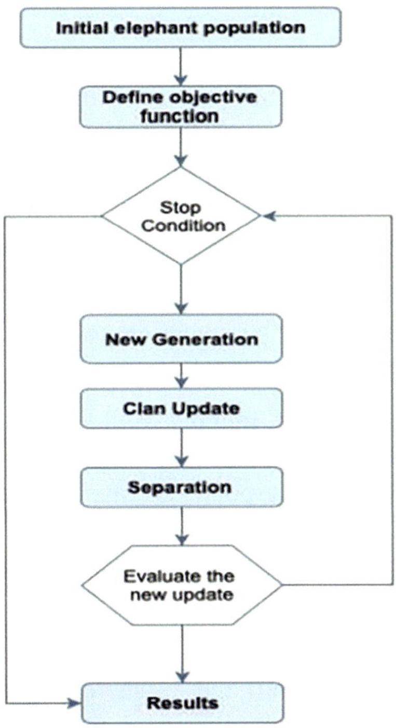

Figure 11.8 EHO flowchart (Gai-Ge Wang et al., 2015).

4. Separating operator: The male elephant will leave and live alone. Matriarch used to identify the worst elephant individual among the elephant clan or group and replace it with a new individual.

5. Evaluate each position based on the position parameter. Increment iteration value to 1. $G < \text{MaxGen}$

   a) If yes, output the best solution.

   b) No, then go to the fitness evaluation step.

The **Bat-inspired algorithm** (BAT). The Bat algorithm, developed by Xin-She Yang in 2010, is a metaheuristic optimization technique that draws inspiration from the echolocation behavior of bats.

Bats locate the obstacles and prey in their path by using ultrasound. They produce an ultrasound, which returns after striking an obstacle in their way. By hearing the reflected sound and from the time interval (when they produce ultrasound and when they receive them back), they can judge the direction and the distance of the obstacle in their way. By detecting the reflection of ultrasonic sound, bats know the position and the type of prey of any obstacle.

The way bats locate their prey:

1. Bats trace their prey by echolocation. They have a keen sense of hearing that guides them to trace their prey even in darkness.
2. Bats form a stream of high-pitched sound during hunting time.
3. When the sound waves produced by the bats hit an insect or other animal, the echoes bounce back to the bat, which assists them to locate their prey.
4. The echoes also guide the bat about the path to take in the air to avoid hitting with one another or objects.
5. In general, the frequency f, ranging from f_{min} to fmax, corresponds to a wavelength series of $\lambda(\text{min})$ to $\lambda(\text{max})$. For instance, a frequency series of 20 kHz to 500 kHz corresponds to wavelengths between 0.7 mm and 17 mm.
6. For simplicity, we can undertake $f \in [0, f_{max}]$. We see that the higher frequencies have shorter wavelengths and travel shorter distances. Typically, bats' ranges are a few meters. The pulse rate can be characterized as a value between 0 and 1, where 0 specifies no pulses and 1 represents the maximum pulse emission rate.

7. The movement of virtual bats is ruled by the succeeding equations, which are stated below [eqn (11.1)– (11.3)].

$$fi = f_{min} + (f_{max} - f_{min})\,\beta, \tag{11.1}$$

$$vt = vt - 1 + (xt - x*)\,fi, \tag{11.2}$$

$$xt = xt - 1 + vt, \tag{11.3}$$

where $\beta \in [0, 1]$ is a random vector drawn from a uniform distribution. Here, x* represents the current global best location (solution), determined in Figure 11.9 as BAT optimization by comparison of all the solutions among

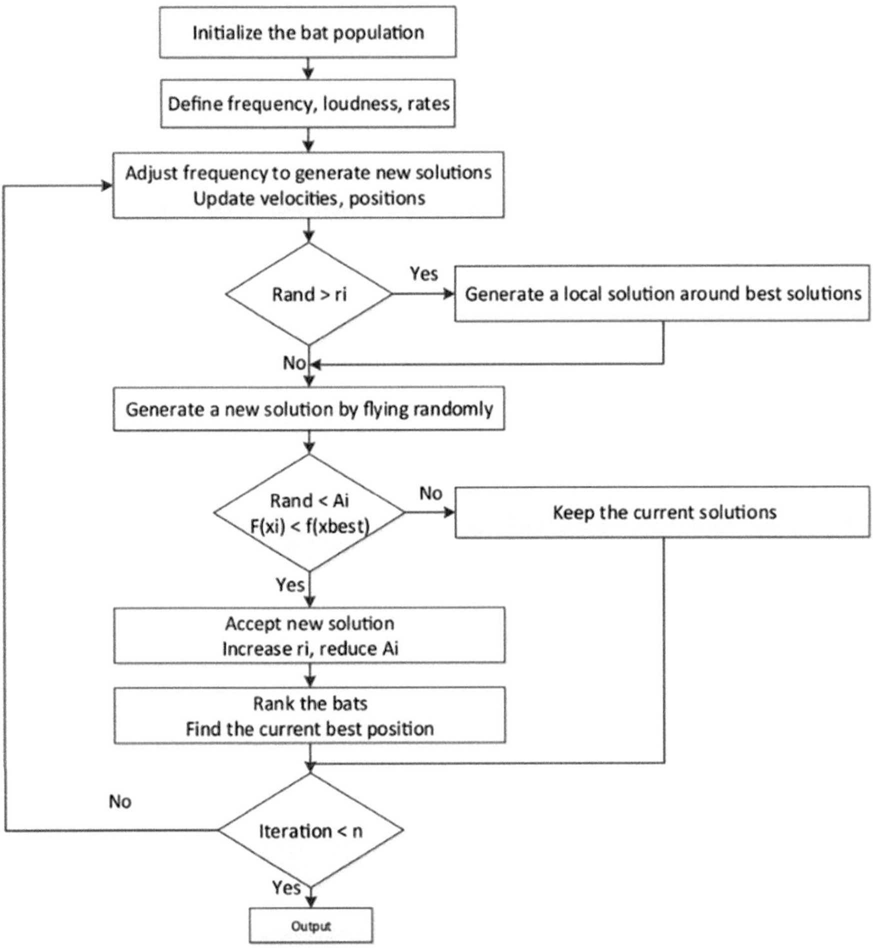

Figure 11.9 BAT optimization flow chart (Xin-She Yang, 2010).

the *n* bats. Each bat is randomly assigned a frequency from the range [f_{min}, f_{max}]. For local search, a new solution is generated for each bat using a random walk: x_new = x_old + εAt.

We now use the following idealized rules for simplicity:

1. All bats use echolocation to sense the distance and distinguish between the food/prey and background barriers.
2. Bats fly randomly with velocity Vi at position Xi, adjusting their emitted pulse frequency and rate ($r \in [0,1]$) based on their target's proximity.
3. Although loudness can vary, we assume it ranges from a large (positive) A0 to a minimum value Amin.

Objective function: f(x) = (x1, ..., xd)T

Initialization:

- Initialize bat population xi (i = 1, 2, ..., n) and vi
- Define pulse frequency fi at xi
- Initialize pulse rates ri and loudness Ai

While (t < Max number of iterations):

- Generate new solutions by adjusting frequency and updating velocities and locations/solutions [eqn (11.1)–(11.3)]
- If (rand > ri):
  - Select a solution among the best solutions
  - Generate a local solution around the selected best solution
- Generate a new solution by flying randomly
- If (rand < Ai and f(xi) < f(x*)):
  - Accept the new solution
  - Increase ri and reduce Ai
- End if
- Rank the bats and find the current best x

End while

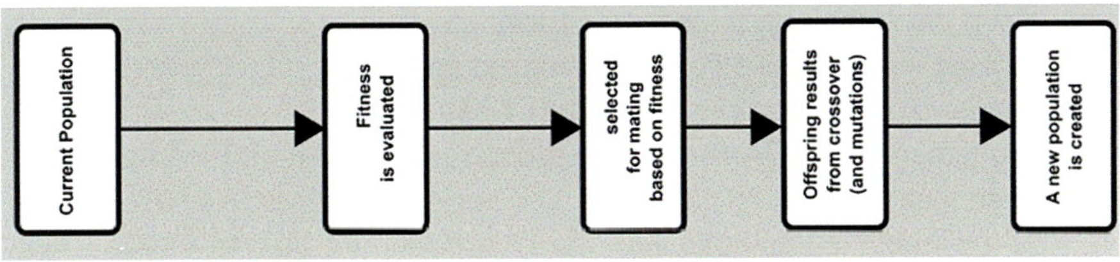

Figure 11.10 Genetic algorithm overflow (Q. J. Wang, 1996).

Post-processing and visualization

The **genetic algorithm** (GA)

Input: Image dataset
Output: Localized “forged regions”
Begin
Input image
If the image is a colored image, convert it into grayscale
Else

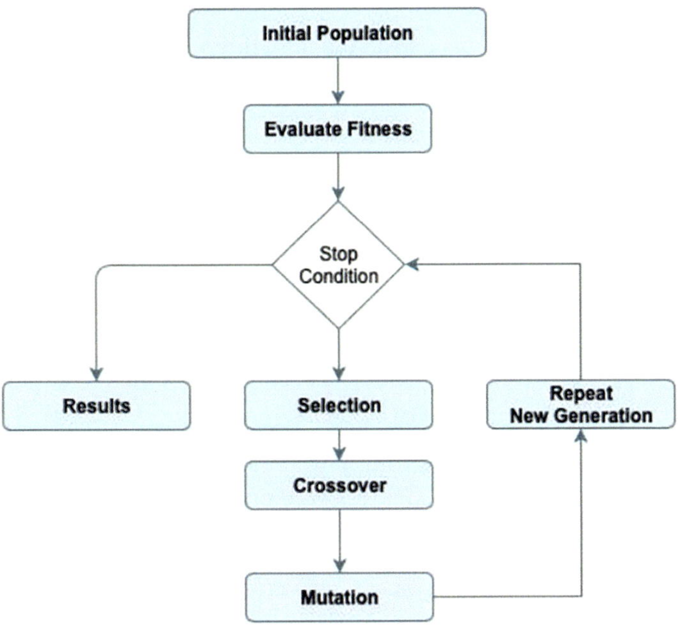

Figure 11.11 Genetic algorithm flowchart (Q. J. Wang, 1996).

Keep the same grayscale image for processing

Extract features based on the proposed approach

Apply extreme learning machine (ELM)

Implement BAT-GA for feature reduction of ELM, and load reduction to manage many images.

If the image is manipulated, apply a bounding box to locate forged regions and find the classifier-based prediction.

Else it will show "image is genuine."

11.5 Experimentation and Results

The proposed technique is tested using MATLAB for localizing forged region using various datasets. The features have been extracted using MATLAB, and the latter features have been processed in Google Collab for the classification process. Dataset images have been tested based on different learning methods.

11.5.1 Image datasets and performance evaluation of ANN and CNN models

The proposed technique was tested using three popular image datasets: MICC-F220, CoMoFoD, and J. Suckling breast cancer image datasets.

- The MICC-F220 dataset consists of 100 color digital images in PNG format.
- The CoMoFoD dataset includes 200 primary images with different views and sites, such as nature, buildings, and city backgrounds.
- The J. Suckling dataset includes 300 pictures, with created copy-move forgeries for research purposes. Additionally, peptic ulcer manipulated images were processed for image forgery detection.

TensorFlow Hub representations have been used to advance accuracy, as Kaggle pre-trained models did not perform well on small datasets. TensorFlow Hub models worked effectively on both small and large datasets. The Table 11.3 illustrated Comparison of efficiency in terms of time taken by bio-inspired algorithms.

Table 11.3 Comparison of efficiency in terms of time taken by bio-inspired algorithms.

Algorithm	BAT	GA	BAT_GA
Time taken in seconds	190.254	191.5478	185.2485

The proposed technique's effectiveness has been evaluated based on commonly employed parameters for copy-move forgery detection:

- Precision (P)
- Recall (R)
- F-measure

Definitions:

- True positive (Tp): It refers to the total number of images correctly detected as forged. At the pixel level, Tp is the total number of pixels correctly detected as forged.
- False positive (Fp): It refers to the total number of original images incorrectly detected as forged.

At the pixel level, the following definitions apply:

- False positive (Fp): It refers to the number of original pixels incorrectly classified as forged.
- False negative (Fn): The total number of forged images that remain undetected is referred to as false negative. Equivalently, at the pixel level, Fn represents the total number of forged pixels that are overlooked.

1. Load the CSV file containing extracted features into a pandas DataFrame.
2. Preprocess the dataset by:
   - Handling missing values
   - Encoding categorical variables
   - Scaling numerical features
3. Define a fitness function to evaluate the performance of each feature subset.
4. Implement the Bat algorithm and genetic algorithm separately.
5. Combine the Bat algorithm and genetic algorithm to create a hybrid algorithm for feature selection.
6. Evaluate the hybrid algorithm's performance on the dataset using cross-validation.
7. Select the optimal feature subset based on performance metrics evaluated during cross-validation (Table 11.4).

Table 11.4 Features subset.

Contrast (Feat1)	Angular second moment entropy (Feat2)	Mean (Feat3)	Inverse difference moments (Feat4)	Auto correlation (Feat5)	Variance (Feat6)	Difference entropy (Feat7)	Contrast (Feat8)	Correlation (Feat9)
41.68201587	41.8068575	5.076269351	4.81455483	0.41685282	0.445415507	455.0642115	41.68230587	41.80687175
41.69710738	41.72504102	4.938056001	4.765869388	0.426069254	0.447564181	460.4765396	41.69735738	41.72505112
41.78117084	41.94613741	4.99965675	4.691445478	0.412312925	0.445170539	449.6162655	41.78207084	41.94603742
41.58286596	41.70013401	5.328743526	5.084924966	0.397548834	0.424829858	463.2351034	41.58286596	41.70003402
37.82563824	38.31343333	7.512558113	6.529370748	0.363548842	0.445163223	596.4575316	37.82563824	38.33333333
Energy (Feat10)	**Entropy (Feat12)**	**Inverse variance (Feat13)**	**Sum average (Feat14)**	**Sum entropy (Feat15)**	**Sum variance (Feat16)**	**Homogeneity 1, 2 (Feat17)**	**Dissimilarity (Feat18)**	**Run percentage (Feat19)**
597.9514	-38.1993	-45.4025	1.68448	1.552704	0.197987	0.112224	0.590571	597.9514
742.2919	-46.0298	-53.4917	1.829119	1.735425	0.134322	0.137458	0.623334	641.2919
636.6489	-51.0055	-57.1789	1.579576	1.365952	0.122023	0.129935	0.622171	636.6489
649.921	-49.6407	-57.1055	1.544124	1.420187	0.152434	0.120087	0.610359	649.921
626.7965	-48.9809	-54.8819	1.537094	1.41767	0.118704	0.12661	0.605852	626.7965

Non-uniformity (Feat20)	Gray level non-uniformity (Feat21)	Run length non-uniformity (Feat22)	Run emphasis (Feat23)	High gray level run emphasis (Feat24)	Low gray level run emphasis (Feat25)	Long run emphasis (Feat26)	Emphasis (Feat27)	Short emphasis (Feat28)
61.7396	56.4676	0.567671	0.315453	0.318827	44.01233	44.01193	12.63817	12.6291
61.8725	57.2124	0.569194	0.299584	0.29983	43.87219	43.87926	12.63768	12.61645
62.2237	56.8471	0.573325	0.29496	0.296752	44.08304	44.08814	12.64343	12.65934
60.8597	56.2857	0.557795	0.317961	0.316514	43.99502	44.0605	12.63123	12.62097
0.609699	0.544348	0.556601	0.32371	0.330102	41.33846	41.28574	11.94656	11.94978
Long run high gray level (Feat29)	**Short run low gray level (Feat30)**	**Short run high gray level (Feat31)**	**GLSZM SAE (Feat32)**	**LAE (Feat33)**	**IV (Feat34)**	**SZV (Feat35)**	**ZP (Feat36)**	**LIE (Feat37)**
195.0578	351.533	119.319	119.5854	2.284796	176.9504	203.6467	568.2547	636.6489
148.8005	302.4375	119.1459	119.0915	2.289522	158.332	182.0684	568.9662	649.921
155.4493	292.4331	119.4621	119.837	2.287747	123.4223	158.4634	563.2492	626.7965
102.5716	181.7596	119.2241	119.3774	2.283755	66.70948	101.6018	518.8956	582.1789
223.4218	395.9502	108.3315	109.1982	2.342568	187.1072	235.5035	388.6504	460.5463

(*Continued*)

Table 11.4 *Continued.*

HIE (Feat38)	**LISAE (Feat39)**	**HISAE (Feat40)**	**LILAE (Feat41)**	**HILAE (Feat42)**	**MGLSZ SAE (Feat43)**	**LAE (Feat44)**	**IV (Feat45)**	**SZV (Feat46)**
195.0578	351.533	301.095	312.6975	11.85971	101.7905	102.2928	190.9865	161.6447
148.8005	302.4375	208.926	291.9901	12.70767	121.2803	121.9969	151.3116	185.1942
155.4493	292.4331	207.4571	249.5617	12.78889	127.4713	127.9316	151.4662	119.5931
102.5716	181.7596	147.5484	147.1823	12.79177	125.3284	125.8799	98.88786	72.21412
223.4218	395.9502	286.0657	329.443	12.77376	125.2043	125.486	225.1967	199.3057
ZP (Feat47)	**LI (Feat48)**	**HIE (Feat49)**	**LISAE (Feat50)**	**HISAE (Feat51)**	**LILAE (Feat52)**	**HILAE (Feat53)**	**FIRST ORDER SD (Feat54)**	**MEAN DEVIATION (Feat55)**
195.0578	351.533	301.095	124.8816	125.3501	2.188042	203.6467	190.9865	161.6447
148.8005	302.4375	208.926	119.134	119.5283	2.279327	182.0684	151.3116	185.1942
155.4493	292.4331	207.4571	117.6449	118.3571	2.297165	158.4634	151.4662	119.5931
102.5716	181.7596	147.5484	117.7086	118.4164	2.296184	101.6018	98.88786	72.21412
223.4218	395.9502	286.0657	110.8013	110.9304	2.335737	235.5035	225.1967	199.3057

Kurtosis (Feat56)	Skewness (Feat57)	Root Mean Square (Feat58)	PWMO (Feat59)	IWLD (Feat60)	GWLD (Feat61)	SWLD (Feat62)	WOD (Feat63)	WLDV (Feat64)
195.0578	351.533	344.7841	400.5706	176.9504	203.6467	190.9865	161.6447	195.0578
148.8005	302.4375	444.0685	525.8477	158.332	182.0684	151.3116	185.1942	148.8005
155.4493	292.4331	370.3785	416.2908	123.4223	158.4634	151.4662	119.5931	155.4493
102.5716	181.7596	366.4453	411.3589	66.70948	101.6018	98.88786	72.21412	102.5716
223.4218	395.9502	433.0995	507.1248	187.1072	235.5035	225.1967	199.3057	223.4218

Label
0
0
0
1
1

Table 11.5 Set operations systems for algorithms.

GLCM	Set1 & Set2	GLCMv & WLD
	Set1 & Set2	GLCMv & FOSf

The features of image pairs have been extracted based on the utilization of various algorithms used to decide the genuineness of the images. The features are assumed as the input to classifiers. The extracted features have the informative knowledge about the input type, which helps in the learning capability of the classifier. The Table 11.5 is about Set operations systems for algorithms & the Table 11.6 is about different set operation possibilities for accuracy prediction. In Table 11.7 best features identified based on BAT optimization algorithm. Also in the Table 11.8 the details about feature selection based accuracy findings have added.

After extracting features from the datasets, all the features have been processed based on the "set operation" concept. Feature subset has been created based on features extracted from GLCM variants, WLD variants, and first-order statistical algorithms. The even, odd, and its randomness and selected attributes for classification accuracy have already been checked (Arun Anoop M. et al., Indian Patent). Here, the "set operation" concepts for feature or attribute selection for classification and accuracy measurement have been checked.

Set operations have been performed before proceeding to the feature matching process and its fused approach.

The following are the set operations used for checking the accuracy of classification.

It is evident that combination methods are not that do not give complete classification accuracy. Genetic algorithm has been utilized for measurement

Table 11.6 Set Operations for proposed system.

GLCMv & WLD	GLCMv UNION WLD
	GLCMv INTERSECTION WLD
	GLCMv DIFFERENCE WLD
	GLCMv CARTESIAN PRODUCT WLD
GLCMv & FOSf	GLCMv UNION FOSf
	GLCMv INTERSECTION FOSf
	GLCMv DIFFERENCE FOSf
	GLCMv CARTESIAN PRODUCT FOSf

Table 11.7 BAT_GA feature set.

Correlation (Feat9)	Long Run Emphasis (Feat26)	High Gray level Run Emphasis (Feat24)	Run Length Non-uniformity (Feat22)	Inverse Difference Moments (Feat4)	Variance (Feat6)	Run Percentage (Feat19)	Short Run High Gray Level (Feat31)	Energy (Feat10)	Angular Second Moment Entropy (Feat2)
41.80687175	44.01193	0.318827	0.567671	4.81455483	0.445415507	597.9514	119.319	597.9514	41.8068575
41.72505112	43.87926	0.29983	0.569194	4.765869388	0.447564181	641.2919	119.1459	742.2919	41.72504102
41.94603742	44.08814	0.296752	0.573325	4.691445478	0.445170539	636.6489	119.4621	636.6489	41.94613741
41.70003402	44.0605	0.316514	0.557795	5.084924966	0.424829858	649.921	119.2241	649.921	41.70013401
38.33333333	41.28574	0.330102	0.556601	6.529370748	0.445163223	626.7965	108.3315	626.7965	38.31343333

Table 11.8 Accuracy performance after feature selection.

Classifier	**Maximum accuracy**	**Best feature columns**	**Number of random chromosomes with number of columns**
LOGISTIC REGRESSION L-BFGS optimization algorithm with GA	94.10	['Feat9', 'Feat26', 'Feat24', 'Feat22', 'Feat4', 'Feat6', 'Feat19', 'Feat31', 'Feat10', 'Feat2']	10,10
	95.744	['Feat37', 'Feat54', 'Feat29', 'Feat20', 'Feat46', 'Feat27', 'Feat63', 'Feat13', 'Feat42', 'Feat49', 'Feat30', 'Feat28', 'Feat1', 'Feat17', 'Feat36', 'Feat49', 'Feat9', 'Feat10', 'Feat53', 'Feat58', 'Feat64', 'Feat62', 'Feat35', 'Feat18', 'Feat2', 'Feat17', 'Feat23', 'Feat47', 'Feat44', 'Feat41']	10,30
K neighbors classifier with GA	95.7	['Feat31', 'Feat3', 'Feat57', 'Feat20', 'Feat45', 'Feat27', 'Feat14', 'Feat56', 'Feat55', 'Feat44']	10,10
Ada boosting classifier with GA	**97.34**	['Feat9', 'Feat31', 'Feat34', 'Feat23', 'Feat55', 'Feat5', 'Feat52', 'Feat50', 'Feat54', 'Feat63']	10,10
LR with GA (31 features selected through BAT)	93.617	['Feat3', 'Feat20', 'Feat16', 'Feat6', 'Feat25', 'Feat27', 'Feat2', 'Feat14', 'Feat26', 'Feat6']	10,10
K neighbors classifier with GA (took 31 features through BAT)	94.68	['Feat15', 'Feat11', 'Feat18', 'Feat9', 'Feat8', 'Feat30', 'Feat8', 'Feat21', 'Feat10', 'Feat26']	10,10
Ada boosting classifier with GA (took 31 features through BAT)	95.21	['Feat18', 'Feat8', 'Feat31', 'Feat3', 'Feat29', 'Feat30', 'Feat9', 'Feat10', 'Feat21', 'Feat3']	10,10
Passive aggressive (took 31 features through BAT)	91.48	['Feat29', 'Feat23', 'Feat16', 'Feat1', 'Feat12', 'Feat14', 'Feat11', 'Feat3', 'Feat4', 'Feat22']	10,10
Ada boosting classifier with GA (took 31 features through BAT)	94.14	['Feat26', 'Feat10', 'Feat28', 'Feat18', 'Feat28']	10,5

of classification accuracy. Here, 64 attributes have been generated based on WLD, GLCM, and First Order Statistics variants. BAT initially processed and selected 31 features as best. Further, GA has processed for arriving at the best features selection. Each feature selection's accuracy has been calculated based on supervised learning-based machine learning classifiers. GA alone has been selected for the best features, and it has calculated the best accuracy better than the combination of bio-inspired algorithms. The model evaluation are illustrated in Figure 11.12 to Figure 11.16.

Finally, we have tried different pre-trained models for our evaluation. It is essential to check cancerous images during transmission to identify the faults. Hence, the main focus of the research has been to extract the VGG16 feature extraction resulting features. CNN is utilized here for features extraction and matching. Lastly, the fully connected layer is connected with the supervised machine learning algorithms to enhance the system to work more to detect forgery during transmission. The exact idea applied here is features extracted using VGG16; the saved features csv file has been processed for supervised machine learning algorithms initially. Later, for getting good results, the received features list has processed firstly in Genetic Algorithm

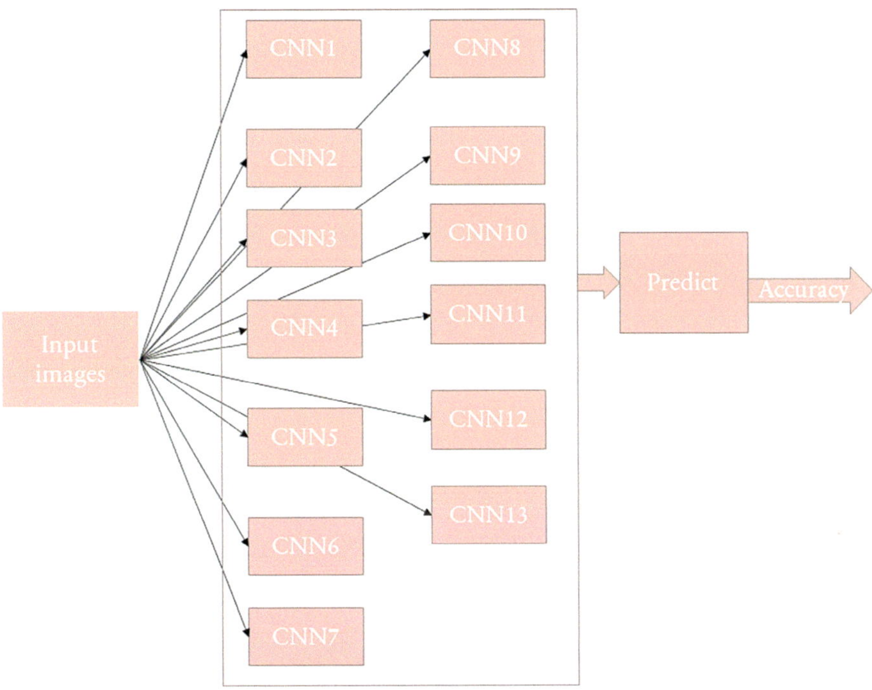

Figure 11.12 Experimental evaluation of pre-trained CNN models.

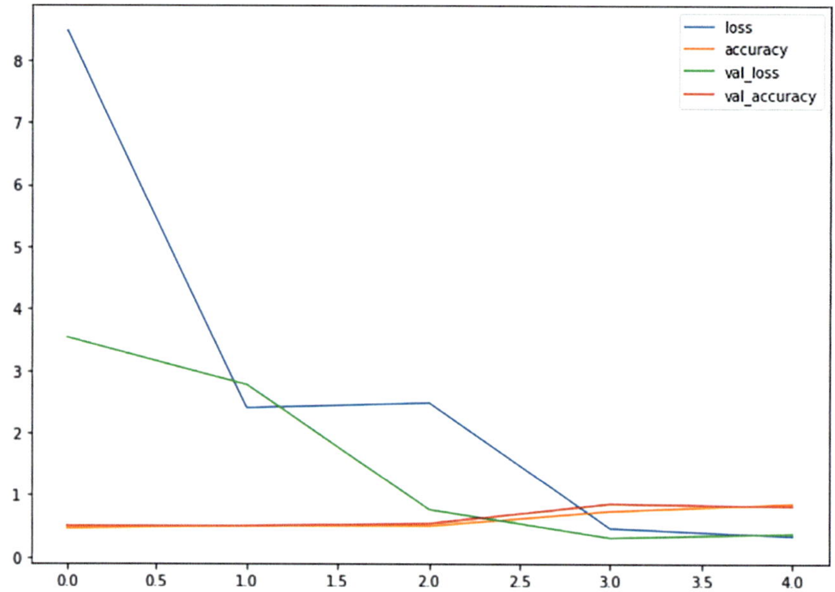

Figure 11.13 Model 1.

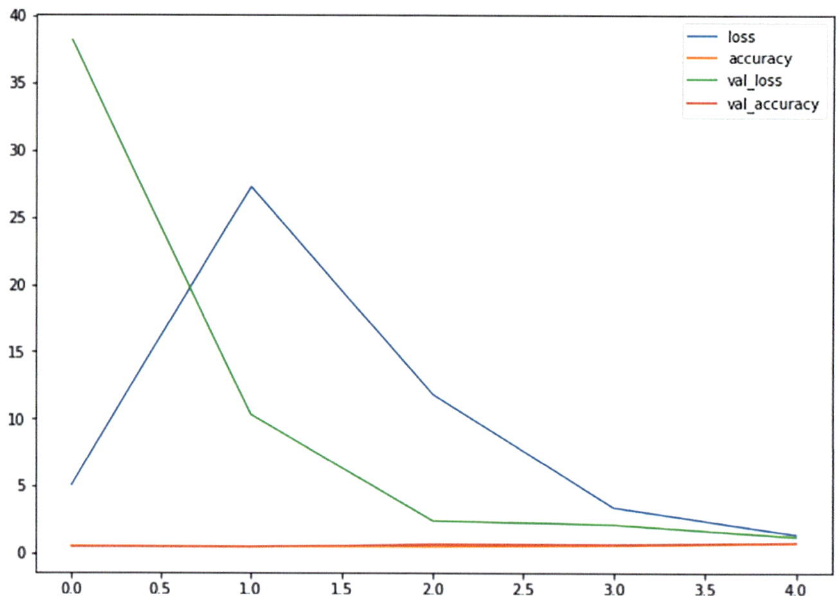

Figure 11.14 Model 2.

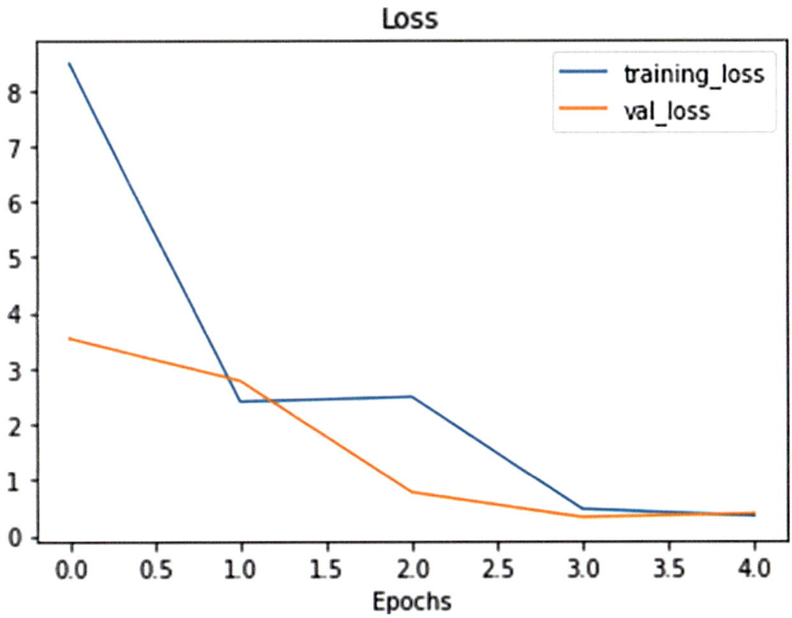

Figure 11.15 Model 3.

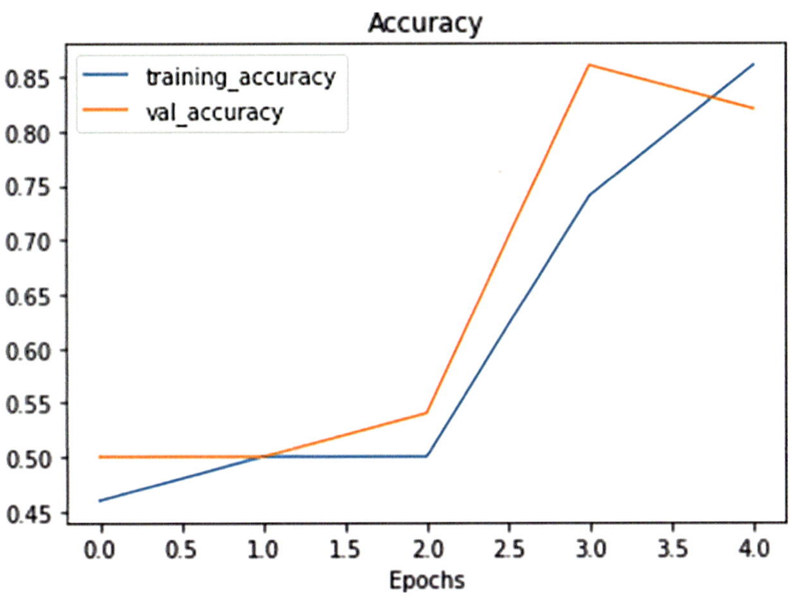

Figure 11.16 Model 4.

and different supervised learning algorithms. Hybrid VGG16-ELM results better than other VGG16-VGG16 CNN. Also, VGG16-GA-ELM, VGG16-GA-SVM, VGG16-GA-RF, VGG16-GA-DT, and VGG16-GA-KNN has processed, and out of these, VGG16-GA-ELM achieved better results than those reported in certain significant journals.

Keras Application VGG16: fit function error. It has been used to avoid overfitting "keras callback early stopping," also, but an error occurred.

RESNET: TensorFlow hub has been used. "Resnet 50 V2 feature vector" has been used. Arguments like model_url and num_classes have been utilized for this evaluation. Hub keras layer method has been used for the download of pretrained model and saved. Model has been created using resnet url categorical cross entropy, Adam optimizer, and epochs 5 has used for processing its accuracy and loss. All the evaluation metrics with different models expressed in Figure 11.17 to Figure 11.22.

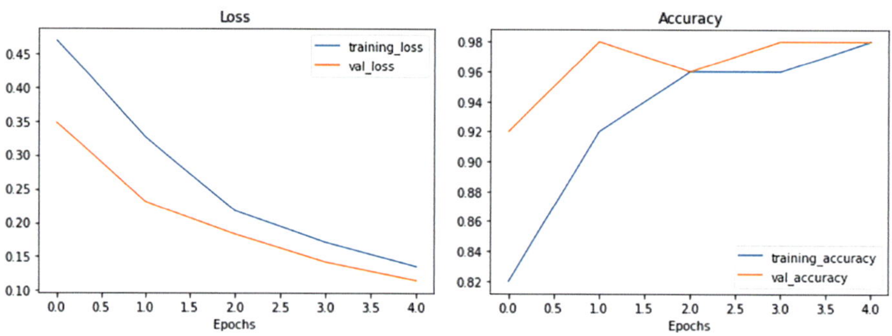

Figure 11.17 RESNET.

EfficientNet: Same process as used in Resnet model.

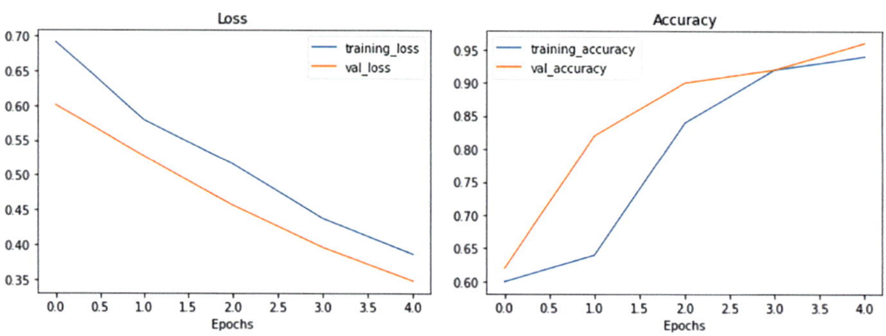

Figure 11.18 EfficientNet.

MobileNet: Same process.

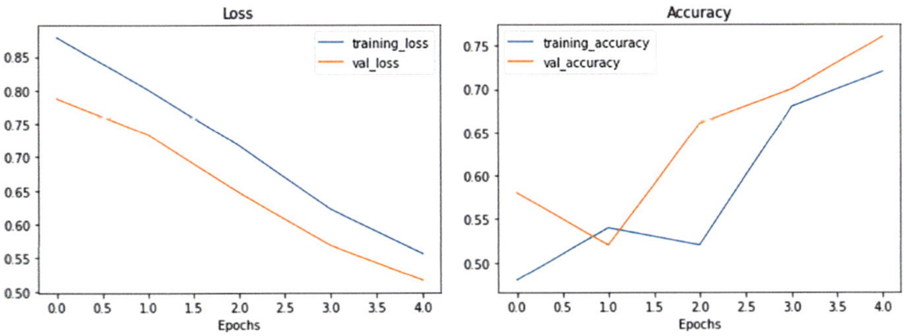

Figure 11.19 MobileNet.

NASNET: Same process.

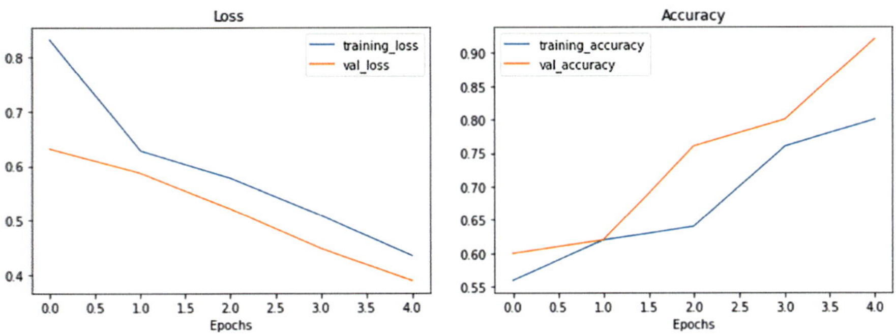

Figure 11.20 NASNET.

Inception: Same process.

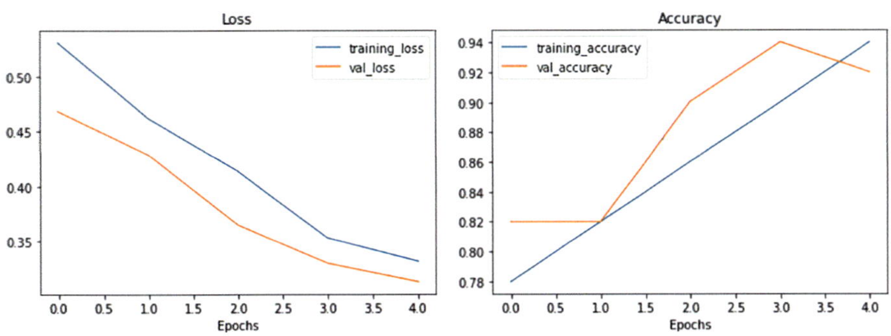

Figure 11.21 Inception.

Inception resnet: Same process

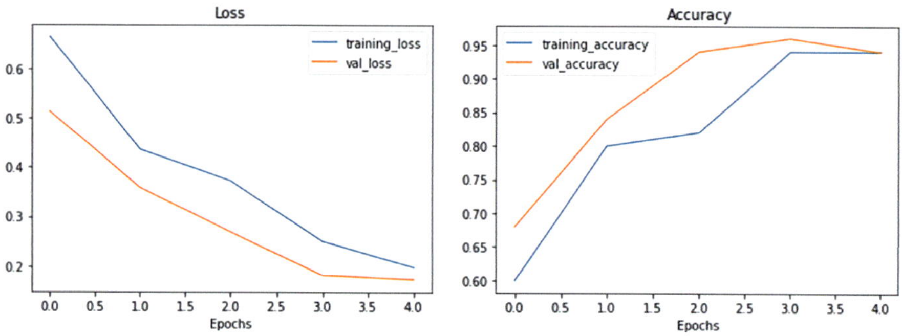

Figure 11.22 InceptionResNet.

Table 11.9 describes about the pretrained CNN models based on Tensorflow Hub URLs for breast cancer detection based on small datasets have processed. In Table 11.10 added the validation accuracy findings based on large and small datasets. And also in Table 11.11, 14 variants of pre-trained CNN models have been used for the accuracy prediction based on large and small datasets. Genuine and forged datasets have been uploaded into the

Table 11.9 Pretrained CNN models based on TensorFlow Hub URLs for breast cancer detection based on small datasets.

Sl. no.	Models	Epochs	VAL accuracy
1	RESNET	5	**98**
2	EFFICIENTNET	5	96
3	MOBILENET V1	5	74
4	NASNET	5	92
5	INCEPTION	5	92
6	INCEPTION RESNET	5	94
7	AMOEBANET	5	ERROR
8	NASNET LARGE	5	ERROR
9	RESNET 100	5	96
10	RESNET 152	5	94
11	RESNET 101	5	94.8
12	MOBILENET V2	5	72
13	MOBILENET V2	5	73
14	VGG16	5	82

Table 11.10 Pretrained CNN models based on TensorFlow Hub URLs for COVERAGE, CoMoFoD datasets detection based on small and large datasets.

Sl. no.	Models	Epochs	Dataset	VAL accuracy
1	RESNET	5	Small	58%
2	EFFICIENTNET	5	Large	**62%**
3	MOBILENET V1	5	Small	60%

Table 11.11 TensorFlow Hub URLs of pre-trained CNN models for breast cancer forgery (Copy Move) detection based on small & large datasets.

Sl. no.	Models	Epochs	VAL accuracy
1	RESNET	5	60%
2	EFFICIENTNET	5	**67%**
3	MOBILENET V1	5	62%
4	NASNET	5	64%
5	INCEPTION	5	62
6	INCEPTION RESNET	5	64
7	AMOEBANET	5	Loss is more
8	NASNET LARGE	5	Loss is more
9	RESNET 100	5	66
10	RESNET 152	5	64
11	RESNET 101	5	64
12	MOBILENET V2	5	62
13	MOBILENET V2	5	63
14	VGG16	5	61

Google Drive for collab analysis work. Later, the "split-folder library" has been used for splitting train, test, and validation folders with ratio .8,.1,.1. After that, different customized CNN models were tested on the dataset, but received only 50% accuracy. Later, it has been processed by using a CNN pretrained model based on URLs of tensor flow feature vectors. The CNN classifier has no magical power to carry a large dataset of images. It is found to be very difficult to manage large datasets after the feature extraction of the CNN process. For that reason, there must be a proposed system that generates features by using a CNN model, and the extracted features must be separated by a dimensionality reduction method for the classification process. VGG16 based features are illustrated in Figure 11.23 & different machine learning evaluations are expressed in Figure 11.24.

filename	1371	1372	1373	1374	1375	1376	1377	1378	1379	1380	1381	1382	1383
m (3).jpg	3.833921	0	0	0	0	0	0	0	0	0	0	0	0
m (4).jpg	9.365171	0	0	0	0	0	0	3.554993	0	0	0	0	0
m (6).jpg	3.146503	0	0	0	0	0	0	0.846128	0	0	0	0	3.953565
m (5).jpg	10.28309	0	0	0	0	0	0	0	0	0	0	0	6.595363
m (2).jpg	14.01242	0	0	0	0	0	0	0	0	0	0	0	0
	16365	16366	16367	16368	16369	16370	16371	16372	16373	16374	16375	16376	16377
	0	0	0	0	0	0	0	0	0	46.40451	0	0	0
	0	0	0	8.57681	0	0	0	0	0	0	0	0	2.736336
	5.83929	0	0	0	0	0	0	0	0	0	0	0	49.43124
	0	0	0	0	0	0	0	0	0	0	0	0	33.59491
	0	0	0	0	0	0	0	0	0	0	0	0	0
	16378	16379	16380	16381	16382								
	0	0	0	0	0								
	0	0	0	0	0								
	0	0	0	14.33443	0								
	0	0	0	20.0395	0								
	0	0	0	0	0								

Figure 11.23 VGG16-based feature extraction.

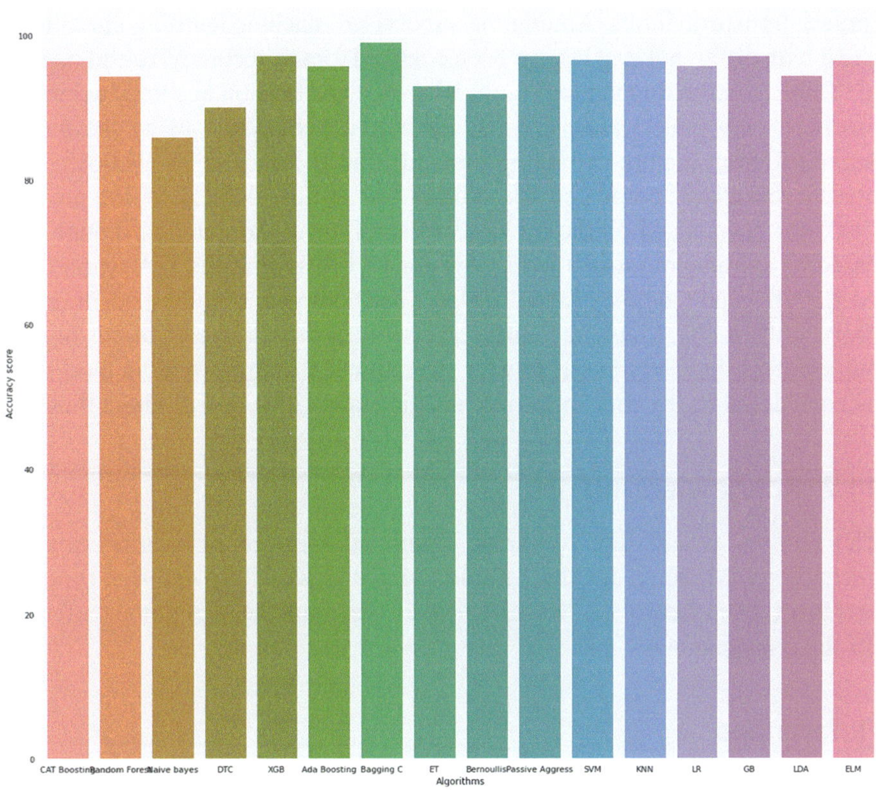

Figure 11.24 Different machine learning evaluation for VGGBATELM method.

Last layer of CNN is removed, later Vgg16 CNN is used for extracting features, and it is processed for bio-inspired GA for features reduction process. Normally, CNN is capable of processing features extraction, optimization, and feature classification processes. As the loss was more than the classification accuracy, that's overfitting, the present research has been processed for extracting features of pre-trained CNN models. After collecting the features csv file, its output has been processed for the classifier's input for the classification process. Genetic algorithm has been processed for the reduction of features and elimination of redundant features.

11.6 Conclusion

Authenticity prediction of an image has turned out to be essential because of the huge misuse of images in different media to change their genuine representation. The proposed approach proved authenticity based on different forgery transformations. Among the supervised machine learning classifiers, ELM with different kernels have been checked for the accuracy. Based on single features extracting strategies, the highest classification accuracy achieved has been between 93 and 96% has been achieved. While using the merging of different feature extracting methods, the accuracy is 97–99.06%. The present research is compared based on different classifiers. Also, the present work has been based on the previous research of the researcher, though not based on significant journal works. Fusion of BAT-optimized GA worked on ALEXNET and vgg16 extracted features for finding out the best accuracy to prove authenticity. Machine Learning performed on extracted features highly outperforms the CNN-based forgery detection. In future, same method may be considered but by forming a mathematical algorithm and different dataset.

11.7 Acknowledgments

The authors would like to thank Velammal College of Engineering & Technology, Madurai, for the completion of the work. No external funding was involved in the present work. And also, we thank the anonymous referees for their suggestions.

References

[1] Afchar D, Nozick V, Echizen I, "MesoNet: A compact facial video forgery detection network," 10th IEEE International Workshop on Information Forensics and Security, WIFS 2018.

[2] Alahmadi A, Hussain M, Mathkour H, "Passive detection of image forgery using DCT and local binary pattern," Signal, Image and Video Processing (2017) 11(1)

[3] Alkawaz M, Sulong G, Rehman A, "Detection of copy-move image forgery based on discrete cosine transform," Neural Computing and Applications (2018) 30(1)

[4] Ardizzone E, Bruno A, Mazzola G, "Copy-Move Forgery Detection by Matching Triangles of Keypoints," IEEE Transactions on Information Forensics and Security (2015) 10(10)

[5] Carvalho T, Faria F, Rocha A, "Illuminant-based transformed spaces for image forensics," IEEE Transactions on Information Forensics and Security (2016) 11(4)

[6] Chen S, Tan S, Huang J, "Automatic Detection of Object-Based Forgery in Advanced Video," IEEE Transactions on Circuits and Systems for Video Technology (2016) 26(11)

[7] Cozzolino D, Poggi G, Verdoliva L, "Efficient Dense-Field Copy-Move Forgery Detection," IEEE Transactions on Information Forensics and Security (2015) 10(11)

[8] Ghoneim A, Muhammad G, Gupta B, "Medical Image Forgery Detection for Smart Healthcare," IEEE Communications Magazine (2018) 56(4)

[9] Hu W, Chen W, Yang C, "Effective image forgery detection of tampered foreground or background image based on image watermarking and alpha mattes," Multimedia Tools and Applications (2016) 75(6)

[10] Jinke X, "Image forgery detection algorithm based on non sampling wavelet transform and Zernike moments," International Journal of Security and its Applications (2016) 10(2)

[11] Li H, Luo W, Huang J, "Image Forgery Localization via Integrating Tampering Possibility Maps," IEEE Transactions on Information Forensics and Security (2017) 12(5)

[12] Li J, Li X, Sun X, "Segmentation-based image copy-move forgery detection scheme," IEEE Transactions on Information Forensics and Security (2015) 10(3)

[13] Li L, Bao J, Guo B, "Face X-ray for more general face forgery detection," Proceedings of the IEEE Computer Society Conference on Computer Vision and Pattern Re...

[14] Li Y, Zhou J, "Fast and Effective Image Copy-Move Forgery Detection via Hierarchical Feature Point Matching," IEEE Transactions on Information Forensics and Security (2019) 14(5)

[15] Liu H, Li X, Yu N, "Spatial-Phase Shallow Learning: Rethinking Face Forgery Detection in Frequency Domain," Proceedings of the IEEE Computer Society Conference on Computer Vision and Pattern Re.

[16] Mahmood T, Mehmood Z, Saba T, "A robust technique for copy-move forgery detection and localization in digital images via stationary wavelet and discrete cosine transform," Journal of Visual Communication and Image Representation (2018) 53

[17] Nguyen H, Yamagishi J, Echizen I, "Capsule-forensics: Using Capsule Networks to Detect Forged Images and Videos," ICASSP, IEEE International Conference on Acoustics, Speech and Signal Processing.

[18] Pun C, Yuan X, Bi X, "Image Forgery Detection Using Adaptive Oversegmentation and Feature Point Matching," IEEE Transactions on Information Forensics and Security (2015) 10(8)

[19] Q. J. Wang, "Using genetic algorithms to optimise model parameters," *Computers and Electronics in Agriculture*, vol. 13, no. 1, pp. 21-32, 1996, doi: 10.1016/S1364-8152(96)00030-8.

[20] Wang, Q.J. (1997) Using genetic algorithms to optimise model parameters. *Environmental Modelling & Software*, 12 (1). 27-34 doi:10.1016/s1364-8152(96)00030-8

[21] Wu Y, Abd-Almageed W, Natarajan P, "Image copy-move forgery detection via an end-to-end deep neural network," Proceedings - 2018 IEEE Winter Conference on Applications of Computer Vision, WACV 20.

[22] You C, Zheng H, Wu X, "Tampering detection and localization base on sample guidance and individual camera device convolutional neural network features," Expert Systems (2023) 40(1)

[23] Yang B, Sun X, Chen X, "A copy-move forgery detection method based on CMFD-SIFT," Multimedia Tools and Applications (2018) 77(1)

[24] Yang F, Li J, Weng J, "Copy-move forgery detection based on hybrid features," Engineering Applications of Artificial Intelligence (2017) 59

[25] Zandi M, Mahmoudi-Aznaveh A, Talebpour A, "Iterative Copy-Move Forgery Detection Based on a New Interest Point Detector," IEEE Transactions on Information Forensics and Security (2016) 11(11)

[26] Zhang Y, Goh J, Thing V, "Image region forgery detection: A deep learning approach," Cryptology and Information Security Series (2016) 14

[27] Zhao H, Zhou W, Yu N, "Multi-attentional Deepfake Detection," Proceedings of the IEEE Computer Society Conference on Computer Vision and Pattern Re.

[28] Zheng J, Liu Y, Yang H, "Fusion of block and keypoints based approaches for effective copy-move image forgery detection," Multidimensional Systems and Signal Processing (2016) 27(4)

[29] Zhu Y, Shen X, Chen H, "Copy-move forgery detection based on scaled ORB," Multimedia Tools and Applications (2016) 75(6)

Index

About the Editors

Dr. Saurav Mallik is currently working as Research Scientist in the Department of Pharmacology and Toxicology, The University of Arizona, USA. Previously, he worked as Postdoctoral Fellow in Harvard T.H. Chan School of Public Health, University of Texas Health Science Center at Houston, and University of Miami Miller School of Medicine, USA. He obtained his Ph.D. degree in the Department of Computer Science and Engineering from Jadavpur University, Kolkata, India in 2017 while his Ph.D. work was carried carried out in Machine Intelligence Unit, Indian Statistical Institute, Kolkata, India while he was Junior Research Fellow and Visiting Scientist. He obtained the award of Research Associateship from CSIR (Council of Scientific and Industrial Research), MHRD, Govt. of India in 2017. Dr. Mallik has more than 350 research publications in different top high impact factor peer-reviewed International Journals, Conferences, a Book Chapters and Books having an H-index of 37. He is working as the active member of Institute of Electrical and Electronics Engineers (IEEE), USA, ACM and American Association for Cancer Research (AACR), USA and Bioclues, India. His research interest includes computational biology, knowledge retrieval and data mining, bioinformatics, biostatistics and machine learning/deep learning.

Dr. Soumita Seth is currently serving as an Assistant Professor in the Department of Computer Science and Engineering of Future Institute of Engineering and Management, Kolkata, India, Affiliated to MAKAUT, Kolkata. Previously, she worked as Assistant Professor in the Department of Computer Science and Engineering of Brainware University, Kolkata (Mar–Aug 2023) and in the Department of Computer Science and Engineering of Pailan College of Management and Technology, Kolkata, India, Affiliated to MAKAUT, Kolkata (Feb 2022– Mar 2023). She is recently submitted her Ph.D. thesis in the Department of Computer Science & Engineering (CSE) from a state-government university, Aliah University (AU), Kolkata, India. Previously, she completed M.Tech. and B.Tech. degrees in the departments of CSE and IT, respectively. She is collaborating on her Ph.D. research with The

University of Texas Health Science Center at Houston (UTHealth), USA. She has academic experience of almost 10 years, full-time research experience of 2 years, and industrial experience of 2 years. Dr. Seth has almost 20 research publications in different top high impact factor peer-reviewed international journals, conferences, book chapters and books having an H-index of 6. Her research interests include computational biology, data mining, bioinformatics, pattern recognition, biological regulatory networks, statistical application on bioinformatics, machine learning/deep learning.

Dr. Ben Othman Soufiene is currently serving as an Assistant Professor in PRINCE Laboratory Research, ISITcom, Hammam Sousse, University of Sousse, Tunisia. Previously, he served as an Assistant Professor of computer science at the University of Gabes, Tunisia from 2016 to 2023. He received his Ph.D. degree in computer science from Manouba University in 2016 for his dissertation on "Secure data aggregation in wireless sensor networks". He also holds an M.Sc. degree from the Monastir University, 2012. His research interests focus on the Internet of Medical Things, wireless body sensor networks, wireless networks, artificial intelligence, machine learning and big data. Dr. Ben Othman has published more than 165 publications in reputed international journals, conferences, a book chapters, and books having an H-index of 31. He serves as an associate editor/academic editor for international journals including IEEE Access, IEEE Sensors, IEEE Internet of Things, Elsevier, Springer, Taylor & Francis, IGI, IET, Telecommunication Computing Electronics and Control, and Wiley. Dr. Ben Othman is a Technical Program Committee Member for more than a dozen international conferences.

For Product Safety Concerns and Information please contact our
EU representative GPSR@taylorandfrancis.com Taylor & Francis
Verlag GmbH, Kaufingerstraße 24, 80331 München, Germany